COMMUNICATION ACROSS THE LIFESPAN

***Edited by** Susan Shaw,*
Ailsa Haxell and Terry Weblemoe

COMMUNICATION ACROSS THE LIFESPAN

OXFORD
UNIVERSITY PRESS
AUSTRALIA & NEW ZEALAND

OXFORD
UNIVERSITY PRESS

Oxford University Press is a department of the University of Oxford. It furthers the University's objective of excellence in research, scholarship, and education by publishing worldwide. Oxford is a registered trademark of Oxford University Press in the UK and in certain other countries.

Published in Australia by
Oxford University Press
253 Normanby Road, South Melbourne, Victoria 3205, Australia

First published 2012

National Library of Australia Cataloguing-in-Publication data

Author: Shaw, Susan
Title: Communication across the lifespan/Susan Shaw; Ailsa Haxell; Terry Weblemoe.

ISBN: 9780195585148 (pbk.)

Notes: Includes index.
Subjects: Interpersonal communication.

Interpersonal communication in children.
Interpersonal communication in adolescence.
Older people—Communication.

Other Authors/Contributors:

Haxell, Ailsa.
Weblemoe, Terry.

Dewey Number: 153.6

Edited by Pete Cruttenden
Typeset by diacriTech, Chennai, India
Proofread by Carolyn Pike
Indexed by Glenda Browne
Printed by Sheck Wah Tong Printing Press Ltd

Foreword

It has been said that 'we are what we eat'. While food and beverage intake has a significant impact on our health and well-being, at least as strong a case can be made in this regard for 'we are who we relate to'. The people we relate to, and how we relate to them, have profound impacts on most facets of life: our personal identity and status; our ability to learn and perform diverse social roles in family, friendship, work and wider social settings; our sense of purpose and security, and our ability to cope with stress and adversity. Communication is the glue that connects us to others, and to ourselves, throughout our lives.

This book is about human communication and human development, topics that are usually treated separately, and is intended to help prepare students entering health, disability and related fields to engage effectively with people from cradle to grave. Effective communication is a necessary condition for successful professional practice. While many additional competencies are required, most require high-level communication skills to put them into effect. In reading the chapters in this book, I was impressed by how well the communication and developmental strands run together, each illuminating the other, sometimes in interesting and novel ways. The contributors come from a variety of backgrounds and the editors have done well in orchestrating their varied perspectives.

Communication is fundamental to being human, and its richness and complexity differentiates us from other animals. Language is of central importance in this regard. While perhaps present in rudimentary forms in some other species, the human capacity for symbolic communication is extraordinary and has profound effects in terms of our ability to learn from experience, including the experience and thoughts of other people. It enables us not only to represent our current situation in our 'heads' and share this with others, but also to retrieve and think about past experiences and to imagine future possibilities. This includes our sense of self and knowledge of our personal mortality. The ability to bring back real or imagined experiences from the past, project future scenarios that may or may not eventuate, and mull over past, present and possible future representations is Janus-faced. The consequences can be positive or negative. Among other things, this carries potential for over-exposure to negative thoughts and feelings that can contribute to our understanding of ourselves and others, but also erode our physical and mental health and strain our relations with people close to us. Understanding these things in ourselves, and the people we relate to in personal and professional contexts, is central to the development of both personal coping skills and our ability to both empathise and engage with others.

Non-verbal means of communication remain important to humans, as they are for other animals. It is easy to overlook just how important they are. I remember having this brought to my attention years ago when I was asked to take over the training of a group of telephone counsellors. While I had sometimes used the telephone when working with patients and clients as a clinical psychologist, this was usually only with people I had already related to in face-to-face situations. I initially found it difficult to fully engage with clients over the telephone. Some of the trainee counsellors were much better at it than I was. I realised that I had come to rely very strongly on non-verbal cues, including body posture and facial expressions. In time I got better at picking up changes in vocal tone and the meaning of pauses and breathing—cues accessible over the phone—and making greater use of reflective listening methods to ensure that I understood what clients were seeking to communicate. Some forms of non-verbal communication, including communication involving touch and smell, are often of particular importance in intimate and some highly emotionally charged situations. There are social and professional boundaries relating to the appropriateness or otherwise of using touch in health contexts.

Someone once said that each of us is like all other people, some other people and no other people. This recognises the universals in our nature as human beings—as well as the culture, gender and other characteristics we share with others—and those things that make each of us unique. Our challenge, in terms of our own sense of well-being and ability to relate genuinely to others, is to value these three realities, and to keep them in balance. This involves, among other things, recognising and celebrating our personal uniqueness, our special connections to some other groups and people, and our common humanity.

During the past 20 years, the populations of Aotearoa New Zealand and Australia, and many other countries, have become much more diverse ethnically. We are in the midst of an 'Age of Migration' with vast numbers of people globally travelling, sojourning and migrating. This increasing globalisation is also played out in cyberspace. Over a quarter of New Zealanders are born overseas. This diversity presents challenges to communication. It is important to be especially mindful of the ways in which we are like all others, some others and no others. There are significant cultural and ethnic differences that present challenges to communication even when the people communicating are doing so in a common language, let alone through an interpreter. Age, gender, education, profession, and health condition and impairments are among other differences that need to be considered. However, at the end of the day, each of us is also an individual and will differ from other people we identify with at a group or collective level. There are dangers of stereotyping when this is overlooked and too much emphasis is placed on presumed group differences.

To underline the importance of communication to professional practice and health outcomes, it is worth noting that poor communication is the leading cause of inadequate care and sentinel events (events that are life threatening, incapacitating or lead to death) in hospital settings. Problems with communication, and the lack of respect that this may reflect or imply, are major reasons for patient and family complaints about the care they receive. Good communication makes a huge difference, enhancing both treatment outcome and patient satisfaction with care from health and disability professionals.

Professor Max Abbott
Dean, Faculty of Health and Environmental Sciences
Pro Vice-Chancellor, North Shore and Community
AUT University

Contents

The Authors xv
Acknowledgments xxiv

Part 1: Communication and Lifespan Development 1

Chapter 1: Introducing Communication and Development 3

SUSAN SHAW, AILSA HAXELL AND TERRY WEBLEMOE

Learning about people and communication 4
Models and elements of communication 5
Communication and human development 6
The organisation of this book 6

Chapter 2: The Antenatal Journey 9

ANDREA GILKISON

Transition to motherhood 11
The narrative of pregnancy 12
Listening to women's narratives 13

Chapter 3: Birth and the Neonate 18

ANNABEL FARRY AND CLAIRE HOTCHIN

Birth 19
Supportive communication 22
First communication following birth 23
Early neonatal communication 24
Communicating with babies 24
Practitioners interacting with babies 26
A Māori perspective 27

Chapter 4: Communicating with Babies and Young Children 30

RAIN LAMDIN AND RACHEL LAMDIN HUNTER

Social and cultural contexts of childhood 31
Social context and learning 33
Understanding communicating and language 35
Getting older: 3 years and on 41
Communication through play 43

Chapter 5: School Age 47

ANNE GREY

Developmental theories 48
Learning theories 50
Māori perspectives on development 51
Theories of language development 52
Communication with school-age children 53
The influence of communication on children's health care 55

Chapter 6: Teens 60

GABRIELLE LE GEYT, JAYNE MERCIER, MORGYN HARTDEGEN, AMBER DAVIES AND AILSA HAXELL

The adolescent brain 61
Psychosocial development 62
Physical development 65
Communicating with teenagers 67

Chapter 7: Early Adulthood 72

CHARLES MPOFU AND AILSA HAXELL

Physical development 73
Risks 73
Cognitive development 74
Social development 75
Emotional adjustment 77

Chapter 8: Middle Years 80

KIRK REED

Defining the middle years 81
Roles in the middle years 83
Managing life events 85

Chapter 9: Senior Years 88

HELEN GAETA AND TERRY WEBLEMOE

Psychosocial theories of ageing 89
The ageing population 93
Socio-environmental theory 94
Communication and ageing 96

Chapter 10: Dying, Grief and Bereavement 102

TERRY WEBLEMOE

- Cultural considerations 104
- How practitioners respond 104

Part 2: Communication and Human Engagement 111

Chapter 11: Communication and Survival 113

CHRIS WEBB

- Communication and survival 115
- Situations of crisis and emergency 116
- Truth and responsibility 118

Chapter 12: Access and Communication 124

MELISSA EVANS AND SUSAN SHAW

- Neurological impairment 125
- Impact of neurological impairment on communication 126
- Visual challenges 128
- Impact of visual challenges on communication 130
- Hearing impairments 131
- Impact of hearing impairments on communication 133
- Intellectual or learning disabilities 135

Chapter 13: Power Relations 140

RUTH DESOUZA

- Oppression 141
- Power 142
- Critical social theory 143
- Organisational and management theories 143
- Social psychological theories 144
- Post-structuralist theories 144
- Empowerment 145

Chapter 14: Culture 157

DENISE WILSON, RAY GATES, JUNIOR SONNY SAMUELA AND TERRY WEBLEMOE

- Cultural difference 158
- Cultural competence 164
- Cultural safety 166

Chapter 15: Social and Interpersonal Dynamics 173

LOUISE MILLER

Boundaries and appropriateness 174
Zone of helpfulness 175
Dual relationships 177
Breaking bad news 178
Truth telling 179
Reassurance 180
Communicating with peers 182

Chapter 16: Touch 187

DAVID NICHOLLS

The culture of touch 188
Touch through the lifespan 190
Touch and communication 191
Touch and professional practice 193
Touch and human well-being 194

Chapter 17: Media 197

GREG TREADWELL

Principles of openness 198
Types of media 201
The business model 203
The effect on news 205
Censorship 206
Access, citizen journalism and the digital divide 208

Chapter 18: Types of Messages 212

BRENDA COSTA-SCORSE

Conversation 213
Chat 214
Gossip 214
Delivering information 215
Nice to know versus need to know 216
Difficult messages 218

Chapter 19: Language and Vocabulary 222
SUE RALEIGH AND SUSAN SHAW

Intention 223
Meaning 224
Interpretation 226
Talking with and past each other 227
Colloquial communication 229
Formal language 230
The repercussions of poor communication 231
Responsibilities 233

Chapter 20: Style and Manner 237
TONY MACCULLOCH

Professional communication 239
Casual communication 240
Intimacy issues 241
Integrity 242
Dysfunctional styles to avoid 242

Chapter 21: Receiving the Message 247
KIRK REED

Interpretation 248
Evaluating the message 249
Options for responding 250
Feedback 253
Complaints 254

Chapter 22: Written Communication 258
KATE DIESFELD

The legal terrain 259
The fundaments of record keeping 260
Elements of a consent form 262
Formal submissions 264
The writing process 265

Chapter 23: The Electronic Message 269
AILSA HAXELL

Technology as more than a tool 270
Mobile phones 272
Text messaging 272
Internet 276
Social networking sites 276
Discussion boards 277
Blogs 277
Twitter 278
Virtual reality environments 279

Chapter 24: Creative Messages 283
DEB SPENCE AND LIZ SMYTHE

Poetry 284
Story 288
Image 291
Sound 292
Understanding as ontology 293

Part 3: Professional Communication 297

Chapter 25: Professional Communication 299
SUSAN SHAW

Communication codes 300
Costs of inadequate communication 302
Professional responsibilities 305
Interprofessional communication 306
Communicating in organisations 306

Chapter 26: Therapeutic Engagement 309
ELIZABETH FINN

Consumers' involvement in their care 310
Communication 311
Communication in a health-care setting 312
Effective communication 313
Barriers to effective communication 315
The therapeutic relationship when things go wrong 317

Chapter 27: Care at a Distance 322

SUSAN SHAW

Physical location 323
Technology 324
Making connections 325
Impact on practitioners 326
Communicating across time and space 328

Glossary 333
Index 341

The Authors

Editors

Susan Shaw, BN, MEd Admin (Hons), EdD, Dip Tchg (Primary), NZRGON

Susan has a background in education and healthcare, having originally qualified as a primary school teacher and then a nurse. She is a registered teacher and a registered nurse. Susan has worked at AUT University since 1992 in several roles including teaching, academic leadership and staff development. During this time she has maintained her clinical practice in surgical, medical and palliative care settings. She is currently Associate Dean (Undergraduate) and a director of the National Centre for Interprofessional Education and Collaborative Practice (NCIPECP) within the Faculty of Health and Environmental Sciences at AUT. Her research interests include quality education and clinical practice, along with the responses of patients and health practitioners towards experiences of chronic illness and disability. Her doctorate investigated nursing education in relation to chronic pain.

Ailsa Haxell, BA, MHSc (Hons), PGCertEd (Management), Dip Nursing

Ailsa is a senior lecturer in the Faculty of Health and Environmental Sciences at AUT University. She has extensive teaching experience in nursing and in health promotion particularly in the area of community development. Ailsa has worked with Auckland Youthline as a counsellor and teacher of telephone counselling skills since the mid 1980s. She is currently completing a PhD on change and the use of emergent technologies through Deakin University in Melbourne.

Terry Weblemoe, BA, MA, RN

Terry has had a lifelong interest in indigenous cultures and health, and has worked as a registered nurse in New York, Florida and Aotearoa New Zealand. In 1990 she migrated to Aotearoa New Zealand, acquired an MA in Anthropology from the University of Auckland, worked in various nursing and education roles, and has been involved in several research projects with Māori. She has been employed as a lecturer at AUT University since 1997. She has developed a strong interest in intercultural communication, and has completed several certificates from the Summer Institute of Intercultural Communication in Portland, Oregon.

Contributors

Brenda Costa-Scorse, BHSc (Nurs), Dip ATE, RGON

Brenda has been involved in emergency medicine and paramedic education for the larger part of her professional life. She is a Senior Lecturer in Paramedicine and Emergency Management at AUT University. Her clinical background is predominantly in emergency medicine, both in hospital and out of hospital in ambulance and commercial ski areas. Brenda is presently undertaking a PhD on injury prevention strategies in alpine skiing and snowboarding. She has a strong belief in strengthening the chain of survival by advancing the educational opportunities for all people involved in out-of-hospital care and emergency management responses. Her recent brief has been developing a tertiary education pathway for medics in the New Zealand Defence Force. She is passionate about ongoing research and contemporary best practice and is a member of the international board for the *Journal of Emergency Primary Health Care.*

Amber Davies, BA, Grad Dip (Psychosocial studies), MHSc in Psychotherapy (Hons)

Amber began as a volunteer with Youthline in 2004. In 2010 she became the team leader of the Specialty Assessment Services, supervising counselling services, triage and research for Youthline Ponsonby. Amber is passionate about building strong communities and supporting young people to reach their potential.

Ruth DeSouza, MA (Hons), Dip Nurs, Grad Dip Adv Nurs Pract

Ruth is a Senior Research Fellow and Coordinator of AUT University's Centre for Asian and Migrant Health Research, and Programme Leader for the Bachelor of Health Science in Health Promotion. Ruth has worked as a nurse (in postnatal, mental health and maternal mental health settings), educator and researcher, and has recently completed her PhD about migrant maternity in Aotearoa New Zealand. She is involved in various governance roles to do with health provision, community sector research, and migrant and refugee settlement.

Kate Diesfeld, BA, JD

Kate is Associate Professor of Social Justice at Te Piringa Faculty of Law, University of Waikato in Aotearoa New Zealand. In Los Angeles, she represented people with developmental disabilities. In the 1990s, she was the Legal Supervisor of the Kent Law Clinic (Mental Health and Learning Disability) at the University of Kent in England. She also represented people with a history of mental illness before the Mental Health

Review Tribunal for eight years. In Aotearoa New Zealand, she was the Director of the National Centre for Health Law and Ethics at AUT University until 2011. With Professor Ian Freckelton, she edited *Involuntary Detention and Therapeutic Jurisprudence: International Perspectives on Civil Commitment* (Ashgate). Her teaching and research interests are disability law (including mental health and intellectual disability), medical law, professional discipline and professional ethics.

Melissa Evans (nee Harvey-Sheils), NZ DipOT, AdvDipOT PG Dip HSc

Melissa has worked as an occupational therapist for over 20 years, and has been a lecturer at the School of Occupational Science and Therapy at AUT University since 2005. Melissa's main areas of interest are stroke rehabilitation and working with the elderly, and she is currently studying to complete a Master's degree.

Annabel Farry, BSc, BM, PG Cert

Annabel is passionate about women understanding their bodies and finding self-empowerment through birth. She completed a degree in physiology at Otago University before undertaking a Direct Entry Midwifery Degree at Otago Polytechnic. She moved to Auckland after graduating and worked as part of a high-risk obstetric team at National Women's hospital. She then began self-employed midwifery practice in Central and South Auckland. After two years, she moved to London and practised as a midwife for one year before travelling through the Middle East to Lebanon where her grandfather was born. She returned to Aotearoa New Zealand in 2000 and completed her postgraduate certificate at AUT University. She continued to practise midwifery in South Auckland. She has birthed two daughters at home and now works full time as a midwifery lecturer at AUT University, taking the occasional client for home births. She is currently completing her postgraduate diploma.

Elizabeth Finn, BPharm, MPharm, PhD, FPS

Elizabeth qualified as a pharmacist and worked in hospital pharmacy for many years before moving into research. She served four years on the Council of the Pharmaceutical Society and she has a special interest in the social aspects of health care, especially communication, education, competence and assessment. Her PhD focused on communication between health providers and consumers. Elizabeth taught at the School of Medicine and Health Science at the University of Auckland and AUT University before commencing her current role as Education Manager for the Health and Disability Commissioner in 2003. This role draws on the provisions of the *Code of Health and Disability Services Consumers'*

Rights and the case work of the Commissioner's office, and involves working with health services providers in all kinds of practice settings to facilitate improvements in the quality and safety of health care.

Helen Gaeta, BSc, MSc (Hons), PhD, SPR, CNS

Helen graduated with a PhD from the Faculty of Medicine, University of Auckland. She has held academic positions at the University of Florida and Columbia University. In 2006 she joined the staff at AUT University. Helen's area of research expertise is the neuroscience of cognitive ageing; in particular, understanding the changes in attention and working memory that occur with ageing and the neural processes that underpin these changes.

Ray Gates, BPhty, Grad Dip (Pain Management)

Ray Gates is an Aboriginal physiotherapist descended from the Bundjalung people of north-eastern New South Wales, Australia. He has been professionally involved in Aboriginal and Torres Strait Islander health issues in various capacities for over 16 years. He is a founding member and current president of the National Association of Aboriginal and Torres Strait Islander Physiotherapists. He is an advocate for the use of physiotherapy in primary health care to address the poor health status of Aboriginal and Torres Strait Islander peoples, and is a strong supporter for the provision of culturally safe health care by non-Indigenous services. He is a member of APA and NAATSIP.

Andrea Gilkison, BA (Soc Sci), MEd, PhD, RCompN, RM

Andrea has been a midwife since 1985. She has worked in many areas of midwifery, but has a passion for supporting women who choose to birth at home or in primary units. Andrea completed her Master's degree in education in Liverpool, UK in 2000 when she was working facilitating tutorial groups in a Problem Based Learning (PBL) curriculum. Her Master's research explored the techniques that PBL tutors used to facilitate learning. Andrea has been lecturing in the undergraduate midwifery programme at AUT University since 2001, and has been instrumental in establishing a narrative pedagogical approach in the midwifery programme. Her doctoral research explored the experiences of midwifery teachers and students who were participating in a narrative-centred curriculum.

Anne Grey, BA (Soc Sci.), MEd (Hons), DEd, Dip Tchg (Primary), Dip Tchg (ECE)

Anne is Programme Leader of the Early Years Programmes at AUT University. She is also Licensee of the AUT University early childhood education centre. Anne's main area of research is teaching practice in early childhood education and leadership in early childhood education. Before teaching at tertiary level, Anne taught in early childhood centres and in primary school. She has also helped to set up community early childhood centres.

Morgyn Hartdegen, BA, BMus

Morgyn began volunteering as a counsellor on Youthline's helpline in 2009, and now works for Clinical Services overseeing the assessment and referral process for people of all ages entering Youthline for a wide range of face-to-face services. She is passionately committed to empowering young people and their communities.

Claire Hotchin, BSN, MA, IBCLC, RGON, RM

Claire has been a midwife for 33 years. She has practised in three countries in home, birth centre and hospital settings, providing continuity of midwifery care across the childbearing year for women and their whānau. Her particular interest lies with supporting women to birth physiologically, breastfeed their babies and enjoy the parenting experience. She now lectures in midwifery at AUT University.

Rain Lamdin, BSc, MBChB, GradDip Adult and Higher Education, PhD

Rain is a clinical lecturer in a postgraduate clinical education programme at the University of Auckland. She is also a doctor at Auckland Hospital working in the Department of Emergency Medicine. Her academic interests include professional socialisation and health professional communication. She has taught professional development, communication and clinical skills in medical education. Her experience as a mother and aunt has greatly contributed to her knowledge of child communication and development.

Rachel Lamdin Hunter, BN, RN Comp, PGCert Child and Family Health, MMS

Rachel is a registered nurse who specialised in child health and then family and women's health, mostly in acute settings. She has also worked in private consultation with families expecting their first child, providing birth support and antenatal education. Rachel now teaches in the Bachelor of Nursing programme at Waikato Institute of Technology, focusing on child and family health, personal and professional development, cultural safety and lifespan development. She also teaches postgraduate students. She credits much of her knowledge to the valuable teaching provided by her three young daughters.

Gabby Le Geyt, BA, MSc (Hons)

Gabby works in London as a rehabilitation assistant at the National Hospital for Neurology and Neurosurgery. Gabby spent 2000–10 dividing her time between working at the University of Auckland's Clinical Trials Research Unit as part of a team investigating a depression prevention mobile phone programme for adolescents (the Adapt study) and as a research assistant in the Clinical Services team at Youthline, Auckland.

Tony MacCulloch, MEd, PhD, Dip Couns, RN

Tony draws on an extensive history of involvement in health care. An initial background in general nursing extended into psychiatric nursing, counselling and nursing education. His Master's research explored educators' experience of challenging dominant hegemony, and in 2001 he was a recipient of the AUT University Distinguished Teaching Award. His PhD research involved a critical analysis of discourses of emotional competence. This interest has emerged from a longstanding commitment to fostering emotional intelligence in health practitioners, alongside his work teaching communication, interpersonal skills and clinical supervision to a wide range of health practitioners. His publications and clinical background reflect a diverse range of interests, although there is a clear critical theory, transformative, emancipatory interpersonal communication theme evident. He is currently co-editor and a frequent contributor to a column published in *Issues in Mental Health Nursing*.

Jayne Mercier, BCS, Grad Dip (Psychosocial Studies), MHSc (Hons)

Jayne has been working with young people at Youthline since 2001 and has most recently held the role of Clinical Services Manager.

Louise Miller, BA, PGDip, RN

Louise is currently working as a clinical information specialist with Northland District Health Board, which provides elective and acute services through hospitals in Whangarei, Dargaville, Bay of Islands and Kaitaia and their community services. Her previous experience in Northland includes being a manager of a hospice and practice nurse for a far north iwi provider. While living in Auckland, she worked for AUT University for 15 years for a range of courses including the diploma in military medicine and return to nursing. She considers herself a generalist, and has worked in coronary care, acute medical, assessment and rehabilitation, acute and community mental health. Her areas of interest and speciality include information management, health legislation, communication, spirituality and complementary therapies.

Charles Mpofu, BEd, MHSc, Dip Ed, Dip CTD

Charles Mpofu is a lecturer at AUT University in the Faculty of Health and Environmental Sciences. He has contributed to various undergraduate papers. His broad research interests are in health law and ethics, quality control and accreditation systems for medical education.

David Nicholls, GradDipPhys, MA, PhD, NZSP

David is Postgraduate Head in the School of Rehabilitation and Occupation Studies at AUT University. Before moving to Aotearoa New Zealand in 2000, David lectured in the School of Physiotherapy at Sheffield Hallam University in England, and prior to that he was a practising physiotherapist specialising in the rehabilitation of people with chronic lung disease. Over the last decade, David's teaching and research interests have developed in postmodern philosophy, particularly the works of Michel Foucault, and in 2008 he completed a PhD thesis titled 'Body politics: A Foucauldian discourse analysis of physiotherapy practice'. David teaches in the undergraduate and postgraduate programmes at AUT and has presented his research nationally and internationally.

Sue Raleigh, MHSc (Hons), PgDipMktg, AND (Med-Surg), RGON

Sue is a Senior Lecturer in the Faculty of Health and Environmental Sciences at AUT University. Sue trained as a registered general and obstetric nurse in 1980 and worked in full-time clinical practice from 1980 to 1999 in a variety of specialties, including intensive care, coronary care, cardiothoracic intensive care, orthopaedics, respiratory medicine, haematology, urology and renal transplantation. Sue started work at AUT in 1999 and completed a Master's degree in 2006. After nine years teaching in the School of Nursing, she moved to the Department of Interdisciplinary Studies. Sue's current teaching focus includes human anatomy and physiology, introductory microbiology and pharmacology to interdisciplinary groups of first year students.

Kirk Reed, M OT, DHSc, Dip OT, NZROT

Kirk is the Head of the Department of Occupational Science and Therapy at AUT University. He is a registered occupational therapist with practice experience in the mental health sector both in Aotearoa New Zealand and the UK. He moved into teaching in 2000. Since then, Kirk has completed his doctorate exploring the meaning of occupation using a phenomenological methodology and his research interests include the contribution participation in meaningful occupation makes to health outcomes, interprofessional practice and the future of occupational therapy in primary health.

Elizabeth Smythe, BA, PhD, RM, RGON

Elizabeth began her health professional career as a nurse, and then trained as a midwife. She took time out to do a BA. Because there were limited nursing/midwifery papers available, she added papers from English literature, psychology, sociology and business. Elizabeth came to see how each discipline had its own way of talking about 'the same thing'. In recent years, she has been supervising health students from across the disciplines in their Master's and PhD theses, bringing her experience as a hermeneutic phenomenological researcher. She is aware that often we struggle with the same tensions and delight in the same accomplishments. It is the little things, like 'listening', that make such a difference.

Junior Sonny Samuela, BIB

Junior is the eldest of five children whose parents migrated from Western Samoa in the early 1960s and settled in West Auckland. After spending time in the hospitality and telecommunication industries, and managing his own security company, he returned to the education world in 2002 to fulfil a lifelong dream to obtain a university degree. He completed a Bachelor of International Business degree in 2006, which heightened his desire to assist other Pasifika students to succeed in their academic pursuits. In 2007, Junior was employed as a Pasifika Student Advisor for AUT University. Junior has completed certificates of proficiency in Psychology and Nutrition in Health Promotion and is currently pursuing a Postgraduate Certificate in Public Health.

Deb Spence, BA, PhD, PG Dip Soc Sci, RN, RM, MCNANZ

Deb Spence has a strong practice background in acute care nursing and teaches nurses at Bachelor, Master's and Doctoral levels. Interests and strengths in relation to her teaching include using the arts to enhance students' understanding and working collaboratively with clinicians to advance nursing practice and support the development of clinically focused research. In 1999, Deb completed a doctoral thesis entitled 'Prejudice, Paradox and Possibility: Nursing People from Cultures Other Than One's Own'. She has also undertaken funded research articulating the nature of advanced nursing practice, and completed a collaborative action research project entitled 'Implementing a Prescribing Practicum in a Nursing Masters Programme'. She is currently involved as a co-researcher in the Australasian nursing e-graduate study, an evaluation of the mental health component of the BHSc nursing at AUT University and an appreciative inquiry into the development and implementation of the integrated student model for clinical learning at the Auckland District Health Board.

Greg Treadwell, BA, MA, NZ Cert Journalism

Greg is a journalist and senior lecturer working in the School of Communication Studies at AUT University. An award-winning journalist, Greg joined academia in 2005. Since then he has taught journalism, specialising in news reporting and new media, at both undergraduate and postgraduate levels. In 2010, he was awarded the Vice-Chancellor's Award for Excellence in teaching. His current research is in new media, media in the South Pacific and the journalism education curriculum. Greg is a member of the Journalism Education Association of New Zealand (JEANZ).

Chris Webb, BEd, DipBusStudies, AdvDipTchg

Chris is currently Programme Leader in Emergency Management at AUT University. Chris came to AUT University in April 2006 and has had the responsibility of developing and teaching a pathway of emergency management qualifications from the undergraduate level through to postgraduate. From 2007, Chris took on combined responsibility for the paramedic and emergency management areas. Prior to that Chris was Corporate and Development Manager with the New Zealand Ministry of Civil Defence and Emergency Management and was responsible for enhancing capability through effective professional development within the emergency management sector. Chris has a background in teaching and human resources. He is a Herrmann Practitioner and a member of the IAEM Global Scholarship Commission.

Denise Wilson, BA (SocSc), MA (Hons), PhD, RN, FCNA (NZ)

Denise (Ngati Tahinga descent) is the Associate Professor of Māori Health in the School of Public Health and Psychosocial Studies at AUT University. She has researched and published in the areas of Māori health and health service delivery, cultural issues, family violence and health workforce development. Prior to beginning her academic career, Denise worked as a registered nurse in acute care and community settings. Currently, Denise is a member of the Ministry of Health Family Violence Advisory Committee, Nga Manukura o Apopo, Korowai Atawhai Advisory Group to the Ministry of Health on Family Violence (providing Māori cultural advice on family violence guidelines development) and Wharangi Ruamano (Māori Nurse Educators). She is a Fellow of the College of Nurses Aotearoa (NZ) and Te Mata o te Tau (Academy of Māori Research and Scholarship) and a board member of the Nursing Network for Violence Against Women International (NNVAWI).

Acknowledgments

A wide range of colleagues have contributed expertise to this book and their involvement is clear as authors of chapters. There are also a number of people and organisations who have been involved in supporting contributors or managing the overall project.

In Chapter 3, our midwifery colleagues consulted with Nga Maia, which is the national body promoting Māori midwives and birthing. More information about this organisation may be found at www.ngamaia.co.nz.

Chapter 6 considers the teenage years and all of the contributors are involved with Youthline. Youthline began in 1970 and is a youth development organisation supporting young people to reach their potential through a range of mentoring, counselling, youth work, training and leadership services. More information about this organisation may be found at www.youthline.co.nz.

Chapter 14 considers culture in relation to communication, and the contributors represent Māori, Aboriginal and Pasifika perspectives. Junior Samuela provided the Pasifika insights for this chapter and a group of his colleagues were also involved and should be acknowledged. They are: Neli Sasulu, Josephine Ng Lam, Vicky Totua and Winston Philcox.

In Chapter 24, Elizabeth Smythe and Deb Spence present insights into creative messages and we are grateful to the various artists and publishers that have provided permission to have their work included in this chapter. We extend our special thanks to Glenn Colquhoun for the use of his poetry.

Debra James at Oxford University Press provided ongoing support and demonstrated a commitment to this project, which we greatly appreciate. We are also mindful of the time and energy that the external reviewers put into considering the work and providing valuable feedback. Ann James at AUT University coordinated contributions and managed deadlines for us. Ann's interest and attention to detail has been central to the smooth running of this project.

Susan Shaw, Ailsa Haxell and Terry Weblemoe
AUT University
July 2011

{PART 1}

Communication and Lifespan Development

Chapter 1 Introducing Communication and Development ... 3

Chapter 2 The Antenatal Journey ... 9

Chapter 3 Birth and the Neonate ... 18

Chapter 4 Communicating with Babies and Young Children ... 30

Chapter 5 School Age ... 47

Chapter 6 Teens ... 60

Chapter 7 Early Adulthood ... 72

Chapter 8 Middle Years ... 80

Chapter 9 Senior Years ... 88

Chapter 10 Dying, Grief and Bereavement ... 102

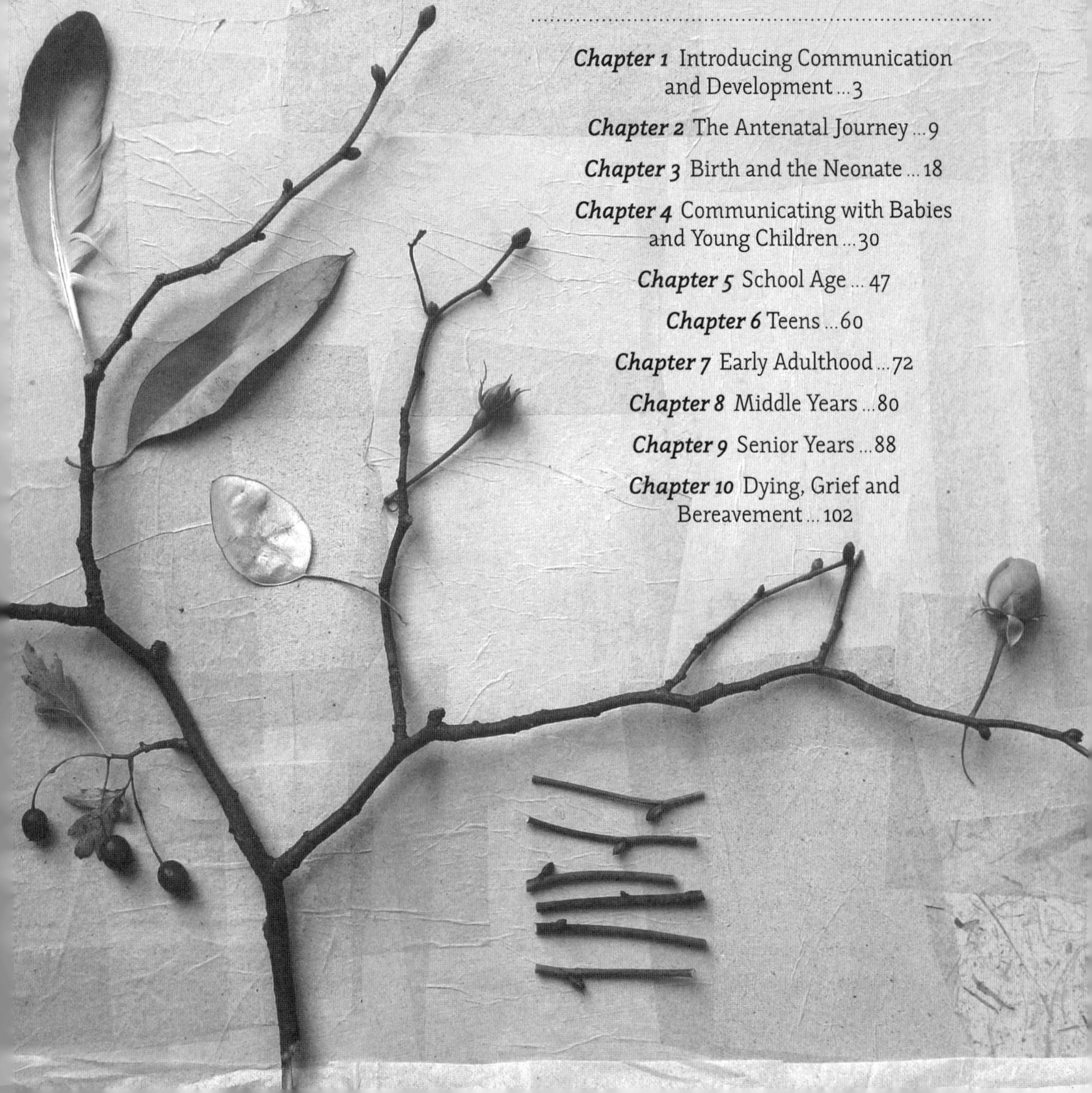

{1}

Introducing Communication and Development

Susan Shaw, Ailsa Haxell and Terry Weblemoe

CHAPTER OVERVIEW

This chapter covers the following topics:

+ Learning about people and communication
+ Models and elements of communication
+ Communication and human development
+ The organisation of this book.

KEY TERMS

Intention
Meaningful
Engagement
Meaning

Good communication is at the very centre of professional behaviour and the provision of appropriate support and care. The judgment of appropriate and good communication rests with the person receiving it, and usually reflects their perspective on what they think matters. While ideas of what information is relevant and important may vary between apparently similar people in comparable situations, the concept and importance of being treated individually and respectfully changes little. Approaching people with the genuine **intention** of appreciating what they need and how they may be helped requires a personal acceptance that people are unique and deserve quality and thoughtful attention. There is no substitute for a genuine interest and desire to interact with others in a **meaningful** way. Social interaction and therefore communication is a fundamental human reality and is inescapably important.

Intention A deliberate attempt to behave in a certain way.

Meaningful A sense of significance, relevance, purpose or importance.

Learning about people and communication

It has long been accepted that people working in the health care and disability support sector need to have an appreciation of human development and communication. Traditionally these two subjects are taught in isolation and students (and practitioners) struggle to apply what they have learnt. We believe that putting these elements together enables students to make connections about how to interact effectively and appropriately with colleagues and those they support. Sound interpersonal **engagement** is at the core of good practice and appreciating the perspectives of others. The knowledge and skill to interact with those around us in meaningful ways is of the greatest importance.

Engagement Being genuinely involved.

In addition to placing communication and human development alongside one another, there are other departures from traditional approaches in this book. Generally books about human development focus on theoretical perspectives, while those about communication include fine details about 'micro skills'. Within this book contributors have taken a range of approaches to presenting their chapters. Some have emphasised theoretical perspectives, while others have highlighted the essence of engagement by providing insights into the process of interacting with others. This varied presentation is deliberate, and we hope that it models a range of approaches to considering and presenting information.

The broad range of communication mediums covered within these pages is another departure from other publications for students within these fields of study. People of all ages are using electronic media to communicate and to access information. At the same time, electronic tools are becoming indispensible in the management and delivery of health care and disability support services. However, it is also important to appreciate the **meaning** of communication in terms of art and creativity, and for that reason Chapter 24 considers art, music and poetry.

Meaning The significance of the message and its delivery and context.

While there are groups of practitioners with roles that involve direct communication with patients or service users, this book is designed to consider communication across the spectrum of service development and delivery. The need for accurate, relevant and appropriate communication is as important for scientists in laboratories as it is for receptionists taking calls from patients and clinical staff discussing bad news with families. The way in which people within all of these roles communicate among themselves is also of great significance. Organisational, professional, cultural and personal understandings and approaches to communication all impact on the quality of services and experience of those interacting with them (Leonard, Graham & Bonacum, 2004).

Communication is embedded in context and culture. In both Aotearoa New Zealand and Australia there are many cultural considerations of particular significance within the health and disability support sector. The details of how to manage particular situations can be found within organisational procedures and processes. Information within this book puts the need for these details into perspective and provides a foundation from which to consider culturally appropriate communication.

Models and elements of communication

There is a great deal of information published about how to communicate with people in different situations, and this includes suggested principles and elements that are enshrined in consensus statements (see, for example, Makoul, 2001). It is our belief that, while there are particular essential elements, practitioners are best served by having a broad appreciation of communication contexts and developing a range of skills that become a repertoire suited to them, their roles and their environments. We do not promote recipe-based approaches to communication as they de-personalise all of those involved and diminish the importance of judgment, reflection and reciprocity.

The teaching of communication skills often relies on borrowed theories or practices from fields such as communication, counselling and business. This book differs from many other health-care communication texts in that it focuses more on the application and adjustment of communication skills than on the presentation of communication models and theories. It is intended as a supporting text for communication skills that are taught and assessed through the actual process of interpersonal communication.

We value and acknowledge the concept of 'helping skills' as discussed by John Heron (2001). To be supporting and enabling—creating more rather than less freedom—provides a way of working in health services not bounded by professional borders. The skills are both facilitative and authoritative, and are chosen primarily for their clarity, simplicity and balance. Heron's six skills for helping clients involve being:

+ supportive
+ informative
+ empathic (cathartic)
+ catalytic
+ prescriptive
+ able to confront with sensitivity.

Communication and human development

The basic premise of this book is that sound communication and a good appreciation of human development are essential to the provision of high-quality health care and disability support services, in their broadest sense. While approaches to communication vary to some degree across the lifespan, we do not believe that there are specific formulae for communicating with individuals according to their age. The use of language needs to accommodate knowledge, connections and connotations that people may have, but this does not mean that there is one procedure for chatting to a 3-year-old and a different guideline for explaining a diagnosis to a 13-year-old. While we present information about lifespan stages and communication, we do not condone reductionistic analyses of communication or approaches to people.

The organisation of this book

One of the challenges for us in developing this book has been how to organise it to enable easy access to information, while demonstrating the integrated nature of communication and development. The book is divided into three parts. The chapters in Part 1 (Communication and Lifespan Development) relate to specific stages of human development. Part 2 (Communication and Human Engagement) includes chapters on how people communicate and the challenges they experience in day-to-day life, as well as within the health care and disability systems. Importantly, this section includes chapters about touch and creative elements of communication, which are often overlooked in communication courses. Part 3 (Professional Communication) considers communication within the context of professional practice, acknowledging the need for it to be responsive and useful for practitioners as well as patients or service users.

CASE STUDY 1.1

A 10-year-old boy, teeth and girls

At the time that the concept of this book was being considered, a particular clinical example came to our attention that clearly illustrated our interest linking communication with lifespan development.

Tom, a bright and sociable 10-year-old boy, attended a dental hygiene clinic and was interested in the whole experience. At the end of the appointment, the clinicians wished him well and one of them casually said to him, 'The girls will think you are great now'.

A week later, Tom confided to his mum that there was something he thought she should know. He went on to 'confess' that he had only made cursory attempts to clean his teeth in the past few days.

His mother was surprised and a bit perplexed given that he appeared to be interested in his teeth and the dental hygiene messages. She asked him why, and he responded that he didn't want girls to think he was great.

While this was rather entertaining for the adults involved at the time, Tom taught us a good lesson: communication needs to be both considered and relevant. We need to be mindful enough to appreciate that 10-year-old boys may not actually want to be noticed by girls!

{ SUMMARY }

Good communication is central in the provision of support and care. The intention of working with people in supportive and enabling ways is shared across health disciplines and roles. Such ways of working are about being adaptive to the uniqueness of each situation. The intention here is to engender a mindfulness that integrates knowledge of communication with an appreciation of lifespan development.

REFLECTION POINTS

1.1 Intention (motivation, message, meaning, emotion)

Valuing people as unique and deserving of quality and thoughtful attention underpins all interactions in the health-care sector.

1.2 Reception (received message, response, feedback)

Who might be the best judge of appropriate and effective communications?

1.3 Perception (style, manner, impression, analysis)

Reflecting on your own life, what were some of the moments you remember about interacting with health practitioners? How did you want to be treated?

QUESTIONS FOR REVIEW

1 What basic intentions underpin effective communications?
2 In the case study above, what was the impact of a lack of consideration for the realities of being a 10-year-old boy?

REFERENCES

Heron, J. (2001). *Helping the client: A creative practical guide* (5th edn). London, England: Sage.

Leonard, M., Graham, S. & Bonacum, D. (2004). The human factor: The critical importance of effective teamwork and communication in providing safe care. *Quality and Safety in Health Care, 4*(13), 185–90.

Makoul, G. (2001). Essential elements of communication in medical encounters: The Kalamazoo Consensus Statement. *Academic Medicine, 76*(4), 390–3.

WEBSITES

Building Relationships and Eliminating Disparities: www.urmc.rochester.edu/fammed/research/center_comm_health.cfm

Health Literacy www.healthnavigator.org.nz/centre-for-clinical-excellence/health-literacy

The Electronic Health Record in New Zealand: www.hinz.org.nz/journal/2004/03/The-Electronic-Health-Record-in-New-Zealand---Part-2/893

{2}

The Antenatal Journey

Andrea Gilkison

CHAPTER OVERVIEW

This chapter covers the following topics:

+ Transition to motherhood
+ The narrative of pregnancy
+ Listening to women's narratives

KEY TERMS

Pregnancy
Maternity care
Childbearing
Conception
Trimester
Antenatal
Narrative

Pregnancy
Carrying a child from conception to birth.

Pregnancy is an extraordinary yet common life event that has a great impact on the lives of the pregnant woman, the father of the baby and extended whānau/family and friends. The experience of pregnancy is always accompanied by an emotional response and involves considerable physical, psychological, social, emotional and relationship adjustments.

The discovery of being pregnant—whether it is the first or subsequent pregnancy, planned or unplanned—may lead to an array of emotions. These include pride and excitement alongside uncertainty or even fear and anxiety about what the implications of the pregnancy might be. There may be feelings of surprise at becoming pregnant, emotional fluctuations, ambivalence and sometimes even denial: 'I can't possibly be pregnant.'

What the impending future might bring and how it will affect their lives are common concerns for parents when they first discover they are pregnant. Concerns may be related to how they will cope with being a mother or a father and how life and relationships might change. Parents' feelings towards the pregnancy can be influenced by many things, including their current relationship, their family situations, study or work situations, plans for the future, financial situations, the timing of the pregnancy, the number of children they already have, and how easy it was to get pregnant. There may be concerns about the mother's health, or that of the unborn baby. The pregnant mother can experience emotions ranging from great joy to despair, depending on her situation, and she may often experience feelings of conflict and confusion about the pregnancy. Over one-third of pregnancies in Aotearoa New Zealand are unplanned (Amin Shokravi, Howden Chapman & Peyman, 2009), so often newly pregnant women will have some unexpected decisions to make when they discover they are pregnant.

After the initial period of discovering that she is pregnant, a woman and those around her have many decisions to make, many of which are guided by the health practitioners she seeks advice from. In Aotearoa New Zealand, midwives are the key health practitioners who work with women throughout their childbearing experience, but many other health practitioners may also be involved in different aspects of **maternity care**. Effective communication is vital for all health practitioners who are communicating with women, especially in this period of her life. To communicate effectively requires excellent listening skills so that communication can be meaningful and sensitive. Parents need to be provided with unbiased information which will enable them to make informed choices about their maternity care.

Maternity care
The care of the woman and her child through pregnancy and for a period beyond birth (postnatal).

Transition to motherhood

Childbearing, the period of time from **conception** until after the birth, has been identified in the literature as a major life event that can bring about many challenges for the woman and her family (Darvill, Skirton & Farrand, 2010). Pregnancy has been viewed as a developmental stage with its own developmental tasks. Both the pregnant mother and father deal with significant life changes and major psychological and social adjustment. According to developmental theories, the pregnant woman prepares for her new role through accomplishment of the developmental tasks during her pregnancy to successfully incorporate a maternal identity in her personality. One well-known theory was developed in the 1960s by Reva Rubin. Rubin (1984) identified four maternal phases that a woman goes through as she adapts to her pregnancy and prepares for her role as a mother (see Table 2.1).

Childbearing The process of pregnancy and birth.

Conception The point during the reproductive cycle at which an egg is fertilised.

TABLE 2.1 *Summary of Rubin's (1984) maternal phases in adaptation to pregnancy*

	Trimester 1	*Trimester 2*	*Trimester 3*
1 Seeking safe passage for herself and her child through pregnancy, labour and birth 2 Ensuring the acceptance of the infant by others 3 Seeking acceptance of self in her role as a mother 4 Learning to give of herself	Concentration on mother's well-being Dealing with physical symptoms	• Concerns about the baby and birth • Responsibility to protect the baby • Baby identified as separate to mother	• Bond established between mother and baby • Safe passage of mother and baby • 'Nesting' behaviour

Another theory of the way that women adapt to pregnancy and motherhood has been proposed by Lederman and Weis (2009), whose framework incorporates several psychosocial dimensions:

+ the woman's acceptance of her pregnancy
+ her motivation to take on the role of motherhood
+ her relationship with her husband/partner

+ relationships between the pregnant woman and her own mother
+ preparation for labour
+ self-esteem and sense of control.

In our society, being in control of what happens in our lives is seen as very important (McAra-Couper, 2007). When a woman becomes pregnant there are some things which she will inevitably not be able to control. It is widely believed that a woman has control over when and if she becomes pregnant through the use of contraception ('birth control'), yet one-third of pregnancies are unplanned and a significant number of women cannot get pregnant at the time that they want to. Conception itself is only partially controllable.

Once she is pregnant, many physical and emotional changes occur that a woman cannot control at all. In one study, Darvill, Skirton and Farrand (2010) found that women who had previously regarded themselves as fit and healthy felt that they had lost control over their bodies in the first **trimester** of pregnancy, due to the onslaught of the physical symptoms and body changes that occurred. According to Darvill, Skirton and Farrand (2010), women sometimes feel more vulnerable to physical harm, and their need to protect the foetus also contributes to their lack of control over their circumstances. As the pregnancy progresses into the second and third trimesters, a mother shifts her focus from her own physical symptoms and self-image to the needs of her unborn baby.

Trimester A period of three months within a pregnancy of nine months.

Parratt and Fahy (2011) critique theories of transition to motherhood, such as those of Rubin and Lederman and Weiss, because they propose that such theories reduce women to a prescribed role: that of being a 'predetermined type of mother' (p. 5). Parratt and Fahy posit that 'transition to motherhood' theory is oriented to stages that are presented as if they were unalterably 'true', when, in reality, they have been predetermined according to socially constructed ideals. Theories about adaptation to pregnancy may devalue the joy and meaning that can be inherent in the here-and-now, moment-to-moment lived experience. If we focus on pregnancy as a developmental stage, then some factors that are of central importance to childbearing women—such as 'inner power' and 'inner knowing', or women's intuition—are excluded as 'not real' or 'non-existent' and therefore become invisible.

The narrative of pregnancy

Health practitioners need to be cognisant of the major life change that pregnancy represents for a woman and those around her, whether the pregnancy is planned or unplanned. The importance of good communication in **antenatal** care is well

Antenatal The period of time before birth.

recognised (Levine et al., 2010) and is fundamental to the Aotearoa New Zealand midwifery partnership model (Guilliland & Pairman, 1995). During pregnancy it is an essential part of communication to develop trust, so that the woman feels comfortable to honestly talk about how she is feeling about the pregnancy, which might be ambivalence, coping with physical changes, body image changes and lifestyle changes. She needs to feel that she can trust the health practitioner so that she can disclose medical and social information of a personal nature.

Pregnancy is not an illness. Communication between health practitioners and the pregnant woman and her partner needs to emphasise accessible and appropriate information that will facilitate informed decision-making for pregnancy and birth. Effective communication encompasses a variety of elements that include development of empathy in the health practitioner–woman relationship, shared decision-making and assurance of satisfaction in the outcomes of the encounter (Levine et al., 2010).

One window to a woman's real feelings is the way she tells her **narrative** (or story/history). The women's individual experience, which becomes apparent when a woman tells her narrative, provides an opportunity for health practitioners to learn about being sensitive to women's individual experiences. It is by recognising a woman's point of view through narratives that health practitioners can provide individualised care and genuine guidance. If a health practitioner relies just on *what* a client says, rather than *how* it is said, then an important aspect of what the client is really trying to convey may be missed, and the health practitioner's response may be routine or standardised (Gilkison, 2011).

Narrative An account or story of an experience or journey.

Listening to women's narratives

As practitioners it is important that we *really listen* to what people tell us. When clients tell us about their experiences, the way they tell their narratives are windows to their view of the world. As a health practitioner it is crucial to acknowledge the feelings that women have about their pregnancy and their thoughts about the future. When a woman tells her narrative (or gives her history), she will connect her experience with her feelings: for example, feelings of joy, sadness, aloneness or anger. When a practitioner *really listens* to those feelings, they acknowledge the centrality of affect and subjectivity in human ways of knowing.

Listening to client's narratives is one of the keys to effective communication. *Really* listening reveals much more than simply listening to the words that people use. We need to 'read between the lines' when we take a woman's pregnancy or maternity history. In Case study 2.1, try to 'read between the lines'.

FIGURE 2.1 *Elements of real listening*

Listening requires cognitive, emotional and intentional presence; sometimes called 'mindfulness'. Notice and understand nuances of language, the range of voice, variations of speech, tones and textures, sounds of joy and anger, mixtures of sadness and laughter, the edgy, uncertain words of fear, the myriad facial and body expressions ... the lengthy silences and continuous stream of words and all the ups and downs of ecstasy and misery.

Think about what is *not* said as well as what *is* said. The parts of stories which a person chooses to omit may tell us about the things which they have overlooked, not seen as important, or they may be too painful to talk about.

Look beyond the surface; a range of possible meanings accompanies each word, sentence and text that extends the range of possible experiences; what stands out in every story is what is meaningful to the listener and to the narrator.

Words matter—think about the words the narrator uses. The words chosen indicate attitudes, beliefs and hold hidden meanings. Listen to metaphors: 'the contractions were like waves', or 'the contractions were like hell'. What do these metaphors tell us about the experience?

Be open to the possibility of anything showing up ... Sit back and wait and listen. We have a tendency to see events or experiences as things which we already understand. We may jump to conclusions too quickly if we assume that we understand the problem.

Source: Diekelmann and Diekelmann (2009), Fiumara (1990), Gilkison (2011), Swenson and Sims (2003).

CASE STUDY 2.1

Emma's narrative

I knew inside me that I was pregnant. I had no idea when my period should have come, but felt like it had been ages. I'd been feeling weird and nauseous. Bill and I had had an on-and-off relationship. We had been living together but we would split up then have these passionate 'getting back togethers'. Gosh, I was only 18 and he was 19. Finally I plucked up enough courage to go to the Family Planning Clinic for a pregnancy test. I took along my jar of urine.

It was 30 years ago, but I can still see that nurse's face and hear her voice. Before she did the test she asked me if I hoped it would be positive or negative. I said 'negative' with a lump in my throat. She was out of the room for an eternity. She came back in and showed me the test. 'It shows you are pregnant,' she said. The room spun around me. All I could think of was how I was going to tell my parents. The nurse was talking to me about things like keeping the baby and adoption. I just wanted to get out of there and go and see my friend. On the bus, I was sure everyone was looking at me and knew. When I told my friend, she just said: 'Wow, you're going to have a baby.'

Interpreting the narrative

Emma's narrative includes phrases that are windows to how she is feeling about discovering she is pregnant. She uses the phrase: *finally I plucked up enough courage.* Emma felt she needed courage to go to the Family Planning Clinic. A person needs courage when they are fearful and Emma was fearful of the result of the pregnancy test, even though she suspected it would be positive. When the nurse asked her what she hoped the result of the test would be, Emma said, *'negative' with a lump in my throat.* She was fearful of going to the clinic, she needed *courage* to go there, and then she feared that the pregnancy test would be positive when she hoped it would be negative. Her emotional response gave her a physical feeling of a lump in her throat.

When the nurse took the urine from the room to do the test, Emma felt that the nurse was gone *out of the room for an eternity.* It was probably only a few minutes, but when a person is highly anxious time sometimes goes slowly, and at other times too quickly. When she heard the result was positive, she said *the room spun around me.* The nurse at this stage was talking to Emma about her choices and some decisions she might need to make. Because Emma was so emotionally distraught, she could not hear a word of the discussion, because all she *could think of was how she was going to tell her parents.*

It is not until the final sentence when Emma remembers her friend's words—*Wow, you're going to have a baby*—that there is a sense of the joy about the pregnancy. Emma has been thinking about the things she fears about being pregnant: telling her parents and her relationship with the father of the baby. It takes her friend's words to remind her that she is not just pregnant; she is going to have the joy of having a baby.

{ SUMMARY }

This chapter has explored some of the developmental theories and concepts that surround adaptation to pregnancy. While developmental theory offers one way of looking at the way a woman might adapt to her pregnancy and the transition to motherhood, some would say that a focus on theory may detract from an understanding of the uniqueness of each woman's individual experience. Women's narratives are windows to their individual experience, and listening to client's narratives is one of the keys to effective communication. If practitioners can learn to *really* listen to narratives—to interpret not only what is said but how it is said—then we can learn a lot about a person's feelings, and in turn provide care that responds to their individual needs. Emma's narrative shows how interpreting the way a narrative was told can uncover what is behind the actual words, and help practitioners to learn how to really listen.

REFLECTION POINTS

2.1 Intention (motivation, message, meaning, emotion)

Listening was described as listening to both what was said and what was not said. What do you think influences what is spoken of and what is not?

2.2 Reception (received message, response, feedback)

Elements of real listening—of listening with 'mindfulness'—involves listening to more than the words or content expressed. What other cues might you listen for?

2.3 Perception (style, manner, impression, analysis)

How might you check if your perception of what was 'not said' is accurate? What risks might this involve?

QUESTIONS FOR REVIEW

1 Do you think the nurse would have had an understanding of how Emma was feeling at the time?
2 What cues might you observe that would show a woman's feelings about coming for a pregnancy test?
3 When you read Emma's narrative, what struck you about the narrative? Were you surprised by anything?
4 What did you notice about the words she used or the way she said things?
5 Were you surprised about the things she did not say in her narrative?
6 How would you handle the situation?
7 How could you provide Emma with the information about her choices?

REFERENCES

Amin Shokravi, F., Howden Chapman, P. & Peyman, N. (2009). A comparison study: Risk factors of unplanned pregnancies in a group of Iranian and New Zealander women. *European Journal of Scientific Research, 26*(1), 108–21.

Darvill, R., Skirton, H. & Farrand, P. (2010). Psychological factors that impact on women's experiences of first-time motherhood: A qualitative study of the transition. *Midwifery, 26*(3), 357–66. DOI:10.1016/j.midw.2008.07.006.

Diekelmann, N. & Diekelmann, J. (2009). *Schooling, learning, teaching: Toward narrative pedagogy*. Bloomington, IN: iUniverse.

Fiumara, G. C. (1990). *The other side of language: A philosophy of listening* (C. Lambert, trans.). New York, NY: Routledge.

Gilkison, A. (2011). *Implementing a narrative-centred curriculum in an undergraduate midwifery programme: A hermeneutic study* (doctoral thesis). AUT University, Auckland.

Guilliland, K. & Pairman, S. (1995). *The midwifery partnership: A model for practice*. [Monograph Series 95/1]. Wellington, NZ: Victoria University Press.

Lederman, R. & Weis, K. (2009). *Psychosocial adaptation to pregnancy: Seven dimensions of maternal role development* (3rd edn). New York, NY: Springer.

Levine, M. D., Marcus, M. D., Kalarchian, M. A., Houck, P. R. & Cheng, Y. (2010). Weight concerns, mood, and postpartum smoking relapse. *American Journal of Preventive Medicine, 39*(4), 345–51. DOI:10.1016/j.amepre.2010.05.023.

McAra-Couper, J. (2007). *What is shaping the practice of health professionals and the understanding of the public in relation to increasing intervention in childbirth?* (doctoral thesis). AUT University, Auckland.

Parratt, J. A. & Fahy, K. M. (2011). A feminist critique of foundational nursing research and theory on transition to motherhood. *Midwifery, 27*(4), 445–51.

Rubin, R. (1984). *Maternal identity and the maternal experience*. New York, NY: Springer.

Swenson, M. & Sims, S. (2003). Listening to learn: Narrative strategies and interpretive practices in clinical education. In N. Diekelmann (ed.), *Teaching practitioners of health care: New pedagogies for the health professions* (vol. 2, pp. 154–93). Madison, WI: University of Wisconsin.

WEBSITES

Choosing an LMC, Kiwi Families: www.kiwifamilies.co.nz/Topics/Pregnancy/Choosing+an+LMC.html
Pregnancy, birth and baby care, Te Ara: www.teara.govt.nz/en/pregnancy-birth-and-baby-care
Your Antenatal Guide, OHBaby!: www.ohbaby.co.nz/pregnancy/your-antenatal-guide

{3}

Birth and the Neonate

Annabel Farry and Claire Hotchin

CHAPTER OVERVIEW

This chapter covers the following topics:

+ Birth
+ Supportive communication
+ First communication following birth
+ Early neonatal communication
+ Communicating with babies
+ Practitioners interacting with babies
+ A Māori perspective.

KEY TERMS

Birth
Whānau
Latent phase
Lead Maternity Carer
First stage of labour
Transition
Second stage of labour
Crowning
Behavioural empathy
Sensitive period
Neonatal
Attuned
Post partum

The **birth** of a new family member challenges parents, **whānau** and those supporting them to interact and communicate in new ways that are appropriate to this everyday yet extraordinary event. Comforting communication between a labouring woman and her caregivers helps to create an environment in which she feels safe to become out of control. Losing control is essential to attaining the powerful primal state of birth.

Birth The process of a baby leaving the mother's body.

Whānau Either family and extended family and significant others, or to be born or give birth.

Birth

Birth is an involuntary process that occurs when a complex hormonal combination is released by the hypothalamus and pituitary gland, which are primitive parts of the brain that humans share with all other mammals.

CASE STUDY 3.1

Responses to hormones

Catecholamines (the adrenalines) are vasodilators. Humans respond to fear, whether it is rational or not, by releasing adrenaline. Adrenaline makes mouths dry, eyes widen, sends blood to the skeletal system and leads to a heightened state of awareness.

Oxytocin is responsible for the contraction of the smooth muscle fibres of the uterus and plays a role in creating a sense of calmness and connection.

Endorphins are the body's own opiates. Their levels in the blood stream increase as labour progresses. Without them, labour would be far more painful, and women would therefore be unable to relax enough to allow progress. Endorphins are responsible for the altered state women experience in labour.

Prolactin is involved with initiating and maintaining lactation. It serves multiple roles in mediating care of the offspring, from 'nesting' to the aggressive response mothers have if their offspring are exposed to any threat.

When there are inhibitions in the birth process, they often originate in the 'new brain' or the neocortex. This is the part of the brain responsible for rational thought and decision-making, and is highly developed in humans (Odent, 1999). Women giving birth are not unwell: they are experiencing a normal life event that can be explained in terms of several stages.

Latent phase The period of time prior to labour becoming established.

Lead Maternity Carer The qualified professional identified as providing primary care for a woman during pregnancy, labour and the post-partum period.

First stage of labour The period of time from when contractions become established until the cervix is fully dilated.

The **latent phase** can go on for many hours, sometimes even days, before regular strong contractions begin. The mother is often nervous, and wise communication can play a major role in supporting her. If her fear levels remain high, so will the levels of adrenaline, causing vasoconstriction and a reduction in uterine blood flow and uterine activity (Mander, 1998). A **Lead Maternity Carer** (LMC) can be very effective during this phase by calming both the woman and her support people. She may do this by reminding everyone that labour can take many hours and to look after themselves and each other. It is also useful to promote a sense of 'everydayness' by seeing the woman at home, reassuring her, and encouraging her to go for a walk, have a bath, hold a hot water bottle, enjoy a massage from a support person or just go to sleep.

The **first stage of labour** begins with the onset of regular and strong contractions that dilate the cervix, and finishes when the cervix is fully dilated. The birthing woman has now moved into an altered state of consciousness. She may be loudly vocalising her sensations or quietly breathing through them.

It is at this point where support people declare themselves. Seeing the person they love experiencing pain can cause a number of responses. Some will try to rescue the person from her experience by reminding her of all the pain relief options available. Others will become hyper talkative to cover up their sense of inadequacy. Others may fall asleep. Some may become angry and try to find answers for what they feel is unacceptable. All these responses are due to fear of pain and a lack of awareness about how long a birth can take. A good support person will be able to continue to 'be with' the woman by responding to her but not reacting to her, while continuing to take care of themselves.

Transition The part of labour between the first and second stages.

Transition is the word used to describe the period of time when the woman's body is moving from the first stage to the second stage of labour. Her cervix is almost fully dilated and she is beginning to feel the pressure of her baby on her pelvic floor. As the baby is pushed down the birth canal, past the last centimetre of cervix and onto the muscles of the pelvic floor, women often become overwhelmed and frightened. Women in transition make statements like:

+ 'I've had enough.'
+ 'I can't do this.'
+ 'This is too intense.'
+ 'Please help me.'
+ 'Get me an epidural.'
+ 'How much longer?'

It is at this point that an LMC will use their wisdom to decide what kind of communication is required to help the woman make it through this transition. She may engage all support people to surround the woman with encouraging, loving and strengthening words. She may step in and ask the woman to make direct eye contact with her and breathe with her through each contraction, thus keeping her in the moment and avoiding panic. She may remind her of the physiology of this stage and that the intensity is encouraging as it suggests excellent progress. She may acknowledge the difficulty of this stage of labour and remind her that these sensations are normal and that they will pass. She may use distractions, focusing her mind on a specific task like emptying her bladder. Helping her to the bathroom and back (she will experience contractions along the way) may take her into the next stage.

The **second stage of labour** is from full dilation of the cervix until the baby is completely born. The high state of despair that can occur during transition passes into a very focused bearing down in second stage, when the woman usually gets an overwhelming urge to push during her contractions. Her sounds become more guttural and lower pitch. With each contraction the baby advances and eventually **crowning** occurs.

Second stage of labour The part of labour between full dilation of the cervix and the birth of the baby.

Crowning When the top of the baby's head becomes visible during birth.

Some women manage the second stage of labour and the actual birth of their baby with minimal guidance; they understand instinctively how to gently ease their baby over this threshold, thus minimising the risk of tearing their perineum. Other women need specific guidance at this stage and may later recall not hearing anything but their LMC's voice gently guiding them to 'push or pant'. This intricate three-way communication between the mother, her baby and her health practitioner is, for most women, the period of most intense sensation. This is also when all four hormones are at their peak levels in both the mother and baby's blood stream. Wide eyed with adrenaline, euphoric with endorphins and replete with oxytocin and prolactin, mother and baby make eye contact and an intense bond forms with their mutual gaze.

CASE STUDY 3.2

The importance of support in labour

In 2007, the Cochrane Review of sixteen trials, which involved 13,391 women in eleven countries, concluded that women who experienced continuous one-to-one support during labour:

- were more likely to give birth without using analgesia or anaesthesia
- were more likely to have a spontaneous vaginal birth
- were less likely to report dissatisfaction with their childbirth experiences
- experienced slightly shorter labours.

Common elements of the care provided by these support people include emotional support, information about labour progress and advice regarding coping techniques, comfort measures and advocacy.

The report does not list any adverse effects and states that none are plausible, so it's clear that continuous support during labour provides definite benefits with no attendant risks. It concludes that 'all women should be allowed and encouraged to have support people with them continuously during labour' (Hodnett et al., 2007)

Supportive communication

It would seem obvious that an event of such personal magnitude involving such extreme sensations and of such a fundamentally private nature would require some support from trusted loved ones; however, just two generations ago women were expected to experience labour alone. Women were isolated from loved ones and birth happened to them in an environment over which they had no control. Many routine interventions were imposed unnecessarily and babies were separated from their mothers for long periods between feeds.

In Aotearoa New Zealand many changes have occurred in the last two decades. It is now respected that because the powerful process of labour produces a new family member, family should be central to the event. Often there will be many family members waiting to meet their new sibling, grandchild, niece or nephew. Family are now expected to play a role in the process—if the mother has chosen to have them with her. The LMC often needs to communicate not only with the mother and the father of the baby but also with other significant family members. There may be a language barrier to navigate, in which case the LMC should use a translator (either a professional or a family member) to keep up a healthy dialogue.

During pregnancy the LMC should discuss labour at length. She should listen to what the woman wants for her labour, share information with the woman and spend time helping her make the choices that will form her birth plan. This plan may change, but it begins the process of mutual trust that is essential to a positive birth experience.

Behavioural empathy Actions that demonstrate an understanding or genuine appreciation of the experience of others.

Experienced LMCs often practice a deliberate empathic response termed **behavioural empathy** (Burleson & Holmstrom, 2008) to encourage a woman to feel safe enough to enter into an altered state of consciousness.

Comforting measures should:

+ be highly person-centred; that is, verbal strategies should acknowledge, contextualise and legitimise the feelings of the distressed other
+ involve statements of positive regard, esteem, admiration for the courage or effort shown, understanding the difficulty of the task and confidence that the other will prevail
+ include non-verbal behaviours such as forward body leans, touches and pats, hugs and hand-holding, focused looks and soothing sounds.

During labour some women become completely internal and do not want any encouraging words or touch. They become completely immersed in their sensations, displaying an instinctive need to find a place of safety. Others are fiercely protective of their internal environment during labour. They will respond to disturbance as though it is a threat to their life. They may swear or make commands like 'Don't touch me' or 'Stop talking' or 'Go away'. While this communication may be unthinkable to the woman in a day-to-day context, there is an altered arrangement during labour. Sometimes support people may experience communication from the mother during labour as hurtful. But, more often, it is clear that there is a sacred transformation occurring; the woman's voice is resonant and powerful. The most respectful approach to supporting women during birth is to believe that the woman knows what she needs. Giving birth is a significant event that can have lasting effects on those involved. It has been said that 'birth is not only about making babies. Birth also is about making mothers—strong competent capable mothers, who trust themselves and know their inner strength' (Katz Rothman, 1996, p. 254).

First communication following birth

Universally, one of the first reactions mothers have after the birth of their babies is a desire to look into their baby's eyes. Already familiar with the voices of their parents, the baby gazes back intently. With loving touch and kind words, this gentle welcome to the world tells the baby they are in a safe place. This time, immediately after birth, is a psycho-physiologically **sensitive period**, which floods the baby's senses with the experience (gentle or rough) of being in the world, helping them to stabilise metabolically, and allowing them to initiate breastfeeding.

Sensitive period
A developmental period where particular impressions are most likely to occur and therefore relevant behaviour learnt.

The optimal place for this transition to happen is skin to skin on the mother's chest. Skin-to-skin contact (SSC) involves gently placing the naked baby prone on the mother's bare chest, facilitating interaction through all the senses: touch, smell, sight, hearing and taste. The ideal environment for this to happen is warm, safe, private and uninterrupted.

CASE STUDY 3.3

Early skin-to-skin contact

Skin-to-skin contact (SSC) stabilises and maintains the newborn's heart rate, respiratory rate, blood pressure and blood sugar. A newborn cannot regulate its own temperature; however, a mother in SSC with her infant will increase or decrease her temperature in response to her baby's temperature, in order to maintain the baby's temperature at ideal levels. Babies who experience SSC with their mothers are less likely to cry. Newborn reflexes help the baby who is in SSC move to the breast (stepping reflex), find the nipple (rooting reflex) and begin suckling (sucking and swallow reflex). Breastfeeding, in addition to providing optimal nutrition, fosters early bonding via touch, responsiveness and mutual gazing (Moore, Anderson & Bergman, 2011).

Early neonatal communication

Neonatal Relating to the period of life from birth to 28 days.

Sensory experiences, both negative and positive, from late pregnancy through the **neonatal** period and into the first three years of life, have a direct impact on how a child's brain develops. Nature and nurture work together; both genes and experience are important. A child's early experiences are critical for their brains to form the connections they need to develop. As experiences are repeated, the connections, pathways and networks in a baby's brain strengthen and become permanent (Rowley, 2009).

Responsive tender care from parents or a consistent caregiver creates effective, loving and lasting parents for an infant. Oxytocin is produced by both mothers and babies and increases bonding, setting the scene for the child to develop lasting attachments with others. Being soothed, comforted and responded to allows the baby to feel that they are welcome, loved and wanted. Happiness, joy and responsive care are the experiences that wire the baby's brain to love and trust others. The mother's capacity to create joy, elation, interest and excitement in a baby is key to early healthy development and lifelong physical and mental health.

Neglect, chaotic environments, violence and abuse (lack of attachment) create experiences of persistent stress, danger and fear, and signal the baby to release adrenaline and cortisol (fight or flight hormones). Cortisol in increased amounts over long periods is toxic to neurons, and growing neurons are most sensitive. A prolonged excess of cortisol causes brain dysfunction and destruction. If the stress response is repeatedly triggered, it becomes the template for brain development. The child that experiences persistent stress lives in a constant state of alertness and arousal, watching for signs of danger. A lack of attachment in the first three years correlates to ongoing life problems marked by impulsivity, easy arousal, the unthinking release of aggression and an inability to establish firm trusting relationships with other humans (Perry, 2002).

Communicating with babies

At birth, babies are already communicating in non-verbal ways. All humans are prepared to send and receive messages long before the development of formal language. What on the surface looks like random behaviour is in fact highly organised. Babies communicate about how they experience the world, using all their senses to get to know their family and their environment. Touch is the first sense experienced and perhaps the last to leave as we die. Smell, taste, balance, hearing and vision follow in a sequence that completes development.

CASE STUDY 3.4

How newborns communicate

Eye contact

A newborn's visual abilities are fine-tuned for eye contact. They recognise faces and prefer to look at faces over any other object. A newborn can see best when an object is approximately 20–30 cm away; the distance a mother's face will be if she is cuddling her baby or breastfeeding. At this distance they can imitate facial expressions.

Hearing and understanding

Although babies are not able to understand words when they are born, they are able to discern emotions. Babies are attuned to the emotions of their caregivers as one of their skills to survive. They understand the feelings of caregivers by listening to tone of voice, looking at facial expressions and feeling the pace of their caregivers' breathing. It is not so much what is said, but how it is said that is being absorbed—not literally but emotionally.

Non-verbal communication signs

Babies are responsive to other people and very expressive in their facial movements and gestures. They have a wide range of facial expressions, including bliss, joy, pain, sadness, fear and curiosity. They use their bodies to communicate. Some of these body movements are reflexive and therefore involuntary (for example, babies startle in response to a loud sound and make a tight fist when something is placed in their palm), while others are developmental; for example, turning their head from side to side and raising it from a prone position.

While babies are all individual, there are some generally accepted behavioural signs of what they are communicating. A happy baby is physically relaxed—they may coo, smile and engage in eye contact. When a baby is tired, they may frown, yawn, rub their eyes and become agitated. When hungry, they lick their lips, open and close their mouth, suck their fists or clothing, turn their head from side to side and become restless. Stressed babies fidget, grimace, look away, become agitated, make jerky or thrashing movements and arch their backs. Crying is a late communication sign for tired, hungry and stressed babies. Crying is always a sign of distress and a need for attention. Extended crying is physiologically harmful. It results in hoarseness, reduced oxygen levels, increased heart rate, disturbed digestion and drained energy. It also floods the baby with cortisol, which negatively affects their developing brain (Ludington-Hoe, Cong & Hashemi, 2002).

Despite being born with the capacity for feeling deep emotions, babies are unable to keep themselves in a state of equilibrium, lacking the skills to regulate either the intensity or the duration of those emotions. Without the assistance and responsiveness of a caregiver, babies become overwhelmed by their emotional states, including those of fear, excitement and sadness. When overwhelmed, and separated from their caregiver, they go into a despair–withdrawal response. If their despair (crying) is not answered, they withdraw. Physiologically, they release high levels of cortisol, become cooler, drop their heart rate and become quiet. A quiet and withdrawn baby may not be one that has learnt to be 'good' but one that is experiencing despair (Grille, 2008).

In order to maintain emotional equilibrium, babies require a consistent and committed relationship with one caring person, usually the mother. As the mother tunes into her baby's internal states, her responses produce a response in the baby. One is not independent of the other, and each has a profound effect on the next response. Healthy attachment is simply the development of that **attuned** relationship. Attunement, in the simplest terms, means following baby's cues. When a child looks, reaches, gestures, makes a sound or uses facial expression, this is a non-verbal conversational turn and our response keeps the conversation going. Engaging a baby in meaningful 'give and take' interactions helps their social, emotional and cognitive development.

Attuned The state of being particularly aware of the needs of others.

Babies are equal partners in communication and have their own spontaneous expressions of themselves. Their emotional experience (for example, pain, pleasure, joy or sorrow) is a total body experience. Babies do not pretend or manipulate. What they communicate is emotionally honest and immediate. They cannot plan ahead, have no concept of time and are not equipped to wait. When people respond warmly and promptly to these expressions, they communicate understanding of what the baby is doing, feeling and even thinking. This acknowledges that the baby's feelings are as important as adults'.

Practitioners interacting with babies

Adult communication needs to be adapted to the needs of newborns. Babies thrive on responsiveness, dependability and warmth. When a baby is responded to with tenderness, warmth and love, their body is flooded with pleasurable hormones and their brain forms the connections that they need to develop into a flexible, responsible, empathetic, loving, independent and intelligent member of society.

The early childhood years profoundly affect adult life and in turn affect society as a whole. Health practitioners have a responsibility to share this important information with parents and whānau. Learning to be a parent means learning a new set of skills. Parents and whānau can be supported in the early weeks by enabling mother and baby to be together and maximising their opportunity to bond. Some parents need more help than others to interact responsively with their babies. Teaching and encouraging parents **post partum** how to recognise and respond to their baby's communication cues, how to soothe their baby, and how to interact lovingly and playfully with their baby supports the family from the beginning.

Post partum The period following birth.

Breastfeeding gives the optimal start for a baby's growth, providing exactly what the baby needs for brain growth, as well as providing the sensory pleasure of being held, gazed at and talked with. Parents need support, energy and resources to be able to cope and respond appropriately to babies. Practitioners need to be alert to any potential problems that make it difficult for mothers to cope—for example, depression or living in a violent situation—in order to provide support and early on build parenting skills.

Practitioners also have a responsibility to role model appropriate communication with, and handling of, newborns. When performing procedures on a baby, they need to touch the baby gently, tell them what they are going to do, monitor their response throughout the procedure and stop if necessary. There is never a reason to handle babies in an insensitive mechanical way that disregards their integrity.

A Māori perspective

Pre-colonial Māori surrounded birth with complex rituals and practices that paid respect to the gods of nature (atua) and encouraged the labouring mother to let go, and to give up control over the process to the gods. For many Māori this rich complexity has been lost along with elements of language and culture as a result of colonisation. Within the language, birth is acknowledged as a fundamental part of life. The word 'whenua' means both placenta and land, the word 'hapu' means both pregnant and subtribe, and the term 'whare tangata' means both womb and ancestral meeting house. This meeting house sits at the centre of the marae (sacred open meeting area), which is central to Māori communities. Respect for whenua (both land and placenta), whakapapa (genealogy), tipuna (ancestors) and whanaungatanga (extended family) keep birth in a normal context, while at the same time respecting it as sacred and otherworldly.

Māori who identify as tangata whenua (people of the land) retain a connection to pre-colonial ways of understanding the natural environment. Māori women have been at the forefront in resisting what they see as the encroachment of science into areas of life governed by forces beyond its control. For Māori, the process of birth is one of the most sacred of all such areas of life. Māori women give birth with less intervention than any other ethnicity in Aotearoa (Ministry of Health, 2010). Encouragement during birth is communicated through karakia (prayer), waiata (song), meri meri (massage), calming words and by loving, present physical contact.

One practice that has become almost mainstream is that of returning the whenua (placenta) to the whenua (land). This communicates a deep respect to papatuanuku (mother earth) for the nurturing of this pepe's (baby's) life into Te Ao Marama (the world of light). While many ethnicities practise this ritual, using a tree to mark a spot for their child to visit in years to come, Māori most often bury the whenua in a place with ancestral connections, showing respect for the tipuna who are acknowledged as having a continued place in this child's life.

{ SUMMARY }

Continuous support during labour by trusted support people and using comforting communication will encourage the mental relinquishment necessary to achieve physiological labour and birth. Newborns come into this world with the ability to communicate and respond. Consistent, responsive, nurturing, positive, rich experiences in the first three years of life are essential for optimal brain development, resulting in flexible, responsible, empathetic and intelligent members of society. The neonate is an aware, dependent, vulnerable human being who is born with the ability to communicate. Optimal lifelong social, emotional and physical functioning depends upon positive early life experiences in a loving and consistent environment.

REFLECTION POINTS

3.1 Intention (motivation, message, meaning, emotion)

While infants may not understand the meaning of words spoken, they are able to interact. What benefits are there to both mother and baby in sharing skin-to-skin contact at birth?

3.2 Reception (received message, response, feedback)

The newborn infant is described as being born with the ability to communicate. How does a newborn baby convey that it is content?

3.3 Perception (style, manner, impression, analysis)

How might health practitioners role model appropriate communications with a newborn infant?

QUESTIONS FOR REVIEW

1 A 4-week-old baby is brought into the busy health clinic by her mother for a 'Well Child Check'. She is late for her appointment. The baby is crying. The mother is stressed. How would you respond to this mother and baby?

2 You have agreed to be your best friend's support person during her labour. She tells you she is scared of being in pain and out of control. How will you respond?

REFERENCES

Burleson, B. & Holmstrom, A. (2008) Comforting Communication. In W. Donsbach (ed.), *The International Encyclopedia of Communication*. Blackwell Reference Online. Retrieved 12 March 2011 from http://www.communicationencyclopedia.com/public/tocnode?id=g9781405131995_yr2011_chunk_g97814051319958_ss50-1. DOI: 10.1111/b.9781405131995.2008.x.

Grille, R. (2008). *Heart to heart parenting*. Sydney: ABC Books.

Hodnett, E. D., Gates, S., Hofmeyr, G. J. & Sakala, C. (2007). Continuous support for women during childbirth. *Cochrane Database of Systematic Reviews*, issue 3, art. no. CD003766. DOI: 10.1002/14651858.CD003766.pub2.

Katz Rothman, B. (1996). Women, providers and control. *Journal of Obstetric, Gynecologic and Neonatal Nursing, 25*(3), 253–6.

Ludington-Hoe, S. M., Cong, X. & Hashemi, F. (2002). Infant crying: Nature, physiologic consequences, and select interventions. *Neonatal Network, 21*(2), 29–36.

Mander, R. (1998). *Pain in childbearing and its control*. Oxford, UK: Blackwell Science.

Ministry of Health. (2010). *Maternal and newborn information 2003*. Report on Maternity. Wellington, NZ. Retrieved 14 December 2006 from www.nzhis.govt.nz/publications/maternityreport03.pdf.

Moore, E. R., Anderson, G. C. & Bergman, N. (2011). *Early skin-to-skin contact for mothers and their healthy newborn infants*. Retrieved 18 February 2011 from www2.cochrane.org/reviews/en/ab003519.html.

Odent, M. (1999). *The scientification of love*. London, UK: Free Association Books.

Perry, B. D. (2002). Childhood experience and the expression of genetic potential: What childhood neglect tells us about nature and nurture. *Brain and Mind, 3*, 79–100.

Rowley, S. (2009). *The early years—how experience shapes the brain*. Retrieved from http://brainwave.org.nz/wp-content/uploads//2009/10/Chronicle-July-2009-English.pdf.

WEBSITES

Centre for Attachment: www.centreforattachment.com

Liggins Institute: www.liggins.auckland.ac.nz/uoa

The Early Years and Brain Development, Brainwave: http://brainwave.org.nz

{4}

Communicating with Babies and Young Children

Rain Lamdin and Rachel Lamdin Hunter

CHAPTER OVERVIEW

This chapter covers the following topics:

+ Social and cultural contexts of childhood
+ Social context and learning
+ Understanding communicating and language
+ Getting older: 3 years and on
+ Communication through play.

KEY TERMS

Family
Attachment
Vocabulary
Play

Communication with babies and toddlers can be rewarding, puzzling or fraught with anxiety, depending on our understanding of the capabilities and needs of children and babies, and also upon our perception of our abilities or experiences. In this chapter we focus on the developing communication of babies and children, and refer to theories of child development where they are directly relevant to communication. We also consider real-life examples of child-focused practice and communication. Life patterns are established in these early years; therefore communicating respectfully and with an understanding of a baby or young child's development is extremely important. This chapter is written with a predominantly Pakeha perspective, influenced by Western theories. We acknowledge the importance of an awareness of differences in communication styles between and across cultures in ethical health-care practice.

There are three points that underpin our views of communication with babies and children. First, the baby or child is a member of a **family**; they come from, refer to, learn within and explore their worlds as part of that family. Second, non-verbal communication is constant and informative. Finally, whether we are child or adult, we are already and always communicating.

Family A close social grouping of people who are related genetically, emotionally or culturally and who provide basic support for one another.

Social and cultural contexts of childhood

How children are perceived in terms of their dependence or vulnerability affects how adults communicate with them and what they expect in return. It is common for adults to consider people as being children until they are in their teen years. Typically, children between the ages of 12 and 18 months are considered babies, while those under 3 or 4 years are deemed toddlers. In Aotearoa New Zealand, children under 5 years are 'preschoolers'. Most children begin primary school at the age of 5 years; however, 6 years is the legal requirement. Socially and legally, children lack certain rights or responsibilities that adults possess. It is common in Western nations to think of working for money or taking care of family members as being the domain of adults, even though in many parts of the world children are expected to carry out caregiving duties and contribute economically to the family.

'Childhood' was not a clear phenomenon until the late seventeenth or early eighteenth centuries. During medieval times, children may have worked for money, attended school infrequently (if at all, depending on their place within the family or society) and carried their own weapons, along with being accountable for any crimes they may have committed (Aries, 1962). The emergence of developmental theory, in which children were held as developmentally incomplete and thus incompetent (in relation to adults), probably contributed to the positioning of children as dependent, vulnerable beings—a common view held today.

Theories that focus upon child development are inevitably formulated by theorists and researchers who are adults. Accordingly, theories of communication development are told from the perspective of the adult 'looking in' on the child's world. Theorists and researchers need to take care to understand and acknowledge their own beliefs about children and how they see themselves in relation to children. It is also important to acknowledge that various theories about development or communication may inadvertently disempower children, negatively influencing working relationships with them or their advocates.

TABLE 4.1 *Assumptions about children and possible effects on communication*

Commonly held assumptions or stereotypes of young children	*Possible effects on communication in practice with young children*
Children are incomplete humans—not fully developed and 'not there yet' as people.	Their wants and needs are seen as less important and may be over-ridden or disregarded.
Undeveloped verbal skills mean they have poor understanding of what is said or what happens to them.	Adults may not bother to explain our actions, procedures or rationales.
Undeveloped verbal skills mean that children cannot communicate or make their needs known to others.	Adults may not seek to understand or acknowledge the ideas, needs or questions of young children.

CASE STUDY 4.1

Human rights and children

Children's rights have been an international work in progress since 1924, initially through the League of Nations and now the United Nations. Human rights frameworks highlight children as rights-bearing individual citizens, rather than the moral property of adults such as their parents or caregivers. New Zealand and Australia became signatories to the United Nations Convention on the Rights of the Child in 1993 and 1990, respectively. The most recent version (United Nations, 2005) has several Articles that indirectly or directly relate to children and their rights within health care:

- Article 5 highlights the responsibilities of organisations to respond to children within the context of their family.

- Guardians, parents and extended family are responsible for the child and, as such, are integral in the decision-making process during the assessment, treatment and care of children.
- Articles 12 and 13 detail the rights of children to express their views and to seek, receive and impart information. This is not written with specific reference to health care; however, it is clearly relevant when caring for and working with young children.
- Article 24 is specifically written to address the rights of children to the access and attainment of health care, including access to information and education regarding their care.

The enactment of children's rights can be complicated when babies and young children are unable to demand that their rights be met. However, communication in health care is as much the right of a child as is access to health-care treatment. It is the professional responsibility of the health-care practitioner to uphold and advocate for such rights.

Social context and learning

Babies and young children are individuals, and learning how to communicate occurs in the context of their individual surroundings. Early family life is a rich setting for development, providing examples of communication including everyday language, intonation, meanings, mannerisms and values. Most communication in very early life is between babies and their caregivers and family members—those most intimately associated with the baby or young child.

CASE STUDY 4.2

Children, family and society

In 2003, New Zealand Members of Parliament undertook an historic vote overturning Section 59 of the Crimes Act 1961, which had provided a legal defence for parents charged with assault after physically disciplining their children. Redress for parents and caregivers to use 'reasonable force' when disciplining their children meant that parents could legally smack or hit their children, when in other such cases of assault they would be charged and convicted. Exactly what constituted 'reasonable force' was difficult for parents, lawmakers, police and judges to agree upon.

Several high-profile cases, in which parents escaped conviction after assaulting children with hosepipes, riding crops or electrical cords, contributed to growing public unease about the detriment caused to children by such treatment. The rights of society's most vulnerable citizens to live free of fear of such correction contrasted with the rights of parents to 'parent as they saw fit', along with anxiety that children would 'run amok' if not disciplined in particular ways. Implicit within each side of the hotly debated argument were contrasting views on the nature of children. However, both discourses acknowledged the crucial role that parents, caregivers and family play in teaching and shaping children as they grow.

One of the most dominant bodies of knowledge regarding the care of babies and communication arose from the child–caregiver work of John Bowlby (1951), following the Second World War. His work followed research carried out with children who were orphaned or otherwise separated from their parents across a variety of settings. Researchers observed that some indicators of developmental progress were delayed or absent in children who had spent long periods of time in unfamiliar or non-nurturing environments, such as hospitals, refugee camps or orphanages. In particular, the absence of intimate caregiver-type relationships was believed to interrupt the growth, development and health of such children. Such studies were linked with research indicating that adult well-being and mental health were related to childhood experience, primarily before the age of 3 years. Later attempts to restore such developmental input for children were often unsuccessful, promoting the view that children had a prime but limited window of developmental opportunity in their early years.

Bowlby claimed that a primary caregiver—specifically, the child's mother—must be available to respond to a young child's needs in order for them to thrive physically, cognitively and socially, and to avoid what he termed 'maternal deprivation' (Bowlby, 1951). This '**attachment**' bond between mother and child provides a secure social foundation from which children are able to safely explore new surroundings. The concept of attachment still features strongly in many approaches to parenting and understandings of child–parent relationships.

Attachment
Emotional affection and social bonds between people.

It is appropriate to acknowledge that this emphasis on attachment came from a Western perspective of what is 'good' or 'normal' child development. Within this context, growing up and becoming an individual, independent of the family, is highly valued. Children are encouraged to explore their worlds beyond the family and to be self-assured. However, these values are not common across all cultures. The research and analysis that underpins these views also requires some analysis. In Aotearoa New Zealand, for example, early childhood services cannot be compared with war orphanages in terms of stimulation and caring relationships between child and educator/carer (Claiborne & Drewery, 2010). Also, the mother role has been used in arguments for reducing women's place in the workforce, and continues to be an issue for women who are in the position to choose whether they wish to work outside the home.

For health practitioners working with babies and young children, an essential element of communication involves liaising with parents, caregivers and family members of the child. This is an ethical and legal requirement as parents must consent to assessment, investigations and treatment on behalf of their children. Parents need to feel heard, understood and validated in their knowledge of and relationship with their child. Children look to their parent to assess the risk of danger or to provide comfort in novel situations (Bretherton, 1992). Supporting parents to communicate with their child builds strength into the family, as the parent will continue the care and support of the child beyond their contact with the health-care professions and systems. Parents help to shape children's stories and memories of health care and in so doing heighten or allay anxieties.

Understanding communicating and language

A particular level of attention and intimacy is required in order for any baby-initiated messages to be understood. The child–caregiver relationship requires each person to be 'tuned in' to successfully interpret the non-verbal cues and signs that are essential means of communication.

The earliest expression of discomfort, fear or pain is found in crying. A baby may demonstrate particular qualities to their cry, such as a shrill pitch or particularly high volume and some individuals cry more than others. However, there are generally common qualities among certain cries in terms of tone, pitch and volume, indicating messages that are common to all babies at some stage.

TABLE 4.2 *Types of baby cries*

Need or reason for crying	*Type of cry*
Pain or discomfort	Loud, sudden, shrill; silence or long pause between each cry while breath is drawn in for the next cry
Hunger	Begins with an uneven, low-intensity, intermittent grizzle; gradually escalates to continuous wail, increasing in volume and intensity
Fatigue or overtiredness	'Grizzling': monotone of a medium even pitch; seemingly continuous but rises over time in pitch and volume if not attended to
Irritation, frustration or boredom	Can sound most like spoken language—some variances in pitch and volume as if conversing in words
Shock, fear or surprise	Preceded by a quick intake of breath and then a shallow shrill cry, similar but less intense than a pain or discomfort cry; also may have a grizzly, uneven quality

The frequency and duration of crying in young babies, while variable, is mediated by the responsiveness of the parent or caregiver to the baby's needs. When a baby's needs are met there is less need to cry. By the age of 2 months, some babies maintain eye contact with caregivers during feeding and other settled wakeful periods. When a person sustains such eye contact while speaking to the baby, and then pauses, it encourages the baby to 'reply', which models conversation. The baby's responses comprise 'cooing' or 'gurgling'. As the anatomy of the mouth and throat mature, the child's ability to make different sounds improves, resulting in babbling, usually between 4 and 6 months. By 4 months, such sounds may include giggling and laughing.

Even while babies are limited to crying, babbling or smiling, they are able to observe and form rudimentary understandings of what they experience through their senses. Babies communicate, noticing and imitating sounds and facial expressions of other people within the first few months of life, most often from their mother or primary caregiver. Table 4.3 describes common examples of early communication. It should be remembered that there is a wide variation of ages in which each stage is reached, so the milestones mentioned here are approximations.

TABLE 4.3 *Baby communication*

Age (approximate)	*Features*
6 weeks	First 'social smile'—a response to expressions from other people
3 months	Seeks eye contact with others
	May take turns to coo or gurgle with another person
6–8 months	May follow a pointed finger or look to where someone is referring or pointing
8 months	Notices other's conversations and listens
	Recognises surroundings and can show joy or excitement in response
	May understand simple instructions: 'No!' or 'Show me'
10 months	Can follow simple directions to give or show a toy to another person.
	May wave in response to a wave or direction

CASE STUDY 4.3

The 'nappy-free' baby

Elimination communication (EC) is a form of early communication that is used by some families with young babies. Parents adopting this method of caring for their baby spend time with the baby in close proximity, learning the baby's cues or body language signs preceding a bowel or bladder movement. Such cues include wriggling, sighing, appearing to struggle or even emitting a particular cry. The caregiver responds by holding the baby in a particular squatting position over the toilet or potty and using a chosen cue or sound (such as 'ssss') to signal to the baby that they can release and 'go'. Anecdotal supporters of this method claim that the saving of costs in nappies and the eliminated need for toilet training at age 2 (a challenging time for some families of young children) far outweigh the effort required to tune into and learn the baby's methods of communication. Such methods of toileting are commonplace across several cultures (Sun & Rugolotto, 2004).

In Aotearoa New Zealand, the success of such methods also depends upon the physical proximity of the primary caregiver (usually the mother) to the baby. Families utilising EC in Aotearoa New Zealand might experience some judgment from others not familiar with this philosophy of communication with babies, while families in which both parents have outside commitments (such as work) may find it difficult to be in the requisite proximity to the child in order for the method to be successful.

This example of communication with babies and young children highlights the range of cultural, functional and human elements that impact on communication with children.

Young children understand before they can communicate clearly (Buckley, 2003). Babbling includes a repetitive sound such as 'bababa' or 'nanana', initially using a limited range of consonants that are easy to pronounce. Babbling may occur in response to sounds or voices heard by the baby, or may be self-initiated. Using their voice purposefully may include 'calling' for the parent or caregiver when in another room. During excited or playful times, babies from about 6 months of age may begin to purposefully demonstrate their feelings by kicking, waving their arms, wriggling or turning away. The onset of crawling, usually between 8 and 12 months, enables babies to physically communicate their interest in, say, a family pet or their reluctance to have their nappy changed.

During the second half of the first year, communicative abilities expand to involve people other than the primary caregiver, including family members, other babies and strangers. After initially guarded responses to new people, some babies will actively seek contact with others. A baby may signal a desire for a toy by seeking eye contact with their caregiver and looking from the caregiver to the toy and back again. Reaching out or pointing may accompany the request, as well as babbling (Buckley, 2003, p. 30). Between 8 and 10 months, some babies will develop use of some early 'words', such as 'ohh!' or 'wow!' Even with murmurs rather than exact words, a questioning intonation can be used to express intent or interest, or ask a question such as 'May I have that?' or 'Where has it gone?' Such early sounds are often deemed by parents to be first words. Other early words may include names ('Mama', 'Dada'), consisting of short repetitive syllables that resemble early babbling. Other first words typically include those which have been spoken more commonly in front of or to the child, such as 'no', 'bye' or 'more'.

Approaching their first birthday, babies can begin to understand directions communicated to them by combining several techniques for interpretation, known as non-linguistic strategies (Buckley, 2003). Non-linguistic strategies include noticing facial expressions, gestures or movements used by the other person, and utilising their emerging knowledge of the context and what usually happens next. For example, a toddler picking up a toy bunny off her bedroom floor and showing it to her grandmother might hear 'Ohhh ... give him a cuddle'. Noticing the grandmother clasping her hands to her chest and putting her head to one side, as well as the facial and vocal expression of tenderness, the child may mimic her actions.

While initially understanding a direction in only one context, a child's understanding will grow to encompass a broader range of settings in which, for example, 'Give him (or her) a cuddle' is appropriate, such as when a friend is hurt in play. Over time, the child will rely less upon non-linguistic strategies and more upon verbal content, as knowledge of word meanings increases and the contexts in which the child finds themselves are extended.

CASE STUDY 4.4

Baby sign language

The use of sign language between mother and baby can be developed before oral communication is possible. Here, a mother (and aunt) describes her experiences.

> I watched my nieces communicate with their parents in their own way. It involved their hands, attempts at words and even simple and more meaningful eye contact. One niece and my sister-in-law could go a whole day without using words, such was their shared understanding and the use of eye contact and body language.
>
> With my own son, from a very early age I used very simple signs to indicate things I wanted him to understand. This included holding up one finger and saying, 'I will be back in one minute' if he was awake and I left him. I wanted him to understand that my leaving was temporary. I knew this went against what the developmental psychology theory said, given he was apparently too young to understand that objects exist even when he couldn't see them.
>
> One of the most important things I did early on, which I think helped our communication, was to make a lot of eye contact with him, always respond to him and talk a lot to him. This verbal and non-verbal communication was an effort to reinforce our ability to connect and communicate. While books

promote specific signs, we have developed our own. This wasn't intentional but intuitive, and the result is that my son has created his own signs. His signs are often obvious—licking his finger and closing his mouth to ask for food. When I am not sure what he is asking or talking about, I offer suggestions or ask him to show me and I learn. Now he is at the age of 2 years, we have little frustration with communicating. There are also other factors involved—he is a socially oriented and calm child. The key has been to pay attention to him and respond when he communicates.

Vocabulary The collection of words and symbols that people use to communicate.

Early baby **vocabulary** is also characterised by words that may be incomprehensible to others, but very familiar to family members. The child who wakes from their nap calling for 'Dahdah!' may be calling a pet named Poppy, yet this is only apparent to those in the child's immediate family. Such adopted terms must be translated for others. Some early words also include run-together phrases such as 'mo-more' ('no more'). A single term such as the exclamation 'mang!' may have a multiplicity of meanings, being used to comment on hearing a hammer being used, to complain that the child has just bumped their head or to signal their intent to shut a door. Children also begin to make noises or sounds when handling or identifying objects or toys. Similarly, using actions to accompany early words helps others to interpret meaning; for example, using 'bep-bep' to refer to a car when accompanied by the forward motion of a hand honking a car horn. The content of children's communication at this early stage is focused on the immediate and visible experiences of the child.

Piaget observed the development of his own children and identified stages of sensori-motor and cognitive development (Piaget, 1962). Piaget noticed a change in babies aged between 6 and 12 months in which they began to clearly notice the absence of an object or person after they had disappeared, which he termed 'object permanence'. Slightly older babies would look and then search for the object or person, clearly holding an image of it in their mind. This early mental representation signifies the beginning of symbolic thinking, in which children come to understand that objects, people and events have particular names or representations in language. Such a shift in understanding is believed to lead to rapid increases in understood vocabulary, coinciding with improved motor control of oral muscles (Buckley, 2003). While their own pronunciation remains messy, young children may notice others' pronunciation; for example, a mother using the toddler's term 'blana' for 'banana' may be reprimanded in no uncertain terms by the toddler!

The number of words understood by very young children is far greater than those able to be uttered by the child—a ratio of approximately four to one in children aged between

1 and 2 years. However, the uttered words also increase rapidly during this period. For example, at 13 months a toddler may have an understood vocabulary of about fifty words, but by 18 months the toddler will be able to *express* fifty words (Menyuk, Liebergott & Schultz, 1995). The ability to comprehend increasingly complex instructions or questions begins with simple one- and two-part instructions ('Pick up that letter and give it to Grandma') from about 18 months of age. Children may begin pointing to objects or bringing them to somebody and 'asking' for them to be named; some may attempt to pronounce the word.

Children's initial realisations give way over time to broader concepts of objects as being similar to some others, part of a greater set of objects, and with particular descriptors. For example, a child will learn in several stages (usually between 18 months and 3 years) that:

> 'This is called Molly.'
>
> 'This is a cat.'
>
> 'Not all cats are called Molly.'
>
> 'Molly is a white cat [not a ginger or tabby cat].'
>
> 'Molly is a cat [part of a large group of animals known as cats] who lives in a house.'

Teaching words or language to very young children can be restricted by their limited capacity to switch attention from one object to another. Caregivers mitigate this by joining the child to explain or use words that are in the child's current area of focus or interest. As children grow, their ability to look up from what they are doing and attend to something different becomes quicker and smoother.

Approaching their second birthday, children may attempt two word phrases, using different intonations to specify their meaning. For example, 'Mum car?' may denote a request to go in the car, while 'Mum car' indicates that the car belongs to Mum. Such early sentences demonstrate telegraphic speech, comprising mostly nouns, verbs and adjectives. Expressive capability in young children is enhanced when caregivers use the child's area of interest to build a conversation, taking turns to speak, waiting for the child to respond and adding to what they have said:

> Hannah (aged 2 and looking at a book): Look!
>
> Mum (aged 31 and feeling about 90): Oh, look! Maisey!
>
> Hannah: Maisey …
>
> Mum: Maisey's off to a party.
>
> Hannah: Party …
>
> Mum: Wearing her dress.
>
> Hannah: Party dress.

Getting older: 3 years and on

The size of a child's expressive vocabulary varies according to the type and amount of language to which the child is exposed. Children who are questioned, prompted to join conversations by taking turns to speak, and given positive feedback to what they say demonstrate a larger vocabulary than children from whom less participation is expected (Hart & Risley, 1980). Parents are encouraged to talk to, listen to and read to their children in order to build their understanding. Likewise, health practitioners who give simple, age-appropriate explanations and information to children—as well as time to process information and to ask questions—promote understanding and the capability to communicate.

Around the age of 3, most children begin to add descriptors, such as shapes or colours, to the objects they talk about. This is not always with accuracy. A 3-year-old still needs time to refocus on what the parent or caregiver is directing them to, while a child of 5 may be expected to follow instructions without having to first 'look up' from what she is doing (Buckley, 2003). Such focusing ability is an important skill for children when entering school and working in a busy classroom. Children also grow in their ability to 'repair conversation' (Buckley, 2003) by clarifying or repeating what they have said if not responded to by others, indicating their understanding that they have not been heard or regarded. Similarly, children learn to interrupt with increasing force in order to contribute to a conversation. While talking is often assumed to be the predominant form of communication, children adopt word use later than other communication methods. From the age of approximately 3 years, spoken language becomes the main form of communication for children.

The vocabulary of a 3-year-old is about 1000 words (Claiborne & Drewery, 2010). Some children use different tones of voice when addressing adults or peers, indicating an early understanding of some of the conventions associated with the social positioning of those with whom they communicate. At about this age, children can begin to respond appropriately to questions posed with the beginnings 'why', 'what', 'where' or 'when'. This is often the age when children begin to initiate stories about events, people or phenomena that are familiar or visible to them. Approaching the age of 5, a child will attempt an answer to increasingly complex questions, such as those beginning with 'how' or 'what if'.

Children at the age of 4 and 5 years are increasingly competent at remembering and relating a story as 'news' to interested adults or others. 'Show and tell' in kindergarten and new-entrant school settings is promoted as a way of developing the child's ability to begin, furnish and conclude a verbal account of an event or phenomenon (Claiborne & Drewery, 2010). Children's understanding of basic language concepts relating to time (when, before, during), space (beside, above) or quantity (too much, all, few) precede an emerging ability to understand and cooperate with increasingly specific or detailed instructions (Buckley, 2003).

Conversation provides a rich opportunity to test out children's understanding and interpretation of others' language. Older pre-schoolers attempt to negotiate or to convince others of their point using an increasing variety of questions and arguments, which is sometimes interpreted as challenging behaviour.

Approaching ages 4 and 5, children are likely to be in increasing contact with children of a similar age, and are able to adjust their language and intonation according to whether they are conversing with adults or younger children. Around this time questions directed to adults such as those beginning with 'why?' or 'what?' are as much an expression of the intent to interact with someone as actually seeking to understand a cause or phenomenon (Buckley, 2003). Children also become increasingly able to keep the attention of the other person with frequent questions. With an increased vocabulary, the child is able to name their feelings and this also contributes to their understanding of others' feelings, identified by non-verbal and verbal indicators. Considering this within health-care practice is important. Supporting children's expression of their feelings and thoughts will help to clarify their understanding of what is happening to them and why. We reiterate this as a moral and legal obligation.

CASE STUDY 4.5

Assessing young children

How do we assess babies and young people when we are unable to communicate with them in adult-to-adult ways?

If you apply the principles in this chapter, your first step may be to consider the best way to initially approach the child or baby. Parents convey to the child their acceptance or approval of your work, and have a primary role in giving permission for assessment. They should always be present and informed about what is going to happen. Surprise or distress in a parent will be noticed by the child and mirrored or reacted to accordingly. Caregivers will require explanations and the opportunity to have questions answered before they give their consent for you to work with their baby. Children should be given age-appropriate explanations and be invited to ask questions. Seeking the approval of a very young child may seem difficult, but must be attempted where possible.

Use your assessment skills to direct your communication with the child. Your ability to use your communication knowledge in forming rapport improves your chances of the child being happy, forthcoming and cooperative with you, the stranger.

Always consider how your body language is perceived by the child. For example, eye contact for you may indicate interest or respect, but be received as a threat, especially by children in unfamiliar surroundings such as hospital departments or clinics. Likewise, your height beside a small child can appear frightening, so sitting or crouching to speak to a child should be considered.

Children's experience of one health practitioner is rapidly applied to others. Children who are upset or frightened in the health-care setting may have had fearful experiences with others. Your way of being with the young child frames future experiences with health-care practitioners—another reason to be mindful of your attitude and ways of being with the child and their significant others.

Communication through play

Play Interaction and activity that is relaxed and entertaining.

Engaging in **play** is indicative of understanding and communicative ability in children as they grow older. Play provides an outlet for the expression and regulation of feelings, wishes or fears, and enables children to begin to understand the perspectives of others. When playing, older children practise talking and using their bodies to express themselves (Santrock, 2009). As a form of communication, play can be used by child health practitioners, caregivers and advocates as a means both for understanding and teaching.

Piaget stressed the role of play and the provision of opportunities for the child to internally process anxiety or conflict and to release tension (Piaget, 1962). Children practise different skills and use even solitary play conditions to literally talk to themselves (initially out loud and, later, silently), instructing, reflecting and even praising or berating themselves. Piaget referred to this as 'private speech' or 'inner speech'.

Vygotsky (1962) believed that, over time, inner speech becomes a taken-for-granted process of thinking that supports social and verbal communication. He believed that children who frequently engage in inner speech demonstrate better social communication abilities than those who do not. Piaget's theory of cognitive development is useful because of the concept of object permanence—a child's ability to remember and convey an image in asking for or searching for something is an example of developing communicative ability. Similarly, the work of Vygotsky and Piaget regarding inner speech provides an example of development facilitating communication skills.

Parten classified the ways in which children played, according to the types and levels of social interaction she observed in a study with children aged 2–5 years (Santrock, 2009), as depicted in Table 4.4.

TABLE 4.4 *Young children's play*

Type of play	Example or explanation	Value to communication learning
Solitary play	Studying a toy or book 'in their own little world'—the child appears uninterested in what is going on around them	Children engage in private speech that contributes to the regulation of emotions
Pretend play	Acting out an event in which children play parts—for example, in a game of 'going to the supermarket' the child may 'be' the mother and request the adult/other children to be the child or checkout assistant; older children will generate stories about less familiar/unpractised events	Children are enabled to practise other perspectives or roles, such as 'being the mum' or 'telling the children off'
Parallel play	Playing alongside others with little interaction or conversation—children may use same or similar toys beside each other	The child's social development via an emerging awareness of other people is promoted
Associative play	Children focus their attention upon one another and play together with little or no organisation or set games	

As children grow older, their increased interaction with other children provides the challenge of having to share or take turns, negotiate understandings with a limited vocabulary, and respond to other's points of view, with a growing capacity to see a situation from another person's perspective. A final stage in Parten's framework, cooperative play, is generally seen in older children where two or more children will play together, rather than simply alongside one another. The communicative potential in children's play is typified in Parten's work by the continuity of children's communication, aspects of which may be missed or misinterpreted by others, including health practitioners.

There is no single theory of child communication. Theories about children arise over time and depend or reflect the cultural and social perspective of that time. We have drawn upon a variety of perspectives to show the richness of the field, but three areas are key:

+ Children are always members of a family, whether the family is visible or not.
+ Non-verbal communication is continuous and informative, and so always should be looked for.
+ Children and adults alike are always communicating with us, even if we do not realise it. Therefore, we should watch and listen to understand and care for babies and children.

{ SUMMARY }

Babies and children develop certain communication skills over time, and health practitioners must understand and tune into the ways in which babies and young children are already (and always) communicating. Conceptions of children as naive, vulnerable or not fully human might make it easy for adults to disregard or limit communication with them. We have shown that children are entitled to be listened to, regarded and invited to participate in their care by aware and trustworthy professionals. Such attention benefits not only the child but also their family members and caregivers.

Health practitioners should uphold the rights of young children to communicate in ways that are meaningful to the children, and be mindful of less obvious aspects of communication. This requires acute listening and observation. Good communication with this age group requires entering the child's world and attending to the multilayered nature of communication. This includes non-verbal intonations, facial expressions and body movements as ways in which children begin to consciously communicate.

The responses and knowledgeable interpretation of adults encourages children to develop and participate in their world. Health practitioners must comprehend the unfolding of children's understanding and expressive capability, at different ages, to grasp the potential in reciprocal communication that goes far beyond the spoken words upon which many adults have come to rely.

REFLECTION POINTS

4.1 Intention (motivation, message, meaning, emotion)

Observe the children in your world. Who are they with? Who do they relate to? How are they communicating? How do their express fear or the need for reassurance?

4.2 Reception (received message, response, feedback)

In watching children play, how do they make meaning of events and how does this change with age?

4.3 Perception (style, manner, impression, analysis)

What might be the effect of using child rights or human rights frameworks to guide health-care practice with babies and young children?

QUESTIONS FOR REVIEW

1. In what ways do health practitioners enlist the support or guidance of family members to understand the needs or wants of young children?
2. What specific strategies can health practitioners utilise to communicate appropriately with babies and young children?
3. How can you use play to communicate with children?
4. What assumptions do you have about children and communication?

REFERENCES

Aries, P. (1962). *Centuries of childhood: A social history of family life*. New York, NY: Knopf.

Bowlby, J. (1951). *Maternal care and mental health*. Geneva, Switzerland: World Health Organization. Retrieved from http://pages.uoregon.edu/eherman/teaching/texts/Bowlby%20Maternal%20Care%20and%20Mental%20Health.pdf.

Bretherton, I. (1992). The origins of attachment theory: John Bowlby and Mary Ainsworth. *Development Psychology, 28*, 759–75.

Buckley, B. (2003). *Children's communication skills from birth to five years old*. London, UK: Routledge.

Claiborne, L. B. & Drewery, W. (2010). *Human development: Family, place, culture*. Sydney, NSW: McGraw-Hill.

Hart, B. & Risley, T. (1980). In vivo language intervention: Unanticipated general effects. *Journal of Applied Behavior Analysis, 13*(3), 407–32. Retrieved from www.ncbi.nlm.nih.gov/pmc/articles/PMC1308147/pdf/jaba00049-0027.pdf.

Menyuk, P., Liebergott, J. & Schultz, M. (1995). *Early language development in full-term and premature infants*. Hillsdale, NJ: Erlbaum.

Piaget, J. (1962). *Play, dreams and imitation*. London, UK: Routledge.

Santrock, J. (2009). *Lifespan development*. New York, NY: McGraw-Hill.

Sun, M. & Rugolotto, S. (2004). Assisted infant toilet training in a western family setting. *Developmental and Behavioural Pediatrics, 25*(2), 99–101.

United Nations (2005). *The United Nations convention on the rights of the child*. Wellington, NZ: Office of the Children's Commissioner.

Vygotsky, L. (1962). *Thought and language*. Cambridge, MA: MIT Press.

WEBSITES

Attachment Parenting International: www.attachmentparenting.org
Development, kidspot: www.kidspot.co.nz/subsection+26+Toddler-Development.htm
Huggies New Zealand: www.huggies.co.nz

{5}

School Age

Anne Grey

CHAPTER OVERVIEW

This chapter covers the following topics:

- Developmental theories
- Learning theories
- Māori perspectives on development
- Theories of language development
- Communication with school-age children
- The influence of communication on children's health care.

KEY TERMS

Holistic
Development
Cognitive
Learning
Nativist perspective
Behaviour

Children of school age are typically between 5 and 11 years of age, who have begun their school years but have not yet entered the adolescent stage. This period is also known as middle childhood. It is a stage of developmental consolidation, because although children are continually learning and developing at this time, there is no rapid development as in the early childhood or the adolescent stages. There are a number of developmental and learning theories, both Western and indigenous, that underpin communication with school-age children. Understanding individual differences among children, and the impact of culture and context, are useful for critically reflecting on communication with school-age children in a way that promotes greater empathy and understanding.

Developmental theories

Holistic An emphasis on the whole person, rather than separate parts.

Development The process of progressive change and growth.

Development is a term that is used to explain the **holistic** growth and change in all aspects of the child's physical, intellectual and social functioning (Brooker & Woodhead, 2010) that occur naturally as a result of the maturational process. Although children's development is a holistic process and each aspect of development is of equal importance to the child (Lindon, 2005), domains of **development** are sometimes artificially separated to enable a deeper understanding of each aspect to be gained. As many of these theories derive from Western thinking and writing, it is important to be aware that these theories can contain 'hidden messages' (Cannella, 1997, p. 59) about children from Western cultures, and sometimes ignore or reflect badly on children from other cultures.

The Western developmental theories explained below outline a general view of the main developmental characteristics of a school-age child, although each theory is specific to a certain domain or aspect of development. To gain this broad perspective, a brief overview is provided on physical development, as well as a discussion on the psychoanalytic theories of Freud and Erikson, and the **cognitive** theories of Piaget, Vygotsky and Bruner.

Cognitive Relating to thought and thinking.

Physical development in school-age children is gradual and regular, and occurs at a much slower rate than in early childhood. Children slowly become taller, heavier and better coordinated. Gross motor skills (such as running and jumping) and fine motor skills (such as writing and drawing) are well developed and continue to improve throughout this period. This enables children throughout the school years to master physical skills such as sports, playing musical instruments, school work and household tasks. Children in developed nations enjoy better health, lower likelihood of childhood illnesses, low risk of infant mortality and increased standards of living, which has enabled many school-age children to participate in sports and cultural activities (Hoffnung et al., 2010). Unfortunately, however, this is often not the case for children in much of the world.

Although psychosocial development is not as readily observable as physical development, there are theories that explain this aspect of development. Psychoanalytic theories form a framework for understanding how the human mind works, and explain how feelings, emotions and imagination contribute to development (Crain, 2005). Sigmund Freud was the first to introduce the notion that behaviour is determined by both the conscious and unconscious mind. Freud proposed that all people need to find a balance between these two drives for well-being to exist. Freud's psychosexual theory focused primarily on sexual development. Freud named the stage of school-age children 'the latency stage', recognising the developmental consolidation that takes place in this period. Because of Freud's emphasis on sexual development, and because his observations were based on a small sample of ill people and were not representative of the general population, today this theory is often negatively critiqued. However, for those working with children, Freud's theory highlights that behaviour and communication may reflect both conscious rational thoughts and unconscious irrational thoughts. To illustrate how these irrational fears may occur, it is useful to reflect on the example of a 7-year-old boy who went to hospital to have his tonsils removed. When the nurse was taking his temperature, he asked if the doctor was going to chop his head off to get out his tonsils (Cook, 1999).

Erik Erikson (1902–1994) built on Freud's theory to construct the psychosocial theory of development. Erikson believed that each individual's identity is the result of interactions with other people and the wider community. He divided the lifespan into eight stages from infancy to old age, with each stage of development involving a crisis or issue that can be resolved either positively or negatively. In most cases, the outcome of each issue would neither be totally negative nor positive, but a combination of both. The crisis or issue that school-age children are involved in is 'industry versus inferiority'. Here, children either develop skills that allow them to feel competent (the positive end of the continuum) or fail to do this and are left with a feeling of incompetence (the negative end of the continuum). In general, throughout this stage the child's sense of competence is developed. It is usual for children to develop a realistic self-image that falls somewhere in the middle of this continuum and involves both positive and negative feelings. For the adult working with school-age children, Erikson's theory emphasises the importance of maintaining a positive environment and interactions to foster a sense of self-worth and competence in children.

Jean Piaget (1896–1980) focused his theory on the cognitive development of children by observing children's thinking and the ways that thinking changed as children matured, and how the maturational process gave rise to **learning**. Piaget believed that children's thinking develops as they interact with their environment by adapting and assimilating new information into their existing knowledge base. He constructed four stages, where each stage is qualitatively different from the stage that precedes it. The stage for school-age children is known as 'the concrete operational stage'.

Learning The process of acquiring skills and knowledge.

Piaget believed that when a child reaches the school age, thinking becomes more logical and organised than previously, but that they still have difficulty in thinking abstractly or reasoning about abstract ideas. This is because Piaget believed that mastery of logical thought developed gradually (Berk, 2008). In recent times, because Piaget emphasised that children's thinking developed in stages, this theory has been critiqued as concentrating more on what children were unable to understand than on their cognitive capabilities. However, it is important to be aware of the limitations to children's understanding. For example, most school-age children can name bones, blood, heart, stomach and lungs when asked about internal anatomy, but cannot explain the location of these organs or what their function is (Rushforth, 1999).

Learning theories

Learning theories refer to the acquisition of knowledge, skills and identity. These theories explain that what is learnt by children is shaped by the relationships that they build, by the cultural values of society, and by the lived daily experiences that form their lives. Moreover, what a child learns is also limited or extended by the economic and social context in which each child lives. In addition, the language a child speaks shapes the child's identity, as well as providing a means of learning (Brooker & Woodhead, 2010).

Vygotsky's sociocultural theory of development provides a different way to understand children's learning and cognitive development. Vygotsky viewed learning and development as a collaborative and social undertaking where children learn from the people who are part of their daily lives, especially those who are more experienced than they are themselves (Wertsch, 1991). Vygotsky believed that language and communication are essential to learning and cognitive development, as it is through language and communication that internal thoughts are expressed. Vygotsky believed each person had a 'zone of proximal development' (what a person can do and understand with help from another person) and a 'zone of actual development' (what a person can do and understand on their own). The process of assisting a person through the zone of proximal development is known as 'scaffolding'. Vygotsky also thought that people, especially children, often talk to themselves in order to guide their own learning. He called this type of communication 'private speech'. Vygotsky explained that each culture had tools that could assist with learning and understanding. In Western cultures these are often books, computers or photos, while in other cultures cultural tools may take the form of legends, songs or dances. Language itself was viewed by Vygotsky as a major cultural tool for learning as language provides the medium for the exchange of ideas between people to build shared meanings about their social, cultural and intellectual experiences (Smidt, 2009). Vygotsky believed that learning individuals are continually extending both their zone of actual development and their zone of proximal development. Vygotsky's sociocultural theory is valuable as it demonstrates the importance of culture and interpersonal relationships for learning, and how individuals learn from participating in a community.

Jerome Bruner, an American psychologist, elaborated on Vygotsky's view of learning. Bruner viewed children as active problem solvers who were motivated to learn quite difficult concepts if those concepts were of interest to them (Smidt, 2009), or had direct meaning for their life, and if those concepts were revisited frequently until understanding was gained. He extended Vygotsky's theory by introducing the term 'scaffolding' to emphasise the role the adult plays to give support, usually in the form of dialogue or communication, to the child's learning and understanding. Bruner also explained learning as being distributed; that is, some learning takes place on an individual basis and some while being part of a social group, and some learning is explicit as a result of direct teaching and some is tacit or absorbed as a result of personal experiences.

Communication involves the processing of information, and the current social environment provides children with an overwhelming amount of information at any one time. The framework that focuses specifically on this aspect of cognitive development is known as the 'information processing' approach. Here the metaphor of a computer is used to explain the human mind. Mental strategies and the flow of information are directed by a central executive area of the working memory (Berk, 2008). In school-age children, information processing becomes more efficient as they are able to pay attention to information for longer periods and can remember and understand complex tasks and topics. They are more selective about the topics they pay attention to, and can switch back and forth between topics as they use various mental strategies more effectively (Hoffnung et al., 2010). This ability to control thought processes is known as metacognition, or the awareness of mental activities and thinking processes (Berk, 2008). This, in turn, leads to greater cognitive self-regulation. The information processing theory is useful to understand communication, as it involves information entering a child's sensory register with mental strategies then employed to enable understanding to take place.

Māori perspectives on development

In Māori culture, theories and concepts of development have been passed down through songs, stories and karakia (waiata, kōrero and karakia) where human development and learning is explained holistically as being a part of the life force (te ira tangata) of the universe (Royal-Tangaere, 1997). From this perspective, each individual, especially each child, is considered to be a taonga, or a gift from the gods. Each individual's learning and development is also connected to the gods as it is believed that the three baskets of knowledge were collected from the heavens by Tane. In order to collect the baskets, Tane climbed Te Ara Poutama, or the stairs that are often depicted in the weaving panels on a marae. Each stair reflects a stage of learning and development that leads onto the next through a learning process of observing, listening and then speaking (titiro, whakarongo, kōrero). Central to the learning process is the concept of tukana-teina, or older sibling–younger sibling, where it is the responsibility of the older or more experienced person to pass on learning to those who are younger or less experienced. As this learning process connects man to the gods, learning is considered a taonga, or a precious gift.

No one aspect of development and learning can be considered in isolation from the others and holism is considered an important principle of human development and learning (Macfarlane, 2007). Moreover, as each individual is connected to the gods, each individual is considered a taonga to be valued and respected (Pere, 1988; 1991). Accepting that there is also a cultural perspective to understanding children's development assists carers to be more empathetic to diversity and difference, and to ensure that communication is culturally sensitive.

Theories of language development

As communication is linked to language, it is important to understand the theories of language development. There is no one theory that gives a clear explanation—several theories explain language development from various perspectives. However, there are particular perspectives from which to consider this. For example, the behaviourist perspective explains language as resulting from environmental learning, while the **nativist perspective** posits that language naturally emerges from the normal process of maturation.

Nativist perspective The view that children build on their innate understanding as they move through developmental processes.

The 'behaviourist' perspective to learning language was outlined by B. F. Skinner. He explained that language occurs through the processes of imitation and reinforcement, whereby children imitate language from those around them and are rewarded, or reinforced, for using these words themselves. It is true that children who are spoken to frequently and who are encouraged to engage in conversations develop strong language skills, but this is no longer thought to be a valid explanation for language development in general. The nativist perspective, outlined by Noam Chomsky, claims that children are born with an innate ability to understand and use language. It is true that children have a remarkable ability to communicate that is not always the result of imitation and reinforcement. For example, children can often make sense of words they have not heard before. Similarly, children who are born deaf, but are surrounded by speaking adults, do not have a sign language to imitate yet invent their own sign systems (Berk, 2008). It can be concluded that children have the ability to acquire language, but this ability requires nurturing if it is to flourish.

In middle childhood, language ability develops significantly, partly as a result of more complex cognitive abilities. By 10 years of age children have a richer vocabulary and are able to choose between words that have a similar meaning but different connotations. This allows children to engage in word play, to tell jokes and to build specialised vocabulary relating to their interests. At this age, children can use language to communicate in different ways, including being able to take another's perspective, empathise with others and to express their own internal fears and emotions in words. This allows children to realise that communication can be a means to understand the world and to resolve conflict, and so language and communication become a means of regulating impulsive emotional **behaviour** (Davies, 2011).

Behaviour
Observable activities, conduct and responses.

The implications of these theories are that although all school-age children should be able to understand communication about health-care treatment, children who are spoken to and read to more often will have a more extensive vocabulary and should be able to understand medical terminology more easily. However, there are many individual differences within this general description of language development in school-age children, so it is important not to stereotype children's language ability.

Communication with school-age children

Communication is a complex rather than a linear process. The importance of culture and context to the communication process must also be recognised as impacting on the meaning, context and purpose of communication, as well as the relationships between those communicating and the influence of the method of communication. Communication also involves a combination of skills that shape the communication process. These skills include language ability (which is influenced by societies and individuals), individual cognitive information processing to find meaning in another person's speech and vocabulary, and the interpretation of the non-verbal components of communication, such as gestures and movements (Vickers, 2006). Skills are needed to communicate effectively, as well as to know which messages are important to communicate (Quality Assurance Report, 1999).

Because of the complexity of communication, and the individual and cultural differences among school-age children, those working with children need strategies for building rapport, explaining, listening and interpreting information. Communication must be respectful of the rights of the child and be conducted collaboratively with the child and family, but should also take account of the child's individuality, age, development, understanding and cultural background, and how circumstances affect the style of communication. Explaining a routine health check to a child may require a different style of communication from explaining about surgery or a serious illness. Health practitioners and the language they use may be unfamiliar to the child, and the environment may contain sights, sounds and smells that are threatening to a child. It is important to consider the child's perspective and to encourage their participation in any communication.

To ensure communication is not threatening to the child, it is first important to build trust between the health care professional and the child by adopting friendly gestures, facial expressions, body language and tone of voice. Carers can get down to the child's level, although not all children make eye contact for individual or cultural reasons. In framing the communication, the professional should explain to the child what has happened, what is happening now, what is going to happen, what this is likely to mean to them, and what is being done to help them (Cook, 1999). It is essential for the carer to explain all key words and phrases in plain language (not medical jargon), ideally in the child's home language, so an interpreter may be needed. If children are given simple, clear information about their illness and the treatment required, they are provided with a meaningful base on which to add new information.

Sometimes it may be necessary for carers to communicate bad news to children. In the past, adults have avoided talking about difficult situations, such as terminal cancer, with children. This has given children an extra psychological burden, and resulted in children losing their sense of competence and control, resulting in depression or excessive fears and fantasies (Beale, Baile & Aaron, 2005). Evidence suggests that terminally ill children as young as 3 years are aware of a diagnosis and prognosis without being told by an adult, and that the avoidance of discussions about death can lead them to feel abandoned (Levetown & the Committee on Bioethics, 2008). It is now thought children should be given honest, accurate information about illnesses and the treatment this entails. In these cases, professionals must be aware that the child needs to know, what the child already knows, how and when the information is best given, and what support the child may need afterwards (Cook,1999).

The following '6 Es' strategy is a guide to difficult communication:

+ Establish open communication with the child and the family.
+ Engage the child at an appropriate time.
+ Explore what the child already knows about the illness and what else they would like to know.
+ Explain medical information in answer to the child's questions, rather than presuming what they want or need to know.
+ Empathise with the child's emotional reactions. The child may be upset and expressing these feelings is necessary before a constructive discussion can take place. In this case, the carer can empathise ('I can see that you've been really worried about this'), validate ('We've been wondering why you've been upset') and clarify ('Can you tell me what

you've been thinking?). Children may prefer to express their feelings in a drawing or through play rather than verbally.

+ Encourage children by reassuring them that they will be listened to and supported. If necessary, explain that although there is no cure for the illness, life still continues. It is not helpful to give the child false hope or reassurance by saying, for example, 'Don't worry—everything will be all right!' (Beale, Baile & Aaron, 2005).

When communicating with children, the information given by the carer addresses two needs. These are the cognitive need to know and understand the information, and the affective/emotional need to feel supported and understood (Levetown & the Committee on Bioethics, 2008). By enhancing awareness of communication strategies when explaining treatment and listening to children's questions and expressions of anxiety, carers can improve the psychological well-being of children.

The influence of communication on children's health care

Several studies demonstrate effective communication is associated with quality of care, which in turn results in better health outcomes. Paediatric health care is improved when children are recognised as having their own cognitive and emotional needs, are respected and are regarded as intelligent, capable and cooperative (Levetown & the Committee on Bioethics, 2008). Studies indicate children have often been passive recipients of health care, and have been given little opportunity to share decision-making with health practitioners. Indeed, it is more usual for health practitioners to ask parents about their child's health than it is to ask the children themselves. Studies show that children over the age of 7 years give a more accurate description of their health, including the pain they experience, than their parents. For practitioners, it is very difficult to accurately assess the extent and nature of pain without description from the child. Some children may not have the vocabulary to adequately describe their pain in words, but may be able to indicate the severity of it by pointing to a face from a continuum of smiles to grimaces. In pain management, it has been shown that patients who control their own pain-relief treatment experience greater pain relief. Children as young as 4 years have been successfully taught to do this. By being listened to, given accurate information about why they are experiencing pain, and by being taught to administer their own pain relief, children experience less negative outcomes as a result of the pain (Levetown & the Committee on Bioethics, 2008).

Asthma among children is common, and studies in the USA have revealed the incidence of children with asthma was greater for children from lower socio-economic backgrounds or ethnic minorities. These children experienced a poorer quality of care than other children because of more barriers to communicating effectively about asthma symptoms, treatment, medication and self-management (Diette & Rand, 2007). The practitioners also experienced difficulties with these children and families because effective communication often took more time than was allocated. Health-care professionals tended to dominate conversations more and listen less to these children and their families. Communication was not child-centred and there were also cultural differences in how symptoms were described. In some cases these factors resulted in the severity of the asthma not being correctly assessed and lower rates of prescription of medication.

Although these children and their families were less able to read information about health, to follow written instructions and to calculate correct doses of medication, the study found when time was taken to explain guidelines for treatment in a one-on-one situation, asthma patients were able to administer their treatment successfully at home. Improved communication was shown to support increased positive health outcomes, while enabling the child to take responsibility for their own health and well-being.

Recently, in accordance with the United Nations Convention on the Rights of the Child, surveys on children's opinions on the quality of their hospital experiences were completed in the USA, Switzerland and Finland. In these surveys communication was noted as both the best and worst aspect of children's hospital experiences. In the USA, 120 children aged 4–20 years were surveyed. They reported they valued relationships with staff and appreciated if nursing staff, doctors and other medical staff listened to them, but confusing communication and not being told about medical procedures were reported as the worst features. These children listed better communication as one suggestion for improvement (Lindeke, Nakai & Johnson, 2006).

In Switzerland, 136 children aged 6–12 years were surveyed on hospital experiences to better understand their priorities. This survey indicated that children do not necessarily have the same priorities and opinions as their parents. The children reported a high satisfaction rate with the nurses (90 per cent), but attitude and relationships were more important to these children than the technical aspect of care. The children appreciated, for example, that nurses took good care of them and explained things to them. The older children commented on their need to feel recognised and reassured, and be able to act on their own behalf. This survey clearly shows children appreciated being asked their opinions on the quality of care they received. This study concluded that children recovered faster if they were prepared for their hospital stay, had explanations about treatment and were supported by being listened to (Chappius et al., 2011).

The study in Finland surveyed 388 children aged 7–11 years about their best and worst experiences of hospitalisation. The children reported that people were one of the best experiences and that the best nurses were pleasant, friendly and nice, and took care of them. Here children described their worst experience as having an unidentified person doing something to them. This study concluded that good communication between nurses, children and their families is linked to increased understanding of treatment and illness (Pelander & Leino-Kilpi, 2010).

These studies all suggest that for hospital environments and treatment to be more child-centred, children's viewpoints need to be heard and children need to be allowed to participate in their own health care. If this happens, children are likely to be less stressed and the treatment more effective.

{ SUMMARY }

By communicating with children in a respectful manner, professionals can positively reinforce children's sense of competence (Erikson's theory). School-age children's thinking and understanding is logical when connected to concrete experiences (Piaget's theory), but is influenced by culture and context (Vygotsky's theory). Children in the school age can process information more efficiently (information processing theory) to make sense of their world (Bruner's theory), and are able to understand quite complex concepts if an adult assists their understanding (scaffolding).

Māori views on child development need special consideration as each child is considered holistically as a special gift from the gods and cannot be viewed in isolation from the family or whānau.

Communication with children is both verbal and non-verbal. Although communication transmits information from one person to another, the way the information is interpreted and understood is influenced by individual, cultural and contextual differences.

Health-care professionals working with children need a range of strategies. Information should be as honest and accurate as possible. Children should be allowed to express their feelings and have these listened to.

REFLECTION POINTS

5.1 Intention (motivation, message, meaning, emotion)

When engaging with children, how might you ask open-ended questions that would scaffold a child's ability to describe their symptoms?

5.2 Reception (received message, response, feedback)

Informed consent in Aotearoa New Zealand is less about age and more about the ability to understand, given the cognitive abilities of a person.How would you know that a child has really understood what you have been telling them without asking a simple yes or no question?

5.3 Perception (style, manner, impression, analysis)

Identify communication skills that children value in their health-care providers. Are these the same or different from ones that you value in a health-care provider?

QUESTIONS FOR REVIEW

1 How is communication affected by social/emotional, cognitive and cultural influences? Use a mind map to illustrate the relationships.
2 What are five strategies you could use to make communication with school-age children more effective?

REFERENCES

Beale, E., Baile, W. & Aaron, J. (2005, May). Silence is not golden: Communicating with children dying of cancer. *Journal of Clinical Oncology, 23*(15), 3629–31.

Berk, L. (2008). *Infants and children*. Boston, MA: Pearson Education Inc.

Brooker, L. & Woodhead, M. (2010). Culture and learning. In M. Woodhead & J. Oats (eds), *The series: Early childhood in focus (No.6)*. The Hague, Netherlands: Bernard Van Leer Foundation.

Cannella, G. (1997). *Deconstructing early childhood education: Social justice and revolution*. New York, NY: Peter Lang.

Chappuis, M., Vannay-Bouchiche, C., Flückiger, M., Monnier, M., Cathieni, F. & Piot-Ziegler, C. (2011). Children's experience regarding the quality of their hospital stay: The development of an assessment questionnaire for children. *Journal of Nursing Care Quality, 26*(1), 78–87.

Cook, P. (1999). Will it hurt? Children in medical settings. In P. Milner & B. Carolin, *Time to listen to children: Personal and professional communication*. London, UK: Routledge.

Crain, W. (2005). *Theories of development: Concepts and applications* (5th edn). Upper Saddle River, NJ: Pearson Prentice Hall.

Davies, D. (2011). *Child development: A practitioner's guide* (3rd edn). New York, NY: The Guilford Press.

Diette, G. & Rand, C. (2007). The contributing role of health-care communication to health disparities for minority patients with asthma. *Chest, 2007, 132*, 802–9.

Hoffnung, M., Hoffnung, R., Seifert, K., Smith, R., Hine, A., Ward, L. & Quinn, A. (2010). *Lifespan development*. Brisbane: John Wiley & Sons.

Levetown, M. & the Committee on Bioethics. (2008). *Pediatrics, 2008, 121*, 1441–50.

Lindeke, L., Nakai, M. & Johnson, L. (2006). Capturing children's voices for quality improvement. *The American Journal of Maternal/Child Nursing, 31*(5), 290–5.

Lindon, J. (2005). *Understanding child development: Linking theory and practice*. London, UK: Hodder Arnold.

Macfarlane, A. H. (2007). The value of Māori ecologies in the study of human development. In L. Bird & W. Drewery (eds). *Human development in Aotearoa: A journey through life*. Boston, MA: McGraw-Hill.

Pelander, T. & Leino-Kilpi, H. (2010). Children's best and worst experiences during hospitalisation. *Scandinavian Journal of Caring Sciences, 24*(4), 726–33.

Pere, R. R. (1988). Te wheke: Whaia te maramatangame aroha. In S. Middleton (ed.), *Women and Education in Aotearoa*. Wellington, NZ: Allen & Unwin.

Pere, R. R. (1991). *Te wheke: A celebration of infinite wisdom*. Gisborne, NZ: Akoako Global Publishing.

Quality Assurance Report. (1999). *Improving interpersonal communication between health care providers and patients*. Bethesda, MD: Center for Human Services.

Royal-Tangaere, A. (1997). Māori human development learning theory. In P. Te Whaiti, M. McCarthy & A. Durie (eds), *Mai i rangiatea: Māori well-being and development*. Auckland, NZ: University Press with Bridget Williams Books.

Rushforth, H. (1999). Practitioner review: Communicating with hospitalised children: Review and application of research pertaining to children's understanding of health and illness. *Journal of Child Psychology and Psychiatry, 40*(5), 683–91.

Smidt, S. (2009). *Introducing Vygotsky: A guide for practitioners and students in early years education*. London, UK: Routledge.

Vickers, P. (2006). Communicating with children and families. In I. Peate & L. Whiting (eds), *Caring for children and families*. London, UK: John Wiley & Sons, Ltd.

Wertsch, J. (1991). *Voices of the mind: A sociocultural approach to mediated action*. Cambridge, MA: Harvard University Press.

WEBSITES

Bristol Royal Infirmary Enquiry, Leadership in the NHS: www.bristol-inquiry.org.uk/final_report/report/sec2chap29_13.htm

Improving services for children in hospital, Healthcare Commission: www.cqc.org.uk/_db/_documents/children_improving_services_Tagged.pdf

{6}

Teens

Gabrielle Le Geyt, Jayne Mercier, Morgyn Hartdegen, Amber Davies and Ailsa Haxell

CHAPTER OVERVIEW

This chapter covers the following topics:

+ The adolescent brain
+ Psychosocial development
+ Physical development
+ Communicating with teenagers

KEY TERMS

Adolescence
Identity
Role
Neurological
Impulsivity
Risk
Resilience

Between childhood and adulthood comes **adolescence**. Transitions in and out of this developmental stage are gradual, usually beginning at age 11 or 12 years, continuing through the teenage years and completing in the early to mid twenties (Turkstra & Byom, 2010). Adolescent communication is frequently stereotyped as comprising slammed doors, grunts and (on good days) monosyllabic responses. However, to gain an understanding of teenage communications, it is useful to consider the major developmental changes occurring in adolescence and how these influence teenage minds and behaviours. This chapter examines some of these processes and their influence on communication, and outlines some ways to enhance communication with this age group.

Adolescence A developmental phase between childhood and maturity.

Adolescence is characterised by considerable physical, intellectual, emotional and psychosocial changes, which allow the young person to attain a sense of independence from parents or guardians and develop their own unique **identity**. There are many processes that support development during this stage, including family, peer affiliation, knowledge seeking and **role** experimentation. Changing biological processes also have a great influence during this stage of life; the adolescent brain continues to develop and mature, which creates advanced cognitive processing and reasoning, and contributes to the emergence of new patterns of behaviour.

Identity The sense of self and individual character that a person has in relation to others.

Role A socially accepted way of behaving and carrying specific responsibilities.

The adolescent brain

Until recently, it was believed that the major 'wiring' of the human brain was achieved during the first three to four years of life, following a dramatic increase in grey matter volume, and that by the age of 10 to 12 years the brain was fully mature. Advancements in neuroimaging techniques have now revealed otherwise. Current research supports the understanding that brain development is not complete until the late teens or early twenties, with the adolescent brain undergoing a great deal of neural restructuring following a second wave of grey matter overproduction in preadolescence (Crone, 2009; Turkstra & Byom, 2010).

The continuing maturation of the adolescent brain underlies advances in cognitive processing, social competence and emotional capacity in teens. The refinement of connections between different brain regions during adolescence is reflected in changes in the way information is processed and communicated. In pre-teens, problem-solving using logical processes is limited to 'concrete operations'; that is, problems that relate to real events and objects (Piaget, 1926). In Piaget's theory of development, teenagers achieve formal operational thought: an accomplishment that allows individuals to consider abstract problems logically and systematically. Thoughtful hypothesis testing also becomes possible; therefore teenagers become increasingly adept at contemplating moral and ethical issues and applying hypothetical reasoning. These skills can be nurtured by facilitating debates, and by encouraging teens to consider multiple perspectives.

Neurological Involving the nervous system.

These **neurological** changes may also provide an insight into a number of teenage characteristics that have in the past resulted in adolescence being discussed as a period of 'storm and stress' (see, for example, the oft-cited writings of G. Stanley Hall, 1904). Physical developments occur in the frontal lobe and the limbic system, regions of the brain that are responsible for self-control, judgment and emotional regulation. In a normally functioning adult brain, these regions plan and coordinate behaviour in a way that takes into account consequences and motivational goals, while regulating and modifying emotional urges to fit into socially acceptable norms. The teenage brain, however, is still developing this ability, which may explain the prevalence of spontaneous actions, poor decision-making, risk-taking behaviour and emotional outbursts in teens. Changes also occur in the way pleasure and reward is processed in the brain—as Steinberg (2005) explains, 'rewarding things feel more rewarding' for teens. Experimenting with drugs and alcohol, for example, is more common in young people than for other age groups. According to New Zealand's Ministry of Health (2010), 30 per cent of 16–24-year-olds reported drug use within the last year, compared with only 16 per cent of New Zealanders aged 16–64. There are many factors explaining the appeal of drugs to young people, including resistance to authority, testing boundaries, peer group affiliation and their use as a coping mechanism. This risk-taking behaviour also correlates with the changing prefrontal regions in the brain that regulate **impulsivity** and decision-making, making biological influences a possible contributing factor. Because of the changing nature of brain structures, drug taking in teenagers can result in long-term consequences; the adolescent brain is not yet fully mature, therefore young people have an enhanced vulnerability to addiction resulting from substance misuse.

Impulsivity The tendency to act without prior analysis.

Communication patterns in adolescence that reflect brain developments may include seemingly irrational outbursts and high-level emotional responses that do not seem to reflect the gravity of a situation. However, due to the advance in cognitive processes, young people may also start to engage in debates and question the decisions and rationale of those around them, including friends, family and teachers, demonstrating an increased ability to negotiate and develop logical arguments. Over time, an increased ability to judge different social situations and adapt their communication accordingly will emerge.

As the ability to consider abstract and moral dilemmas grows, young people may also explore different philosophies, religions and subcultures, and openly reject the values of family. These explorations may be commonly expressed through art, poetry, music or other creative media. These explorations are also heavily influenced by peers, as outlined below.

Psychosocial development

Psychosocial development refers to the development of the self with particular reference to the social context. Psychosocial processes become particularly important during this developmental stage, with adolescents experimenting with different roles, establishing a sense of identity, and achieving a greater social awareness and ability to communicate efficiently in different social situations. As young people start to experience a sense of independence from their parents or guardians, peers become an increasingly important and defining feature of their lives. The importance of identity formation during adolescence was recognised by psychologist Erik Erikson (1968), who discussed this developmental stage as being characterised by a 'crisis' of identity versus role confusion, where the adolescent tries out a number of ways to express their personality and values. If negotiated successfully, the adolescent will eventually develop a stable identity, separate from their family, that can function in wider society. If not negotiated successfully, a firm sense of adult self will not emerge, leading to an over-reliance on the opinions and approval of others (Erikson, 1968).

Newman and Newman's (2003) revisions of Erikson's stages of psychosocial development contemplate an additional stage of adolescence, with early adolescence (12–18 years) concentrating on group identity versus alienation, where the acceptance of the group is paramount and is achieved through looking, thinking and acting the same as one's peers. Newman posits that 'identity versus role confusion' occurs from 19 to 22 years of age.

Understanding the processes involved in achieving identity within a group can provide insight into the different levels of adolescent communication and behaviour. Peer pressure, for example, may encourage behaviours or responses that reinforce the group identity. Loyalty to the group may limit communications on certain levels, and there may be an element of in-group, out-group dialogue. To the outside observer, this may result in what appear to be radical changes in personality as the adolescent conforms to these group norms, or a number of peer group changes as the adolescent also questions whether group norms fit his or her developing identity. Alongside neurological development, peer processes and role experimentation may also play a part in spontaneous actions involving **risk**, and the testing of boundaries. Substance use, for example, may reflect the increased importance of peer affiliation and intergroup processes. Group affiliation can also be communicated non-verbally through choice of clothes, music and activities.

Risk The possibility of injury, loss or death.

As peer affiliation becomes more important, adolescent communication may be characterised by increased time spent sending text messages and interacting on social networking sites. A corresponding decrease in communication with family and other adults may also occur as the adolescent strives to become independent. Those around the young person may observe this in the form of a greater need for privacy, boundary testing and rejection of family norms and values. Further friction is created when parental boundaries directly impinge on the ability to conform to group norms; for example, disallowing body piercings and imposing curfews. Although communication with parents tends to reduce during the teenage years, external approval remains important in the process of identity formation. Teens may, therefore, demonstrate heightened sensitivity to the evaluations and opinions of others and react strongly to criticism and comments that challenge their sense of self (Steinberg, 2005).

The preference for peer communication can also be seen in young people's interactions in help-seeking settings, where research shows that many young people do not access formal support due to fear of lack of confidentiality or not wanting to make a fuss, and prefer to use peers as a source of wisdom (Watson et al., 2003).

However, it is important to note that this withdrawal from adults may not emerge in isolation within the adolescent. Predominant stereotypes of adolescents are negative, with teenagers frequently cast as lazy, selfish and, at worst, criminals (Giroux, 2009; Cohen, 1972), which potentially makes it difficult for adolescents to engage with and place trust in an adult world.

When given an opportunity to be heard, what young people ask for is acceptance: 'Just accept us as we are more' (McCreanor, Watson & Denny, 2006), and to be heard on their own terms (Haxell, 2008).

CASE STUDY 6.1

Feeling misunderstood

A 17-year-old female enters counselling with depressive symptoms, truancy, suicidal ideation and harming behaviours, and regular drug and alcohol use. Family relationships are strained and the young woman relies solely on her same-sex partner as a confidant and support. She feels generally mistrusting of adults, while fear of reprimand for her behaviour (truancy and drug and alcohol use) and uncertainty about confidentiality also prevent her from seeking support from those around her.

To assert her identity she reveals her sexual identity to her family, which increases her sense of feeling misunderstood. This revelation also disconnects her from her peer group, although risk-taking behaviours provide a level of peer affiliation. She continues to feel disconnected and isolated, both at home and at school.

In counselling, the confidentiality policy is explained. The counsellor communicates with empathy in a calm and reassuring manner, without judging or reprimanding the young woman's behaviour. The counsellor also works with the client in a holistic way, focusing primarily on her strengths rather than solely on her risk. This increases the young woman's sense of self-efficacy and encourages her to engage more in activities she enjoys, such as drama and singing. This allows her to connect with a pro-social peer group and have her sense of identity affirmed.

Moments of irrational thinking are sensitively challenged, particularly the idea that ending her life is the only way to change her situation. Through talking, role-play, music, song writing and poetry, the young woman learns more abstract ways to view her situation and manage her seemingly extreme reactions to situations, as well as identifying and being able to express internal feelings.

Physical development

Alongside significant neurological and psychosocial changes, adolescents are also undergoing massive physical development during puberty and subsequent sexual maturation. Changing hormones mean adolescents experience an increase in sexual drives (Udry, 1988), along with an increase in thinking about sexual behaviours and a change in the meaning of them within the individual and from society (Steinberg, 1999).

According to Brooks-Gunn and Paikoff (1993), there are four main developmental challenges of adolescence with regards to sexuality:

+ accepting one's body is changing
+ accepting feelings of sexual arousal
+ understanding that sexual activity is voluntary
+ ensuring that all sex is safe sex.

As with all developmental processes during adolescence, this does not occur in isolation and is influenced by both neurological and psychosocial development. As discussed earlier, changes in the pleasure and reward processes in the brain may influence decisions to have sex. Ultimately, physical changes will be communicated in the adolescent engaging in sexual activities. Youth 07 data notes that 38 per cent of young males and 35 per cent of young females who participated in the survey have had sexual intercourse (Adolescent Health Research Group, 2008). However, Erikson (1968) suggests that the ability to develop intimacy in relationships does not occur until the ages of 18–24 years, when the young person can express feelings, wishes, needs, goals and fears. In this way adolescents may experience physical readiness for sexual relationships before the ability to communicate about and negotiate sexual relationships is fully developed. This may be evidenced by the mediation of peers in intimate relationships, and risk taking in sexual practice.

Continuing development of identity may also result in the questioning and testing of sexual identity, with the Youth 07 survey indicating that about one in twenty New Zealand secondary school students identify an attraction to the same sex or to both sexes (Rossen et al., 2009). The physical changes in the body at this time can also lead to young people feeling self-conscious about their bodies and an increased need for physical privacy. This is often communicated non-verbally through increased hiding of the body; for example, discomfort with getting changed in front of parents or peers where previously there was no issue. Respecting a young person's need for physical privacy is therefore very important at this time.

CASE STUDY 6.2

Teen issues in textspeak

Youthline provides a free live text counselling service for young people. Below are some generic examples of the types of communications received from youth, demonstrating the key developmental concepts they experience.

Developing abstract thinking skills

YP: im grounded. My mum h8s me and i h8 her.

YL: that sux, howcome ur grounded.

YP: its just cos I was late home the otha nite, and its totally unfair, cos i was helping my friend

YL: does ur mum kno the reason why u were late

YP: no she just went mental at me and grounded me

YL: Thats tuff aye? wn u haven't had a chance 2 explain ur story.

YP: yeah, my friend is goin thru some real serious stuff

YL: Do u reckon ur mum wld think differently if she knew why

YP: maybe. shes prob still gonna be angry

YL: Any idea why she mite be angry

YP: She was prob worried about me cos i didn't tell her i was with my frnd.

Impulsivity

I don't see how its eva gonna change and its pointless tlking 2 u. I may as well just not be here

Importance of friends

I am seeing this guy and i really lyk him but my frenz think he is a dik. Not sure if I should dump him.

all my frenz r callin me emo and im not I just like different music from them

Concerns about confidentiality and trust

R u guys gonna tell ne1 what I txt u?

How will I know if i get to tlk 2 the same person next tym?

Sexual identity and development

My gf wants 2 hav sex and im not sure if I want 2. How do u know n ur ready?

ive been lookin at my friends body when we r getting changed for phys ed class. Does that mean im gay?

Communicating with teenagers

The huge developmental, physical, social and emotional changes occurring during adolescence have an impact on how young people engage with those around them; equally, successful communication with teenagers involves both an understanding and an appreciation of a young person's development. The frustrations that an adult might feel at a teenager's seemingly irrational or thoughtless decisions can be balanced with an understanding of the changing underlying processes. The knowledge that teenagers may experience increased impulsivity and heightened emotional arousal should guide responses when communicating in difficult situations with teens. A calm, reassuring approach is more likely to lower arousal and encourage reasoning than a confrontational stance, which may challenge the young person's sense of self and provoke defensive retaliation.

While many adults feel uncertain around teenagers, from a young person's perspective adults can appear to have a lot of power to make decisions about their life or curb developing independence. Communications with adults or professionals in regard to personal issues, therefore, may be subject to a period of wariness or testing to establish trust. This will possibly involve questions from the young person, silence or even acting out behaviours, such as being overly rude and saying things aimed at shocking the adult to check out their response. Appreciating that when young people are pushing limits and boundaries they may also be testing care and acceptance may help adults get through what can feel like periods of rejection.

This can be a very vulnerable and private time for some adolescents as they try on different identities to see which ones fit. They can easily feel shamed and withdraw if their expressions are met with disdain or dismissal. To permit sincere communications with teens, adults need to take time to build rapport and be curious about the young person's emerging individual identity. Sometimes it can be difficult to explain how one feels, and being asked this outright may result in the young person becoming conscious of being put on the spot in having to explain themselves. An alternative way of exploring what's important in the life of a young person is through showing an interest in the individual's culture and their motivations. An entry point into difficult subjects can be had, for example, by asking if there are song lyrics that express how they feel.

Young people's sensitivity to how they might be perceived by adults is accompanied by their developing ability to analyse situations, which means that teens are fairly adept in judging when someone is not being genuine. Genuineness is about communicating on the level of the young person, but without using language that is unfamiliar to the communicator or that they do not feel comfortable using; for example, slang. A teenager will know when people are trying too hard and this will decrease rapport. This also means the communicator asking when they do not understand the young person's way of talking, rather than pretending that they know—which is disempowering—or adopting the unhelpful attitude that there is a 'generation gap' and 'teenagers speak a different language'. Being genuine may also involve letting the young person know some personal information such as likes and dislikes. Even with established rapport and genuine communication, adults may still need to be the one to raise sensitive topics, such as sex, and speak directly and plainly about the subject. Discomfort on the part of the adult is likely to make the young person uncomfortable and disinclined to engage in conversation.

Theories of psychosocial development emphasise role and identity formation. It is important, therefore, to consider whether communications support positive or negative identity formation when working with teens. By concentrating on faults and failures, a problem-focused approach risks reinforcing the problem as being an inherent part of the young person's identity. Think back to Hall's portrayal of adolescence as a time of 'storm and stress'. This idea of young people in a permanent state of turmoil suggests that conflict with parents is inevitable and risks leading to disengagement. A more constructive form of communication takes a strengths-based approach. A strengths orientation encourages the young person to recognise their competencies and strengths, and supports these as part of their identity (McLaren, 2002). Positive approaches like this have the potential to encourage connectedness and supportive relationships; this approach is also understood to foster **resilience** in teens (Youth Mentoring Network, 2011), or the ability to bounce back from difficult situations. Regular and positive communication with teens can also support positive role identification by providing pro-social role models (for example, youth workers and mentors).

Resilience The ability to recover from stress or injury.

Holding a strengths-based approach does not mean that communicating with a young person solely involves providing positive affirmation. A strengths-based approach with youth involves encouraging the positive things they are doing while sensitively challenging risk-taking or anti-social behaviours (Ministry of Youth Development, 2007). Adults who have realistically high expectations of young people's behaviour and a firm belief in what they can achieve will support the young person to have equally high expectations of themselves. Young people may enter relationships with a deficit approach. They may experience a limited sense of self or lack hope for their future. In this way, a key task for the strengths-based practitioner is to assist the young person to find their strengths and remain focused on the young person's potential—despite personal and contextual challenges—and, often, holding hope for the future before the young person can see this for themselves. Aronowitz (2005) referred to this process as 'envisioning the future' (p. 205), which in turn builds resilience.

CASE STUDY 6.3

A strength-based approach in health promotion

Working with young people inside of a strengths-based approach challenges service providers to consider young people not only as recipients of a service, but also as central to the provision of that service.

In providing an online discussion board, young people can post a question and have it answered by others who may have worked through the issues for themselves.

Topic: What's it like going to family planning clinic?

> I've made an appointment with family planning as I want to start using contraception, but I'm terrified that someone will see me going in. I feel like there will be a big red arrow hanging over my head. Everyone will know I'm having sex.
>
> And what happens when you go in? It's all a bit nerve-racking for a shy person (well, the shyness is currently in remission). I'm ok talking about this stuff with my boyfriend but talking about sex with anyone else makes me squirm.
>
> Any advice?
>
> Posted by Sarah

Re: What's it like going to family planning clinic?

> Hey Sarah—i know it seems scary—i've been there! but trust me, the people that work at family planning are really used to people like us (or like I used to be) (i dont think ANYTHING would surprise them). I found them really supportive.
> They talked with me and my friend bout lots of options. Did you know u can take a friend? or the boyfriend if you want. They don't mind at all, they figure they are helping twice as many people in one go!

Don't worry about people seeing you go in, yeah they may see you go in, but if the clinic is on a floor in a bigger building, no one will know where you are going, and even if they do bother to stop and think about it (and i doubt they would—most ppl are too wrapped up in there own stuff), they probably wouldnt care.

Pay it forward; if you discover its OK ... tell someone else or post on here

Posted by Ellie

{ SUMMARY }

Developmentally, a young person is coming in to their own. They are learning about who they are, how they relate to others and how they want to be in the world. When working with young people it is important to establish a trusting and accepting environment that encourages the person to reflect on possibilities, rather than simply telling them what they should be doing. In other words, the focus should be on creating more rather than less, of working with strengths rather than deficits, and of growing resilience rather than failure.

REFLECTION POINTS

6.1 Intention (motivation, message, meaning, emotion)

Think about what it is like when someone focuses on your strengths rather than your weaknesses. What impact does this have on how hopeful you feel about the things you can accomplish?

6.2 Reception (received message, response, feedback)

How might establishing boundaries and limits also demonstrate caring?

6.3 Perception (style, manner, impression, analysis)

Establishing trust, being genuine and having a positive regard for a young person's strengths are all part of building rapport. What behaviours demonstrate these attributes?

QUESTIONS FOR REVIEW

1 What are the developmental tasks for adolescence?
2 How is resilience fostered in young people?
3 What is involved when taking a strengths-based approach in working with young people?

REFERENCES

Adolescent Health Research Group. (2008). *Youth'07: The health and wellbeing of secondary school students in New Zealand. Initial findings*. Auckland, NZ: University of Auckland.

Aronowitz, T. (2005). The role of 'envisioning the future' in the development of resilience among at-risk youth. *Public Health Nursing, 22*, 200–8.

Brooks-Gunn, J. & Paikoff, R. L. (1993). 'Sex is a gamble, kissing is a game': Adolescent sexuality and health promotion. In S. G. Millstein, A. C. Petersen & E. O. Nightingale (eds), *Promoting the health of adolescents: New directions for the twenty-first century* (pp. 180–208). New York, NY: Oxford University Press.

Cohen, S. (1972). *Folk devils and moral panics: The creation of the mods and rockers*. London, UK: MacGibbon and Kee.

Crone, E. A. (2009). Executive functions in adolescence: Inferences from brain and behavior. *Developmental Science, 12*(6), 825–30.

Erikson, E. (1968). *Identity, youth and crisis*. New York, NY: Norton.

Giroux, H. A. (2009). *Youth in a suspect society. Democracy or disposability*. New York, NY: Palgrave MacMillan.

Hall, G. S. (1904). *Adolescence: Its psychology and its relation to physiology, anthropology, sociology, sex, crime, religion, and education* (vols. I & II). Englewood Cliffs, NJ: Prentice-Hall.

Haxell, A. (2008). Cn I jus txt, coz I don wan 2b heard: Mobile technologies and youth counselling. Paper presented at the Ascilite. Hello! Where are you in the landscape of educational technology? Retrieved from www.ascilite.org.au/conferences/melbourne08/procs/haxell.pdf.

McCreanor, T., Watson, P. D. & Denny, S. J. (2006). 'Just accept us as we are more': Experiences of young Pakeha with their families in Aotearoa New Zealand. *Social Policy Journal of New Zealand, 27*, 156–70.

McLaren, K. (2002). *Building strength*. Ministry of Youth Affairs. Available from www.youthaffairs.govt.nz.

Ministry of Health (2010). *Drug use in New Zealand: Key results of the 2007/08 New Zealand Alcohol and Drug Use Survey*. Wellington, NZ: Author.

Ministry of Youth Development. (2007). *Youth development strategy Aotearoa: Action for child and youth development*. Wellington, NZ: Author.

Newman, B. & Newman, P. (2003). *Development through life* (8th edn). Pacific Grove, CA: Brooks/Cole.

Piaget, J. (1926). *The language and thought of the child*. New York, NY: Meridian Books.

Rossen, F. V., Lucassen, M. F. G., Denny, S. & Robinson, E. (2009). *Youth'07: The health and wellbeing of secondary school students in New Zealand: Results for young people attracted to the same sex or both sexes*. Auckland, NZ: The University of Auckland.

Steinberg, L. (1999). *Adolescence* (5th edn). New York, NY: McGraw-Hill.

Steinberg, L. (2005). Cognitive and affective development in adolescence. *Trends in Cognitive Sciences, 9*(2), 69–74.

Turkstra, L. S. & Byom, L. J. (2010, December 21). *Executive functions and communication in adolescents*. Rockville, MD: The ASHA Leader.

Udry, J. R. (1988). Biological predispositions and social control in adolescent sexual behavior. *American Sociological Review, 53*, 709–22.

Watson, P. D., Clark, T. C., Denny, S. J., Fa'alau, F., Ameratunga, S. N., Robinson, E. M. et al. (2003). A health profile of New Zealand youth who attend secondary school. *New Zealand Medical Journal, 116*(1171), 1–9.

Youth Mentoring Network (2011). *Panui whakamarama: How to assist your mentee to build resilience*. Retrieved 13 January 2011 from www.youthmentoring.org.nz.

WEBSITES

Information for Teenagers; Child, Youth & Family: www.cyf.govt.nz/info-for-teenagers
New Zealand Aotearoa Adolescent Health and Development: www.nzaahd.org.nz
Youthline: www.youthline.co.nz

{7}

Early Adulthood

Charles Mpofu and Ailsa Haxell

CHAPTER OVERVIEW

This chapter covers the following topics:

+ Physical development
+ Risks
+ Cognitive development
+ Social development
+ Emotional adjustment.

KEY TERMS

Risky behaviour
Post-formal thought
Epistemic thinking
Dualistic thinking
Relativistic thinking
Fluid intelligence
Crystal intelligence
Reproductive technologies
Emotional intelligence

The early adulthood period is presented here as the ages 18 to 40 years. Although developmental psychologists tend to give an age range of 20 to 40 years, the age range adopted here takes into account the context of Aotearoa New Zealand where at age 18 young people assume various legal and social obligations that are associated with entry into adulthood. Individuals at this stage of their life are likely to be at the peak of their physical and cognitive capacities and focused on career advancement and intimacy.

Physical development

Physical development is perhaps the most noticeable aspect of development in human beings. It is about changes in the structures and physiological features of the human body. In terms of physical functioning, young adults are considered to be at the peak of their strength and energy in the middle adult years. Most body functions are fully developed by the time a person is in their mid-twenties. The peak of physical health and fitness occurs on average at approximately age 30 and the vast majority of young adults have no chronic conditions or impairments (Thies & Travers, 2009).

Brain development is an aspect of physical development that has implications for cognitive development during this period. The frontal lobe, which is responsible for reasoning, continues to develop in early adulthood. Knowledge about frontal lobe development is particularly important in terms of judgment and planning, intellectual capacities and problem-solving.

Risks

Within this age group, injuries are a major reason for medical visits. In Aotearoa New Zealand the most significant causes of death among young people are motor vehicle accidents and suicide. Among young adults aged between 25 and 44 years, unintentional and intentional injury (40 per cent combined) is the major contributor to mortality (Ministry of Health, 2001).

Motor vehicle accidents are one of the most common reasons for mortality among young New Zealanders (Fergusson, Swain-Campbell & Horwood, 2003). Drivers aged 20 to 24 are over-represented in traffic accidents and the same trend has been reported in Australia (Fergusson, Swain-Campbell & Horwood, 2003). It is important to note that there is a gender imbalance in this over-representation in favour of males, and this has been attributed to their tendency to engage in **risky behaviour** (Ministry of Health, 2001).

Risky behaviour
Actions that may lead to injury or death.

Cognitive development

Post-formal thought Cognitive processes that emphasise relativism and the non-absolute nature of information.

Epistemic thinking Reflecting on how one arrives at facts, beliefs and ideas.

Dualistic thinking A tendency to see things as binary opposites; for example, as black and white, good or bad, or right or wrong. In addition, such ways of seeing assume that these are permanent states and are independent of one's own thinking.

This aspect of development is about changes in thinking, reasoning, memory and other intellectual capacities.

Advancing beyond what Piaget had labelled 'formal operational thinking' is a concept loosely referred to as **post-formal thought**. One of the distinguishing features of adults is the movement away from models of thinking where facts, beliefs and ideas are acquired, and towards a model of thinking that is personally considered and involves justifiable conclusions. This is a stage that Perry (1998) describes as **epistemic thinking**: a time of reflection on how people arrive at their beliefs. This marks a shift from **dualistic thinking**—where such beliefs might be described as true or false, right or wrong, or good or bad—to appreciating that beliefs held by others might differ yet still be valid for that person. **Relativistic thinking** involves an acceptance that what is 'true' or 'right' or 'good' varies greatly among people. This thinking is flexible, accepts diverse opinions and leads to an acknowledgment that there may be multiple truths. Pragmatism—doing what is possible given the limitations—also has been identified as a characteristic of adult thought (Shaie, 1978). This is based on the idea that young adults are at a period where they make use of skills previously obtained to achieve career goals, domestic goals and other life goals. This places an emphasis on context and relativity.

CASE STUDY 7.1

Margaret

Margaret is a 22-year-old woman born into a very religious family in Aotearoa New Zealand. Margaret describes herself as single on her Facebook page, but with lots of friends, both male and female. Margaret's friends describe her as a very social person who likes being with others and partying. Her parents are concerned for her, as she has twice called them needing transport home in the middle of the night. In each instance, she was worried about drink driving, as the plan to have a sober driver in the group had failed. Margaret identifies that she finds it hard to say 'no' to her friends, especially if she has been drinking, and that she finds it hard to be as 'good' as she knows her parents would like her to be.

To ensure that Margaret maintained the family's religious values when she was growing up, she was rarely allowed to play with other children. They discouraged her from joining clubs or participating in social events with her peers. Therefore, school and university were the only places when she was around people from different cultures and with other values.

Recently, Margaret attended an entrepreneurship workshop and was inspired to work with a partner to set up a podiatry practice. Margaret is worried about not being able to say 'no' to her business partner about obtaining a loan to establish the practice. Margaret is also reluctant to discuss this aspect of the business with her family.

Labouvie-Vief (1985, 2003) emphasises that young adults need to function in a world that is complex, and where there are multiple options or paths that could be taken. This requires the development of thinking that is unique to the circumstances of such situations. Labouvie-Vief also points to how the emotions play a part in decision-making: that there may be discrepancies between how a person feels about something and the logic of a situation. Such discrepancies become more organised and integrated with maturity and with the increased exposure to decision-making that early adulthood brings. In Case study 7.1 Margaret can be identified as moving towards relativistic thinking modes in considering how she is beginning to make choices; that is, she is just beginning to develop insight into how her emotions are influencing decisions.

Relativistic thinking Considering information according to its relationship with other known facts.

Rather than focusing on the process of decision-making, Horn and Cattell (1967) investigated types of intelligence in adults that they referred to as crystal and fluid intelligence. **Fluid intelligence** can be viewed as the ability to think and reason abstractly, and to solve problems independently of any related previous experience. **Crystal intelligence**, by contrast, relates to the accumulation of knowledge and skills acquired with experience (Horn & Cattell, 1967). Fluid intelligence starts to decline at around 30 years of age, while crystal intelligence continues to increase through middle adulthood. Horn and Cattell argued that this pattern was physiological rather than subject to context or culture. This increasing crystallised intelligence can be explained by the continued exposure to a wealth of experiences and skill acquisition.

Fluid intelligence The in-born ability of an individual to think and reason quickly and responsively.

Crystal intelligence The ability to think and reason based on experience acquired during life.

Social development

In reference to early adult development, Erik Erikson's theory of psychosocial development proposed that the main task is either to flourish in the achievement of intimacy, or to avoid the crisis of isolation as a result of failing to achieve intimacy (Erikson & Erikson, 1997). The outcome of navigating these two opposing forces has a bearing on achieving a mature personality and successful later development. The key issue here is seeking identity through intimacy and adjusting this identity when new relationships are sought. It is important to note that Erikson's concept of intimacy was not limited to relationship partners, but also referred to the capacity to make meaningful and lasting relationships. These include relationships with friends and colleagues, and could even be applied to developing a love for one's work. In Case study 7.1 it can be seen that even though Margaret is not in a long-term intimate relationship, she has friends, has maintained connections with family and is considering commitments towards career advancement.

CASE STUDY 7.2

Maiuu

Maiuu Fafo is a 23-year-old New Zealander whose parents come from Samoa. He was sent to Aotearoa New Zealand at the age of 17 by his grandmother to find a job and to financially support his extended family in Samoa.

Maiuu is very clear that his priorities lie in fulfilling his grandmother's wishes of being a breadwinner for the extended family. He tells his New Zealand-born friend Brian that he is finding it very hard coping with this pressure. Brian tells Maiuu that these issues don't really matter and that he should find a girlfriend. If this girlfriend is good then the next step is to find a flat where he would live with her while they are deciding about marriage and having children. Brian is baffled by Maiuu's response when he says that his family in Samoa will not approve of these ideas. Maiuu is similarly astounded by Brian's apparent selfishness and disrespect for elders.

Maiuu remembers his grandmother told him that if he has problems he should contact other extended family members in Aotearoa New Zealand, but he is not sure they would understand the pressures he is under. In addition, he knows these other members of his family have responsibilities for disciplining him if he misbehaves. He decides not to discuss his concerns with them.

Young adults find themselves making life decisions that are similar across many societies. These commonly involve career development, choosing a partner and establishing a family. However, contemporary New Zealand society is so diverse that within any community or group there will be people from a wide range of backgrounds who live with various expectations about their behaviour, how they use their time and how they plan for the future. Along with these differences are many expectations about the role and influence of family members. Case study 7.2 presents Maiuu as he is entering into adulthood in Aotearoa New Zealand, which is in some ways similar but in other ways quite different from his life in Samoa. He is increasingly aware of these contradictory demands and the inability of his previous methods of problem solving to resolve the stresses he experiences. Trying to meet the expectations of the differing groups that he interacts with creates additional stressors on him as he moves towards adulthood.

Erikson's theory of psychosocial development emphasises entering relationships, establishing long-term commitments, living with a partner and perhaps considering starting a family as key transitions for young adults.

Fertility is at its peak in the early adulthood years. The twenties are said to be the best times for pregnancy and giving birth because foetal and maternal risk increase after the age of 30 (Thies & Travers, 2009). However, women are increasingly participating in the paid workforce. This means that such decisions require balancing many considerations, such as the loss of income and the pressures of establishing careers, in conjunction with studying and perhaps the legacy of some student debt. These issues all contribute to many women deciding to defer when they have children.

In 2008, Statistics New Zealand reported the median age for women giving birth to their first child was 28 years. Advances in **reproductive technologies** have contributed in supporting the possibility for having children later in life; however, this raises further ethical and legal issues in addition to social and physical considerations.

Reproductive technologies The use of medical and surgical techniques to assist with fertility and conception.

Emotional adjustment

Young adults encounter many issues that make demands on their emotional adjustment. These adjustments occur within the context of both personal and professional relationships.

Erikson contributed to the understanding of emotional development during early adulthood when he noted that a strong sense of personal identity is critical to the development of intimate relationships. Erikson also noted that those with a poor sense of self tend to be associated with less committed relationships, and a higher likelihood of suffering emotional isolation and loneliness, which may lead to depression (Erikson & Erikson, 1997). Developing emotional competence and the capacity for clear communications, therefore, is useful in fostering resilience in early adulthood.

To help foster resilience, Goleman (1996) provides a model for enhancing **emotional intelligence**. The focus is on developing:

1 self-awareness—learning how to read one's emotions and recognise their impact while also using 'gut feelings' to inform decisions
2 self-management—controlling one's emotions and impulses as appropriate to changing circumstances

Emotional intelligence Insight into emotional needs and skills of self and others.

3 social awareness—developing awareness of and sensitivity to others' emotions while navigating one's social networks
4 relationship management—having the ability to inspire, influence and develop others while negotiating conflict.

The link between cognitive and emotional development in the form of emotional intelligence has also been researched in relation to its positive impact on learning among Australian adolescents (Downey et al., 2008).

In both case studies introduced in this chapter, it is apparent that the areas of cognitive, emotional and social development are clearly interrelated.

{ SUMMARY }

Early adulthood is a period when individuals begin (and are often expected) to take various social responsibilities, such as seeking an intimate partner, having children and establishing a career. A number of theories can be used to describe and explain physical, psychosocial and cognitive aspects of development in the early adulthood age group. However, concepts must be considered in relation to the wider social environment of the individual. Understanding the experiences of people in relation to their period of life and the wider context in which they live assists in ensuring that communication is appropriate and meaningful.

REFLECTION POINTS

7.1 Intention (motivation, message, meaning, emotion)

Having autonomy is often considered a hallmark of what it is to be an adult. Should autonomy always be respected?

7.2 Reception (received message, response, feedback)

Think about when you have been stressed, anxious, unwell or in pain. How receptive are you to learning at these times? Having educated someone about his or her condition, how would you check if information shared has been understood?

7.3 Perception (style, manner, impression, analysis)

In interactions with practitioners, what expectations do you hold about how you would like to be treated?

QUESTIONS FOR REVIEW

1 What are the dangers of assuming that young adults are at the best years of their health?

2 What conflicts between emotional and cognitive development may people in this age group experience?

3 What part do physical and social development play in risk-taking behaviour?

REFERENCES

Downey, L. A., Mountstephen, J., Lloyd, J., Hansen, K. & Stough, C. (2008). Emotional intelligence and scholastic achievement in Australian adolescents. *Australian Journal of Psychology, 60*(1), 10–17.

Erikson, E. & Erikson, J. M. (1997). *The life cycle completed* (extended version). New York, NY: W. W. Norton.

Fergusson, D. M., Swain-Campbell, N. R. & Horwood, L. J. (2003). Risky driving behaviour in young people: Prevalence, personal characteristics and traffic accidents. *Australian and New Zealand Journal of Public Health, 27*(3), 337–42.

Goleman, D. (1996). *Emotional intelligence: Why it can matter more than IQ*. New York, NY: Bantam Books.

Horn, J. L. & Cattell, R. B. (1967). Age differences in fluid and crystallized intelligence. *Acta Psychologica, 26*, 107–29.

Labouvie-Vief, G. (1985). Intelligence and cognition. In J. E. Birren & K. W. Schaie (eds), *Handbook of the psychology of aging* (2nd edn) (pp. 500–30). New York, NY: Van Nostrand Reinhold.

Labouvie-Vief, G. (2003). Dynamic integration: Affect, cognition, and the self in adulthood. *Current Directions in Psychological Science, 12*, 201–6.

Ministry of Health (2001). *The burden of disease and injury in New Zealand*. Wellington, NZ: Author. Retrieved from www.moh.govt.nz/moh.nsf/pagesmh/952?Open.

Perry, W. G. Jr. (1998). *Forms of intellectual and ethical development in the college years: A schema*. San Francisco, CA: Jossey-Bass.

Shaie, K. W. (1978). Toward a stage theory of adult cognitive development. *Journal of Aging and Human Development, 8*(2), 129–38.

Statistics New Zealand (2008). Births and deaths. March 2008 quarter. Retrieved www.stats.govt.nz/browse_for_stats/population/births/BirthsAndDeaths_HOTPMar08qtr.aspx.

Thies, K. M. & Travers, J. F. (2009). *Growth and development through the lifespan*. London, UK: Jones and Bartlett.

WEBSITES

Births and Deaths: March 2008 quarter, Statistics New Zealand: www.stats.govt.nz/browse_for_stats/population/births/BirthsAndDeaths_HOTPMar08qtr.aspx

Burden of Disease and Injury in New Zealand, Ministry of Health: www.moh.govt.nz/moh.nsf/pagesmh/952?Open

Demographic Trends 2009, Marriage, civil union, and divorce, Statistics New Zealand: www.stats.govt.nz/browse_for_stats/population/estimates_and_projections/demographic-trends-2009/chapter3.aspx

{8}

Middle Years

Kirk Reed

CHAPTER OVERVIEW

This chapter covers the following topics:

+ Defining the middle years
+ Roles in the middle years
+ Managing life events.

KEY TERMS

Life roles
Transition
Crisis
Life events

The journey through the middle years can be explored by considering the common developmental tasks as outlined in the work of Erikson (1994) and Havighurst (1972). Another view can be found in the **life roles** that are generally experienced by those in their middle years. Communicating effectively with people at this stage of their life requires a respectful understanding of their perspective, the journey they are on and the issues and challenges they are likely to be experiencing.

Life roles The set of rights, obligations and behaviours associated with various tasks and positions (for example, learner, parent and employee).

Defining the middle years

From a Western lifespan perspective, Erikson (a psychologist) and Havighurst (a physicist and educationalist) identified some developmental tasks that tend to be associated with the middle years. Havighurst (1972) identified that in the middle years, which he described as being from 30 to 60 years, the key tasks include: selecting a mate; starting and rearing a family; managing a home; getting started in an occupation, and reaching and maintaining a successful career; finding a congenial social group; and achieving adult and civic responsibility. He also indentified that the middle years include adjusting to having ageing parents, assisting teenage children to become responsible and happy adults, and accepting and adjusting to the physiological changes of middle age.

Erikson (1994) described middle age as being from 35 to 65 years and called this life stage 'generativity versus self-absorption'. He stated that middle age is when a person tends to be occupied with creative and meaningful work and with the issues that surround family life. One of the significant tasks of the middle years is to perpetuate culture and transmit cultural values through family, while working to establish a stable environment for family and the community. During this stage of life, Erikson identified that significant relationships are within the workplace and family, and that a sense of strength comes through the care of others and the production of something that contributes to the betterment of society. He called this 'generativity', which he described as a response to a sense of fear of inactivity and stagnation. As goals, relationships and family life change, a person may be faced with major life changes—a mid-life crisis—and struggle to find meaning and purpose to life. Erikson argued that if a person did not successfully get through this life stage then they could become self-absorbed and stagnant.

From the work of Havighurst and Erikson, it is clear that there are some common key developmental tasks associated with the middle years, namely: management of a career, negotiating and maintaining a relationship, expanding caring responsibilities, managing a household, adjusting to ageing parents and coping with the physical changes of ageing. At this stage of life there are a range of health issues that are common, which may include: heart disease, stroke, chronic illness, work-related illness, respiratory disease, alcohol and other drug misuse, and depression. In addition, screening for conditions such as breast cancer and prostate cancer, and risk factors associated with chronic heart disease are recommended. These health issues are, of course, different for each individual, but managing and coming to terms with physiological and cognitive changes is an inevitable part of growing older, especially towards the end of the middle years and into older age.

Transition The journey from one place or position to another.

As people enter their middle years with a great many hopes, goals and ambitions, some of these go unrealised as a person settles into the daily round of activities. At around age 40 some adults experience a mid-life **transition** or 'mid-life crisis', where a reassessment of their personal goals and aspirations takes place. Up to this point they may have hung onto their personal story that their life would be a success in every way. There was plenty of time to get a better job, start a family, write a book, take an overseas trip or purchase a fast car. But at some point a person may begin to realise that time is rapidly running out to do all these things. Some adults who go through a mid-life transition do so very well and accept their life as it is. Others refuse to abandon their goals and train for a new job or take a positive step to getting what they set out to. Still others become depressed or turn to alcohol or other drugs as a means of escape when they realise their goals and aspirations may never be achieved.

CASE STUDY 8.1

Kath

Kath is a 42-year-old woman living a long way from her family networks. She is married, and she and her husband own their own home and have a 3½-year-old son. She works full time, gets up at 5:30 am to commute an hour to work and picks her son up from day care at 5.30 pm. Kath has a strong commitment to her career in a large company; she enjoys the challenge of her job but is beginning to realise that when her son goes to school she may have to reduce her hours or resign from her job to manage getting him to and from school. She has a number of friends who live locally, but she does not see them often as she needs the weekends to rest and spend time with her family, and also catch up on household chores. She has few leisure interests outside of her family and home, simply because she does not have enough time in the day. In the past 18 months she has had some health problems and has had her gall bladder removed. Kath is beginning to realise that the health of her parents is beginning to deteriorate, which she finds difficult when she lives so far away from them and cannot be there when they need her.

Roles in the middle years

Depending on a person's life stage, they will take on varying roles. Nine roles were identified by Super (1980). From his perspective as a psychologist he presented explanations that may account for the roles that most people engage in most of the time. These nine roles are: child, student, leisure user, citizen, worker, partner/spouse, homemaker, parent and retiree. In the middle years, and for any particular individual, some of these roles may be absent or insignificant; however, most of these life roles will be present to one extent or another. Super also identified four key areas in which these roles may be acted out: in the home, workplace, school or community. These are all important parts of the environment or context in which people live out their lives, and the environment may significantly influence or impact on a person's roles. For example, an employer may expect their employee to work late or at the weekends to get tasks done, and this may become a routine part of a person's life. This in turn may impact on their leisure time roles and cause conflict with their spouse or partner.

It is important to consider if a person's roles indicate balance. If there are either significant gaps or roles that are too demanding, they may impact on health and well-being. A person in their middle years is likely to have one or more of the roles identified by Super. It is worth considering from the person's perspective what their involvement is in these roles, the meaning the role has and how one role impacts on other roles. Super's roles may be explored in relation to the middle years in the following ways:

+ Child—as life progresses, a person in their middle years may take on more responsibility for caring, looking after and supporting parents, particularly if their parents become frail or need assistance. It is likely that a person in their middle years will still socialise with their parents and have obligations at family events or during holidays or festivals.
+ Student—during the middle years a person may take on the student role and engage in ongoing learning, professional development or higher education. Becoming a student in this stage of life might be linked to career aspirations and advancement, retraining to find a worker role that is more aligned to self-identity, or the need to retrain or upskill because of job loss. The student role is likely to be in conjunction with balancing other life roles; for example, a person might attend an evening course purely for personal interest. It is likely that those in this life stage who engage in higher education will have been successful in this environment in the past, although for some this might be their first time experience, and it may take some time to become familiar and comfortable with the demands of a formal education setting.

+ Leisure user—activities and leisure time may have been curtailed while raising a family and spending more time in the worker role. Leisure time may start to increase in the middle years as children leave home and there is more spare time. It is likely that leisure interests will change in response to a mid-life crisis or decreasing health or physical ability associated with ageing. There may be more time and resources to engage in new leisure activities.
+ Citizen—in the middle years, a person may feel the need to contribute to their local community and give 'something back'. A person may take on civic roles such as city councillor, become a member of a governance group such as a board for a school or non-profit organisation, or join a community group.
+ Worker—this role is likely to be predominant and stable during the middle years, and work commitments and responsibilities may increase due to length of time in the job and promotion. Job loss or redundancy may have a significant impact on a person's sense of identity and self-belief.
+ Partner/spouse—it is likely that a person in the middle years is in a committed relationship or is seeking their second or third long-term committed relationship as a result of the loss of their partner or the dissolution of their marriage or civil partnership. Significant time and energy may be devoted to maintaining the relationship and spending time with their partner.
+ Homemaker—this is likely to be a significant role in the middle years, due to home ownership and management, home renovation, and maintenance of the home environment. These are all likely to take up a considerable amount of time. As a person ages, they may choose to do less around the home or in the garden, and employ someone else to do these tasks while they focus on work or leisure. A person in their middle years may make changes to the physical environment of their home to ensure easy access, downsize the family home or move house in preparation for retirement and/or older age.
+ Parent—during the middle years the role of parent may change as children leave home and 'make their way in the world'. The 'empty nest syndrome' may be experienced where parents mourn the loss of their children as they leave the family home and establish relationships and a home of their own. There may be increased responsibility as a grandparent as a person's children start to create their own family.
+ Retiree—some people in their middle years may take early retirement or may be made redundant. This is a significant change and some might take a long time to deal with the sense of loss. As a result in the change of worker role, a person may reorganise their life to accommodate the loss of the worker role by taking on a part-time job or increasing their leisure interests. Others may begin planning and preparing for retirement, reducing the hours spent in work as they move to the next stage of their life.

Managing life events

While the list above gives a broad and general view of the types of roles a person may have in their middle years, it is by no means comprehensive. As life progresses, a number of events beyond the person's control may take place. This can range from the loss of a partner or spouse or job loss due to the economic climate to deterioration of personal health or a mid-life **crisis**. In order to cope with these **life events** Reese and Smyer (1983) suggest eight factors to consider when working with a person to manage life events. It is important to consider the person in context and work with them to identify the following:

Crisis A significant point of change with potential risks of loss or harm.

Life events Situations or experiences that are significant for the change related to it.

1. Trigger—what set off the event? Was the event expected or anticipated? Was the trigger internal or external to the person?
2. Timing—how did the timing of the event impact on how it was experienced or managed?
3. Control—how much control did the person have over the event, both when it happened and the way it was managed or progressed?
4. Role change—what impact has the event had, or will have, on life roles?
5. Duration—how long did the event last? Was the change permanent or temporary?
6. Previous experience—had the person experienced a similar life event in the past? How has this previous experience impacted on the current event?
7. Concurrent stress—what are the other stressors in the person's life and how have these demands impacted on the current event?
8. Assessment—did the experience have a positive or negative impact? Did this change over time?

While on first appearances this might simply appear to be a list of factors to work through with the person as a means to understand the life events they are experiencing, it is important to make sure that this is done with respect and empathy. Developing a sense of rapport with the person will allow them to feel comfortable and enable them to tell their story in detail. A person in this age group may relate better to someone they connect with their family, rather than a professional. It is therefore important to clarify roles and purpose when talking with them. It may also be useful to adapt language and vocabulary so that it is relevant to their age. Carefully listening to responses will provide cues about how they are going about managing their life event. Be aware that a person may become upset and this must be responded to in a respectful and sincere manner.

CASE STUDY 8.2

Drew

Drew is a 35-year-old gay man living in the inner suburb of a large city. He has a wide circle of friends, who he sees as often as he can, plus a broad range of interests, which include travelling overseas, networking with his friends, jogging, going to the gym, spending time on the net and cooking. He spends most of his weekends with his friends and they often go to bars or clubs. He sees his family from time to time, but this is usually at family events such as birthdays. His father has a long-term illness and lives away from the family home, so his mother lives alone. He tries to support her usually by calling or visiting once a week, but he does not have much time to see her.

He has a successful job and has been studying to update his knowledge. There has been some talk of restructuring at his workplace and he may be made redundant, but he is not too concerned if he loses his job because he feels like a new challenge. He feels like he is well positioned to get a more senior job and that working somewhere else would help him with his career goals. Drew has recently ended a long-term relationship and is looking for someone to settle down with. His general practitioner has warned him that his blood pressure is high; he knows he should do something about this but he is not worried as he knows he is still young and has plenty of time to make those kinds of changes to his lifestyle when he gets older.

{ SUMMARY }

The middle years are generally considered to be between a person's thirties and retirement and is a time when a person is highly productive and secure, and has a high sense of achievement. Health-care students need to be aware of the roles and responsibilities that are typical in the middle years, but also need to be aware that typical patterns may not apply to every individual's circumstances. These roles and responsibilities can be disrupted due to internal and external factors, such as feeling unsuccessful or having a sense of loss as family leaves home or if the person is made redundant. Having skills and knowledge in understanding a person's life roles and how they manage life events will enable a student to gain an understanding of a person in their context so interventions can be tailored to address the needs of the individual.

REFLECTION POINTS

8.1 Intention (motivation, message, meaning, emotion)

How are the key developmental tasks of the middle years similar to or different from your own life stage?

8.2 Reception (received message, response, feedback)

What would be the ideal role balance for someone in their middle years?

8.3 Perception (style, manner, impression, analysis)

What connections can you make in the case studies of Kath and Drew to the key developmental tasks of Havighurst and Erikson?

QUESTIONS FOR REVIEW

1 Using Super's life roles, can you identify the roles of someone you know who is in their middle years?
2 In what ways does a mid-life transition/crisis resemble an adolescent coming to terms with their identity and place in the world?
3 How would you alter your communication style in order to work with someone that is older than you?

REFERENCES

Erikson, E. H. (1994). *Identity and the life cycle: A reissue*. New York, NY: Norton.

Havighurst, R. J. (1972). *Developmental tasks and education*. New York, NY: Longman.

Reese, H. W. & Smyer, M. A. (1983). The dimensionalisation of life events. In E. J. Callahan & K. A. McCluskey (eds), *Life-span developmental psychology: Non formative life events*. New York, NY: Academic Press.

Super, D. E. (1980). A life-span, life-space approach to career development. *Journal of Vocational Behaviour, 16*, 282–98.

WEBSITES

Agewell: www.agewell.org.nz
Growing Up in New Zealand: www.growingup.co.nz
ThirdAge: www.thirdage.com

{9}

Senior Years

Helen Gaeta and Terry Weblemoe

CHAPTER OVERVIEW

This chapter covers the following topics:

+ Psychosocial theories of ageing
+ The ageing population
+ Socio-environmental theory
+ Communication and ageing.

KEY TERMS

Gerontology
Geriatrics
Activity theory
Disengagement theory
Abandonment theory
Continuity theory
Socio-environmental theory
Ageism
Fluid intelligence
Crystal intelligence

The concept of people in their 'senior years' is commonly reflected in the image of a retired person receiving a state pension. Although this is the case for the current generation of 'seniors', the pension is a fairly modern concept that has its underpinnings in the rise of industrialisation in Europe, especially in Germany. In 1879, Otto von Bismarck, Chancellor of the German Empire, abandoned free-trade policies and adopted protective tariffs on home industries to provide revenue for the German government. The adoption of tariffs proved to be very profitable for German industry, generating an increase in employment opportunities in the urban areas where industry was established. This created an influx of German workers from the countryside to these urban areas. The shift in the working population from agricultural to industrial coincided with the rise of socialism in Europe, a political position that Bismarck opposed. In order to keep the socialist movement at bay, he decided that German workers needed to have a stake in the political affairs of the state of Germany.

The same political influences that were reforming Europe were also impacting on New Zealand. In 1898, the Liberal government led by Richard Seddon, introduced a small means-tested pension to destitute older people over the age of 65 years. Like Bismarck, Seddon was influenced by the plight of the workers, especially the welfare of ex-miners on the West Coast. In 1939, the first New Zealand Labour Prime Minister, Michael Joseph Savage, spearheaded the legislation that was the forerunner of the current 'New Zealand Superannuation Scheme'. This entitled people from 60 years of age to an income- and asset-tested pension, consolidating the notion that 60 years marked the onset of the 'senior years'. Alongside these developments, the fields of **gerontology** and **geriatrics** emerged.

Gerontology The study of social, psychological and biological aspects of ageing.

Geriatrics The study of diseases of ageing.

Psychosocial theories of ageing

Activity theory provides a perspective on ageing that links activity in social roles with life satisfaction (Havighurst et al., 1968, 1969). Optimal ageing involves staying active, maintaining social involvement and finding replacement roles for those activities lost through retirement (Maddox, 1968; Neugarten, 1971). Within this view, failure to age successfully is a failure of motivation on the part of the individual. One of the weaknesses of this perspective is that it makes implicit assumptions about the relationships between people's action and their roles (Gubrium, 1973). Proponents of activity theory assume that people control the types of roles available to them, as well as the activities necessary to the performance of those roles. They assume that people have the capacity to construct and develop appropriate sets of activity goals. However, it is hard to see how this can be so for the elderly who are financially challenged, and the elderly deprived of social support. Another

Activity theory A deterministic approach that sees the older person as responsible for making their own decisions and adjustments to their changing situation.

problem is that it assumes it is better to be active than inactive, and that life satisfaction and activity are positively related. However, research studies have shown there is not a uniform relationship between activity levels and life satisfaction (Lemon, Bengston & Peterson, 1972; Maddox, 1974). Furthermore, it does not take into account that reduced activity is necessary for some elderly because of declining health, and that this does not mean that life satisfaction must decline.

Disengagement theory A belief that ageing involves withdrawal and severing of ties between a person and others in society.

Disengagement theory is an explicit theory based on research conducted by Cumming and Henry (1961). There is a focus on the self and a reduced involvement in organised social structures. Successful ageing is seen as acceptance of, and a desire to, reduce social interactions. The disengagement process is seen as mutually satisfying for the older person and for society. It ensures that society maintains optimal function by preserving social equilibrium and enabling self-reflection for the older person. It provides an orderly transfer of knowledge, capital and power from the older to the younger generation, ensuring that a vacuum is not left when valuable older members of society die. Changes in an older adult's biological and cognitive abilities are not perceived as a threat because the disengagement process prepares one for the anticipated decline that comes with old age. Opponents of the theory claim that it is context-free and biologically homogeneous. Prasad (1964) conducted a study of retired industrial workers and showed that none of the aged men in the study showed any desire to disengage. A number of studies showed that disengagement from employment often worked against an individual's best interest (Glanz, 1983, 1985; Ruffini & Todd, 1979). Furthermore, it was often wasteful or dysfunctional because experienced and productive individuals were being pressured to withdraw or narrow their activities after retirement. Other studies found that when there was disengagement from active life it was usually for health reasons, not ageing per se (Lowenthal, 1968; Mass & Kuypers, 1974).

CASE STUDY 9.1

Disengagement

It was just a sudden decision that I made, but what triggered it was the death of my oldest sister ... so I made up my mind then that I was going to put in my resignation right there and then. I was just thinking I needed to spend some time with my grandchildren. But before I left the office I was asked by the office if I would just do a little project part-time for them for three months, so I thought 'yes' ... and that was the start of my consultancy. Now I'm gradually weaning myself away from the workforce again, taking a couple of days off a week, and that's something that's much more desirable for my stage of life.

Ministry of Social Development (2009)

Abandonment theory was conceived to explain the increasing loneliness and neglect that characterises old age for some people (Burgess, 1960). It aims to explain inevitable and universal negative features of the ageing process. The view is that older people experience a downwards direction with respect to lifestyle, which is accompanied with increasing levels of abandonment and social isolation.

Abandonment theory The perspective that ageing is linked to decreased social engagement and increased isolation.

It suggests that being old means enduring a degree of social deprivation. Baum and Baum (1980) argue that this view has its origins in industrialisation, which has no use for older people. Knowledge and skills are the modern currency and these change quickly in modern Western civilisations. Thus the services of older people are of little economic value, making them outdated and less 'useful'. Status, therefore, is lost in a culture that prizes youth, beauty and success. Prior to the formalisation of abandonment theory, Barron (1961) suggested that the aged become a 'disprivileged minority group'.

Abandonment theory also implies that financial deprivation, through loss of income, accompanies ageing. Furthermore, old age brings psychological and physical segregation of the elderly, particularly when they live in institutions, retirement villages and nursing homes. These views of the elderly are still prominent today, even though most older people in Aotearoa New Zealand stay in their own homes, with less than 10 per cent in supportive environments. In addition, changing demographics and the high cost of housing is shifting asset wealth from younger to older adults. Thus the older adult is increasingly seen as a valuable consumer, contrary to the notion of financial impoverishment.

CASE STUDY 9.2

Abandonment

When I was looking for a job, I'd just go into these recruitment consultants. It was a joke. They were staffed with young kids. If I did manage to score an interview, I'd know immediately. I was told there is virtually no chance to get a job at my age ... just so annoyed by the attitude of 'these kids' that say 'you are not qualified' or 'your skill set is not quite what is required'. Only once, and that was the job I got, I thought, 'I've got a chance here'.

Ministry of Social Development (2009)

Continuity theory was formulated to explain development across the lifespan. Its importance for ageing is that it links the person's past to their present. To this extent, Erikson's (1980) developmental theory of the eight stages of life can be considered a continuity theory. Erikson claims that a person must successfully pass through all prior seven stages to successfully pass through the

Continuity theory The view that ageing is a continuation of the earlier part of life, a component of the natural cycle of life.

eighth stage of life, where synthesis of all prior developmental stages enables the older adult to reflect and accept, with satisfaction, the passage of their life. An individual who achieves this attains what Erikson termed 'ego integrity'. With ego integrity comes wisdom, though Erikson does not expand on what he means by wisdom. An individual who does not achieve 'ego integrity' will experience despair and fear of death.

Continuity theory posits that stability guides psychological development throughout the lifespan. In other words, personality, values, morals, preferences and basic patterns of behaviour are relatively constant through the lifespan, regardless of the life changes an individual experiences (for example, widowhood, illness or loss of income). A major criticism of continuity theory is its deterministic nature. This means there is little, if any, flexibility for change from early behaviours or attitudes as the individual is pre-programmed to age in a particular way. To overcome this inflexibility, new interpretations of continuity have been formulated to encompass evolution and adaptation, reducing the emphasis on stagnation. Newer perspectives still claim that there are basic structures that persist over time (personality traits), but that capacity for change can be incorporated into a person's history. Atchley (1989) states that adults 'employ concepts of their past to conceive of the future, and structure their choices in response to the change brought about by normal ageing' (p. 183). A substantial number of research studies have supported continuity theory (for example, Ross, 1977; Maddox, 1968; Palmore & Kivett, 1977). However, many of these studies have used cross-sectional and short-term designs for data collection. Thus only inferences can be made about the stability of personality over time.

All of these socially based perspectives of ageing have been developed against the backdrop of industrial economies in the Western world. Although most of the research has originated in North America, the underlying principles can be generalised to all Western capitalist industrial models. Activity theory, disengagement theory and abandonment theory are strongly influenced by notions around the usefulness of citizens to economic productivity. During the period in which these perspectives were being developed, only 10 per cent of the New Zealand population was over 65 years old. By contrast, 65 per cent of the population was between 15 and 64 years old. Thus older adults were not needed in the workforce, given there was a plentiful supply of efficient economic units to meet the productivity needs of society. However, the declining birth rate and increasing life expectancy is changing the population demographic. Concomitant with the changing demographic is a shifting perspective of ageing and a need to revise social theories of ageing. The impact of the ageing population is expanded in the next section, followed by a presentation of a newer social theory of ageing that incorporates the changing population demographic and its linkage to recent economic developments.

The ageing population

A common feature of all Western societies is that life expectancy is increasing and birth rates are falling. Consequently, the population is ageing. It is estimated that by 2026, more than 20 per cent of New Zealand's population will be over 65 years, compared with just 12 per cent in 2006. From the late 2040s, this age group will comprise more than 25 per cent of the population (Statistics New Zealand, 2009).

Over the next 50 years or so, the percentage of New Zealanders older than 65 years will approximately double. After this point, the transition from a young society with high mortality rates to an older population with low fertility rates and greater life expectancy will be complete, and a more stable demographic will have been reached (assuming projected fertility rates do not change).

This changing demographic has implications for the labour market that will begin to be felt from 2011, when the baby boomers (those born between 1946 and 1965) begin to turn 65. A shrinking workforce will need to support a larger, more dependent population. In 2000, there were 25 retirees for every 100 workers in Aotearoa New Zealand. If labour force participation rates of the older population stay constant, by 2050 there will be 70 retirees for every 100 workers. This creates a fear that a shrinking working-age population will be obliged to finance the pensions, health care and other services required by a rapidly increasing elderly population, which will lead to higher taxes on a workforce that is already over-burdened with high personal debt.

One approach to managing the impact of the ageing New Zealand population is to maximise the potential of older workers by extending their working lives. For older workers, employment is generally regarded as having positive effects on physical and mental health, as well as providing greater social connectedness and interaction (Ministry of Social Development, 2006), consistent with the perspective expressed in activity theory. According to Statistics New Zealand (2009), 17 per cent of people aged 65 years and over were in the labour force in 2006, up from less than 7 per cent in 1986. This is one of the highest rates of employment for older people in the OECD. Thus the increasing proportion of older adults comprising the population, the need to constrain government spending in support of the ageing population, and the need to retain a skilled workforce are changing the discourse around ageing. Consequently, previous social theories of ageing—that were driven by expansion of the industrial economy where young adults predominated—now need to be revised to accommodate changing Western economies, which are being driven by technological expansion and the need to retain a skilled workforce.

This does not negate some of the perspectives expressed in activity, disengagement or abandonment theories. Instead, it demonstrates how social theories of ageing are very context dependent. A satisfactory theory of ageing needs to take social context into account. A more recent perspective on ageing is to explore the synergies between the older adult and their interactions with their environment.

Socio-environmental theory

Socio-environmental theory An understanding of ageing based on the assumption that the environment of older adults is built on interrelationships between individual and social context.

Socio-environmental theory is predicated on the dynamic interaction between the individual's resources and social resources. The individual context refers to the person's health, financial, intellectual and social support resources, which influence the person's choices and impact on whether they socially withdraw or stay active. The social context refers to the social norms created around the ageing environment and the social resources made available to older adults in the way of housing and local support (Gubrium, 1972). The socio-environmental model states that the life satisfaction of older adults results from the interactions between the social environment available to the older adult and the personal resources of the older person. Furthermore, older adults follow a different ageing trajectory based on different degrees of resources available to them.

The socio-environmental perspective does not dismiss earlier social theories of ageing. Rather, it encompasses them, claiming that abandonment, activity and disengagement theories have both internal and external constructs that vary among individuals. For example, the internal components are a person's tendency to behave in a fixed way towards others and events in the environment. By contrast, the external components are the social expectations of the way older adults should behave. As long as the internal and external constructs are congruent, life satisfaction and high morale will be experienced by the older adult.

This framework proposes that older adults consider the expected social norms of their social situation and accept or reject them based on their personal resources (see Case study 9.3). The environment is defined in terms of physical space, psychological space and economic resources. Furthermore, actions to change social norms can be taken by individuals or by organisations (for example, Grey Power New Zealand, a lobby organisation that promotes the welfare and well-being of citizens aged over 50 years).

The dynamic interaction between individual resource and social environment implies that older adults are heterogeneous with respect to capabilities, resources and motivation. It further implies that ageing individuals can bring about social change by their actions. This reciprocity between individual and social resource sets up a feedback mechanism for the person that enables them to monitor their social effectiveness. For example, a person who experiences abandonment may work to change the social norms that enabled abandonment to occur.

CASE STUDY 9.3

Socio-environmental narrative

Mary is 64 years old and retired. She was a senior manager for a financial company. She is married and her husband continues to hold a senior management position. She has three adult children. Two are married and between them they have five children. The third and youngest is currently living in Italy. Mary and her husband met as students at university. They worked hard at their careers in business and built substantial wealth. Mary worked throughout her pregnancies and returned to work within months of each birth. Mary and her husband could afford to employ home help and childcare to help raise the children and run the home. Mary did not need to retire, but chose to when the firm was about to undergo restructuring. The firm was keen to retain her services, but Mary is interested in literature and theatre, and her career and family never allowed her time to pursue either of these interests satisfactorily. Mary's motivation to retire was to be able to read the books she never had time for, to go to theatre and not feel guilty because she should have been preparing for a meeting in the morning, and to spend time with her grandchildren as they grew up.

Because of Mary's employment history, there was an assumption that she would be bored 'hanging around the house'. It was assumed she would take up voluntary work in community-based activities. She would have plenty of time and she was well qualified to do this. Mary resisted this as it was not what she planned for her retirement. She was made to feel guilty for staying home and reading books when she could be helping in the community. She experienced incongruence between her personal resources and her social environment. This caused her a degree of dissatisfaction and some disengagement from her previous social circles. However, she was able to resolve the incongruence by spending time with her grandchildren and involving herself with their activities; for example, sports clubs and theatre groups. In this way, she was seen as meeting social norms and was able to fulfil her own needs.

The socio-environmental framework is designed to allow flexibility for variations in individual motivations, attitudes and activities among different contexts. An individual may be highly motivated to be active in one social context but not in another. In this model, a person in good health and with sufficient financial resources may still be dissatisfied with their environment; for example, if they are forced to retire from work they enjoy. The key to this model is the degree of congruence or incongruence between personal norms and resources and those of the wider society. The degree of life satisfaction and morale depends on the balance between context-dependent congruence and incongruence (Deci & Ryan, 1987).

Social theory, assumptions and communication

Over the past 200 years, a considerable amount has been written by younger people about older people that objectifies them, minimises their experience and dismisses them from the important issues, such as the ability to compete for rewarding and self-fulfilling employment and to make valuable contributions to society. Some of the above academic arguments have coloured society's attitudes about ageing, retirement and older individuals to the point of considerable society-wide environmental and institutional prejudice, aptly named '**ageism**'. Like institutional racism, those who are not affected by the results of prejudice do not recognise its pervasiveness, while those who are affected are keenly aware and may even adopt the beliefs of their oppressors.

Ageism
Discrimination on the basis of age.

The view that seniors have outlived their usefulness is in direct contrast to the view of the older person as gaining wisdom and possibly to achieving status as a community elder—a view held by many non-Western cultures, as well as our own pre-industrial society. While Erikson may have never defined wisdom, other theorists such as Maslow (1999) have expanded on his concept of generativity as a shift over time from more concrete subsistence-achievement goals to those that are more social or self-actualising.

Experience working with 'seniors' suggests that no one is more aware of these conflicting views than seniors themselves, and that empowerment is key to communicating with seniors. The goal of therapeutic communication is that of respect, empowerment and a 'personal acceptance that people are unique' and deserving of quality and thoughtful attention. Without preconceived ideas of what seniors are or should be like, communicating with them is often a very enlightening and entertaining experience.

The very first consideration when communicating with seniors is that not all individuals age at the same pace, nor do physical, social and psychological aspects deteriorate at the same time. More so than at any other age, it is important to discover and adjust communication and practice to the individual's capabilities, avoiding assumptions based on chronological age.

Communication and ageing

Physical domain

While there is great variation in how people age—based on genetics, environment and behaviour—eventually some deterioration of some senses will occur, while others may remain acute. There may be some physical hearing loss with age, but more frequently there is a deterioration of the ability to distinguish conversations from background noise. This can interfere with clear communication, particularly if the communicator has a soft, high voice, mumbles or gives directions in a noisy room. Consider speaking in a low clear tone, and not necessarily more loudly, and being sure that the receiver of the message can see the face of the person sending the message.

With exposure to the sun's UV rays, the lenses in the eye yellow and become less flexible over time. This can effect colour perception, depth accommodation and the ability to focus on small objects. Even with corrective lenses, this can inhibit reading small print or deter much-loved activities like handicrafts, repair or artwork—even driving for groceries or meeting with friends. When giving written instructions (including, for example, information on drug labels), consider whether the individual will be able to read them, or whether they would like to receive and retain the information in a different way.

Social domain

Everyone is a product of their environment, from their thoughts to the generational periods they have lived through. These events shape the way individuals perceive their world. While it is common today to have a fascination with the 'new', our seniors are often the experts in experiencing and adapting to change. What may seem new to the younger generation may appear to be an 'old concept in a new coat' to someone who has seen many changes. This can create false assumptions in both generations. To be able to communicate meaningfully, it is necessary to always assess and correct assumptions, and to appreciate how older people see their world.

There is some suggestion that as individuals mature, they may shift on an introversion–extroversion continuum of social expression (Myer-Briggs Foundation, n.d.), often moving to a more balanced position. Those that preferred solitary pursuits and achievements may become more social or family oriented, and those who have spent considerable time in the public arena may seek fulfilment of individualistic activities. It is more helpful to discover what retirees want for this and the next stage of life than it is to assume that they are naturally 'disengaged'. The socio-environmental framework can be helpful to remind us that behaviours and attitudes about how seniors should 'act' is strongly influenced by social, cultural, institutional and financial considerations.

Cognitive domain

Raymond Catell (University of Indiana, 2007) informs us about fluid and crystal intelligences. It has been suggested that older adults may have reduced **fluid intelligence**; that is, they are less able to store large amounts of novel information in short-term memory, such as swotting for an examination.

Fluid intelligence
The in-born ability of an individual to think and reason quickly and responsively.

Crystal intelligence The ability to think and reason based on experience acquired during life.

On the other hand, seniors have a larger capacity for practical, **crystal intelligence**, such as making complex financial predictions and decisions based on years of experience. This has considerable impact on understanding how adult learners learn, and this is even more the case with senior adult learners. Because seniors already have considerable understandings from life's experiences, what they often need is the appropriate connections between the new and the old information. A good communicator can discover what the senior already knows and together they can make the connections to new information.

Emotional domain

Once a person has reached 25 years of age, most adults agree that they do not 'feel' any differently as they age. Regardless of our chronological situation, we experience fear, self-doubt, companionship, romantic love, silliness, loneliness and excitement. Often the difference with maturity is in the appropriate control or expression of emotion—or the 'emotional intelligence' (Goleman, 1996). While emotional intelligence is frequently discussed as one of multiple intelligences (Gardner, 2004), it is also a skill in that it needs to be learned and practised. Thus there can be considerably variability, depending on the senior's skills. One individual may be what we might consider inappropriately expressive about their feelings or distress, while another may be stoic to the point of self-harm. It is important to discover and distinguish the internal feelings from the various expressions of feelings in order to support them emotionally.

Emotional support can take many forms of communication, including touch. With our society's glamorisation of physical youth and devaluation of ageing, isolated seniors often speak of not having been touched, cuddled or had their hand held for months at a time. We are already aware of the effect of babies in orphanages being 'untouched'; it is not surprising that adults need touch as well. The willingness to communicate respect, trust, admiration and friendship non-verbally through appropriate touch can often be just as healing as any medical procedure.

{ SUMMARY }

The notion that the onset of the 'senior years' occurs between the ages of 60 and 65 has its origins in the industrialisation of the Western world. Influential social theories proposed to account for ageing development include activity theory, disengagement theory, continuity theory and abandonment theory. Activity theory is the most popular perspective of successful ageing and is indicative of the current prevailing social view in Aotearoa New Zealand.

However, a demographic change towards an ageing population and economic considerations have caused a shift in the way older adults are perceived. This has given rise to a socio-environmental account of ageing that encompasses a dynamic relationship between individual and social contexts. The degree of congruence or incongruence between these two contexts contributes to the sense of life satisfaction and morale the older adult experiences, which can vary greatly.

When communicating with older people, it is important to show respect, to empower the individual, to acknowledge that people do not age at the same pace, and to take into account varied changes in the physical, social, cognitive and emotional domains.

REFLECTION POINTS

9.1 Intention (motivation, message, meaning, emotion)

Most of the theorists presented in this chapter suggest the elderly relate in particular ways more because of *interpersonal* and societal factors rather than because of *intrapersonal* or internal factors. Do you think that this is specific to this age group?

9.2 Reception (received message, response, feedback)

Reflecting on elderly adults that are known to you, in what ways might either disengagement or abandonment theory explain how this person relates to others?

9.3 Perception (style, manner, impression, analysis)

Assuming communication is a two-way interaction, can abandonment and disengagement occur concurrently? In what ways might you alter this dynamic?

QUESTIONS FOR REVIEW

1. How has Western industrialisation influenced thinking about older adults?
2. How does economic theory impact on attitudes towards older adults?
3. Which of activity, disengagement, abandonment and continuity theory is fundamentally different from the other three and how is it different?
4. What are the problems that socio-environmental perspectives of ageing were designed to overcome?

REFERENCES

Atchley, R. C. (1989). A continuity theory of normal aging. *The Gerontologist, 29*, 183–90.

Barron, M. I. (1961). *The aging American*. New York, NY: Cornell.

Baum, M. & Baum, R. C. (1980). *Growing old: A societal perspective*. Englewood Cliffs, NJ: Prentice-Hall.

Burgess, E. W. (1960). *Aging in western societies*. Chicago, IL: University of Chicago Press.

Cumming, E. & Henry, W. E. (1961). *Growing old: The process of disengagement*. New York, NY: Basic Books.

Deci, R. I. & Ryan, R. M. (1987). The support of autonomy and the control of behavior. *Journal of Personality and Social Psychology, 53*, 1024–37.

Erikson, E. H. (1980). *Identity and the life cycle*. New York, NY: Norton.

Gardner, H. (2004). *Frames of mind: The theory of multiple intelligences*. New York, NY: Basic Books.

Glanz, D. (1983). Higher education for retirees: The Israel experience. *Gerontology, 6*, 32–6.

Glanz, D. (1985). Aging and education in Israel. *Educational Gerontology, 8*, 101–5.

Goleman, D. (1996). *Emotional intelligence*. London: Bloomsbury.

Gubrium, J. F. (1972). Toward a socio-environmental perspective on aging. *The Gerontologist, 12*, 281–4.

Gubrium, J. F. (1973). *The myth of the golden years*. Springfield, IL: Thomas.

Havighurst, R. J., Munnichs, J. M. A., Neugarten, B. L. & Thomae, H. (1969). *Adjustment to retirement*. Assen, The Netherlands: Van Gorcum.

Havighurst, R. J., Neugarten, B. L. & Tobin, S. S. (1968). Disengagement and patterns of aging. In B. L. Neugarten (ed.), *Middle age and aging* (pp. 162–72). Chicago, IL: University of Chicago Press.

Lemon, B., Bengston, V. & Peterson, J. (1972). An exploration of the activity theory of aging: Activity types and life satisfaction among in-movers in a retirement community. *Journal of Gerontology, 27*, 511–23.

Lowenthal, M. F. (1968). Social isolation and mental illness in old age. In B. L. Neugarten (ed.), *Middle age and aging* (pp. 81–99). Chicago, IL: University of Chicago Press.

Maddox, G. L. (1968). Persistence of life-style among the elderly. *Middle age and aging* (pp. 181–3). Chicago, IL: University of Chicago Press.

Maddox, G. L. (1974). Aging and individual differences. A longitudinal analysis of social, psychological and physiological indicators. *Journal of Gerontology, 29*, 555–63.

Maslow, A. H. (1999). *Towards a psychology of being* (3rd edn). New York, NY: J. Wiley & Sons.

Mass, H. S. & Kuypers, J. A. (1974). *From thirty to seventy*. San Francisco, CA: Jossey-Bass.

Ministry of Social Development. (2006). *To work, or not to work? Findings from a survey of 65-year-old New Zealanders*. Wellington, NZ: Author.

Ministry of Social Development. (2009). *Maturity matters: New choices for older people. Findings from the focus groups and interviews of the Turning 65 Project*. Wellington, NZ: Author.

Myers-Briggs Foundation. (n.d.). *Type in personal growth*. Retrieved from www.myersbriggs.org/type-use-for-everyday-life/type-in-personal-growth.

Neugarten, B. L. (1971). Growing old along with me! The best is yet to be. *Psychology Today, 5*, 45–8.

Palmore, E. B. & Kivett, V. (1977). Change in life satisfaction. A longitudinal study of persons aged 46–70. *Journal of Gerontology, 32*, 311–16.

Prasad, S. B. (1964). The retirement postulate of the disengagement theory. *The Gerontologist, 4*, 20–3.

Ross, J. (1977). *Old people, new lives*. Chicago, IL: University of Chicago Press.

Ruffini, J. L. & Todd, H. F. (1979). A network model for leadership among the elderly. *The Gerontologist, 19*, 158–62.

Statistics New Zealand (2009). *The impact of structural population change* (Structural change and the 65+ population articles). Wellington, NZ: Author.

University of Indiana (2007). *Human intelligence: Biological profiles*. Raymond B. Catell. Retrieved from www.indiana.edu/~intell/rcattell.shtml.

WEBSITES

Ageing and Life Course, World Health Organization: www.who.int/ageing/en

Aotearoa Ageing 2005: A Bibliography of New Zealand Research on Ageing 2001–2005: www.retirement.org.nz/aotearoa-ageing-2005-a-bibliography-new-zealand-research-ageing-2001–2005

Grey Power New Zealand: www.greypower.co.nz

{10}

Dying, Grief and Bereavement

Terry Weblemoe

CHAPTER OVERVIEW

This chapter covers the following topics:

+ Cultural considerations
+ How practitioners respond.

KEY TERMS

Grief
Palliative
Hospice
Bereavement
Spiritual

A 'good death' has been defined as the freedom (of patients, families and caregivers) from avoidable distress and suffering that is reflective of clinical, cultural and ethical standards (Institute of Medicine, 1997). Central to the concept of a 'good death' is that a person is allowed to die with dignity, on their own terms, and in a relatively pain-free manner (Dyer, 2006). To die with dignity means that the patient has as much control over their situation and choices as is reasonably possible. It also means that procedures, equipment and situations that cause the individual to experience feelings of a loss of function, respect, dignity or mana are absent or minimised. Inherent in the philosophy is that the individual will have reached some kind of emotional resolution with **grief**, the dying process and end-of-life issues, including how they wish to be remembered.

Grief The journey of coming to terms with loss.

Palliative Relating to the alleviation of symptoms rather than the cause of them.

Hospice An approach to palliative and end-of-life care that emphasises holism and healing but does not focus on cure.

Canadian physician Balfour Mount is credited with coining the term '**palliative** care'. He based his pioneer Canadian **hospice** movement on the founding work of Cicely Saunders in England and Elisabeth Kübler-Ross in the USA. Cicely Saunders, who founded the modern British hospice movement, envisioned the hospice as a place of care where the communication between hospice workers and families involved respect and dignity, and where residents would be as free from pain as possible (Foster, 2007). Her work as both a nurse and physician at St Joseph's Hospital in London and her subsequent writings developed the fundamental concepts of 'death with dignity', a 'good death' and the idea of hospice as a place of rest and pain relief. In these specialised facilities, patients could receive physical, emotional and spiritual assistance with their end-of-life issues, surrounded by friends, family and health-care workers trained to take care of their special needs. While originally hospice was conceived as a community-based facility, palliative care is now an integral part of many Western societies. They have diversified to serve different needs and communities, such as in-home hospice services or specialised units within hospitals. Australasian paediatric examples include the Royal Children's Hospital in Melbourne and the New Zealand Starship Hospital (Hospice New Zealand, 2005).

In studying grief, Kübler-Ross (2009) proposed five distinct stages. These stages are not necessarily a simple progression from one stage to the next, but might also include both jumps across stages and recycling through stages. Of particular importance is that not everyone reaches a stage of acceptance, and some people doubt that ultimate acceptance is ever truly reached. The five Kübler-Ross stages are:

1 denial
2 anger
3 bargaining
4 depression
5 acceptance.

Bereavement The experience of losing a person who was emotionally close.

Bereavement can be defined as the experiencing the loss of a loved one through death (Berk, 2010, p. 659). That experience has both components of intense physical and psychological distress, which we call grief, as well as culturally accepted responses or specific expressions of that pain and loss, which we call mourning. While there are several other theorists who suggest different models of stages of grief and bereavement, the grieving process can be considered to have a number of tasks that need to be addressed or resolved. These tasks include:

1. accepting the reality of loss
2. working through the pain of grief
3. adjusting to life without that person
4. developing a sustaining internal link to the missing individual and rebuilding the mourner's life without them (Worden, 2002).

Cultural considerations

Many individuals—particularly older patients or those from some cultures who have avoided Western hospitals as 'houses of death' (Durie, 1994; Macdonald & Park, 2007)—may have considerable 'worries' about what will happen to them while in medical care. This is true of the South Pacific, which is becoming more multicultural, with patients and staff drawn from a wide range of cultural traditions with varying links to their heritage and beliefs. These contextual issues impact on communication at the most fundamental level. For example, older adults may feel intimidated by staff who are considerably younger than they expect, or they may be concerned about understanding or being understood by staff members with distinct language accents and different cultural backgrounds.

Aotearoa New Zealand is unique in that it has both government-funded Western medical health-care providers and Māori health-care (*Kaupapa Māori*) providers, who differ significantly in the cultural and social aspects of health-care provision. It is interesting to note that many Asian and new immigrant groups in Aotearoa New Zealand have found Māori health-care provision attractive and more suited to their needs. That said, one cannot stereotype about cultural needs, as individual and family preferences can demonstrate both considerable differences and eclectic mixes of cultural influence.

How practitioners respond

Many people are apprehensive about interacting with those facing death. They experience discomfort and anxiety, worrying that they have not received sufficient communication training (Peterson et al., 2010), and that discussing end-of-life issues, or poorly breaking bad news (Taft, 2009), will cause stress. Unfortunately, the silence and lack of adequate communication around these patients can create emotional and **spiritual** harm, and inhibit the patient from receiving adequate information and resolving grief (Kaakinen, 1992), especially in long-term-care facilities.

Spiritual Of belief and understanding beyond physical and cognitive experience.

Within many traditions, communicating with the dying is entrusted to the older, more socially or spiritually experienced members of the group, such as kuia/kaumatua (Māori elders) or counsellors and ministers. Practitioners working in health-care services who do not have this experience or expertise tend to focus on machinery and schedules, and distance themselves professionally and emotionally from communication and spiritual care (Hurtig & Stewin, 1990; Peterson et al., 2010). This avoidance is thought to be rooted in personal unresolved issues of mortality (Peterson et al., 2010). Patients have reported significant psychological and physical suffering resulting from 'stereotypical assumptions and behaviours' within health-care practitioners' interactions that do not recognise their individual situation (Janssen, 2010, p. 251).

New and even long-term professional health-care workers often feel anxiety about communicating with people who are dying and those around them. Research shows that not only do staff feel undertrained in sensitive communication, but also that inadequate communication in general is demonstrably the most common basis for customer complaints within the health-care industry (Health and Disability Commissioner, 2009; Healthcare Commission, 2007). Unfortunately, hard-and-fast rules or guidelines are not very useful in this area, where emotional distress can cloud effective communication for the health-care provider, the patient and their families (Rogers, Karlsen & Addington-Hall, 2000). Typically, personal grief or grief for a loved one is managed in the same way that a particular individual has coped with loss in the past. Their coping strategy is influenced by many different unique and cultural perceptions and learned behaviours. The keys to therapeutic communication for health-care professionals in these situations are:

1. having some resolution with one's own feelings about death and dying, and being comfortable around grief
2. having some skills in principles of 'active listening', 'presencing' or 'qualities of authentic being-with' the dying (Seno, 2010, p. 385)
3. having some familiarity with theories of age-related stages, cultural variations and empathetic abilities to be able to appreciate the world view of another person who may react cognitively and emotionally different from yourself.

CASE STUDY 10.1

'Being with'

During my first year as a nurse in a hospital's 'new graduate programme', I worked in the isolation wards. Working these wards meant that staff cared for the same patients for weeks or months, and often formed close relationships with individuals who would eventually die. In most cases the isolation is intended to keep immuno-compromised patients from contracting common bacteria, viruses and other illnesses from the patient's environment, including from contact with the health-care staff. Isolation meant that everyone had to wash, glove and gown-up to enter the room. This extra effort often meant that staff economised on their trips into a room, therefore patients could feel quite socially isolated.

One of my most poignant memories is of a very athletic, successful-looking American businessman who had been diagnosed with terminal pancreatic cancer. He was in his early forties and had a wife and two young children, about 4 and 6 years old. The patient's wife demanded that ward staff not tell her husband that he was dying. This posed an ethical dilemma for the ward staff because we were concerned about the healthy progress of grieving for this family if there was to be no communication about his prognosis.

Many staff members spent as little time as possible in the room with this man, because it was so awkward to care for him and not to discuss his illness or its outcome. When the family first came to visit, the senior nurses tried to take the wife aside and to convince her to let us communicate with her husband about dying. The wife responded to these attempts by becoming quite loud and hysterical. Her voice could be heard all over the ward, distressing others. She stopped bringing the children to visit, and her own visits became less frequent and more stilted. The whole ward was unhappy and distressed.

One day he turned from the window just as I was about to leave the room, looked me in the eyes and asked: 'Am I going to die?' Caught unprepared and forbidden to answer, all I could think to do was 'be with' him in the moment, and share with him how I sincerely felt. I turned back to face him and quietly tears streaked down my cheeks. I stood silently facing him, unashamed of my tears for as long as he held my gaze. As I watched, understanding solidified on his face. He turned back to the window, and then I left.

He became morose and uncooperative in general and specifically angry and sullen if I entered his room. In the following weeks, he alternated between lying unresponsively in a darkened room with occasional bursts of shouting and anger, including throwing a food tray against the wall. His wife was furious and demanded to discover who had told him and upset him so.

> About 10 days before this man died, he turned on the lights in his room, and I could hear him steadily talking to his wife as I worked the other side of the hallway. He spoke lowly and confidently, eventually comforting her as she wept. The next day she brought her two young children in to visit; they had not seen their father for quite a while. I could see, as I passed the room on my other duties, the children sitting on his bed one under each arm, as he soothingly spoke with all of them. After this, the whole family came to visit frequently, and stayed with him as he daily became more and more drowsy.
>
> I visited him again before he died, hoping that he had found his peace. Nothing was spoken out loud. He had always been a strong man and in control of his life, but he again looked me steadily in the face and then slowly smiled.

Individuals in highly emotional and dependent situations often become increasingly sensitive to non-verbal communication (Arnold & Boggs, 1989), particularly attitudes of the people to whom they are increasingly dependent upon. For this reason it is important that health-care professionals working in these areas not be emotionally distant, but be approachable and non-judgmental, have good knowledge of their subject and have good verbal skills (Bailey, 1998).

Active listening (see Chapters 21 and 26) and an emphasis on 'being with' patients and those close to them—rather than 'doing to' or focusing on being busy and occupied with physical tasks—forms the basis for effective and meaningful communication with people experiencing dying, grief and bereavement.

{ SUMMARY }

Communication with patients and families in end-of-life situations is critical and often the most therapeutic tool available to health-care professionals. Therapeutic communication can assist with both bereavement and the grieving process of dying patients, but it needs to be uniquely individualised. The appropriate starting point for such communication is always first gathering information through active listening, then providing appropriate information and a non-judgmental environment for patients to express their fears, wants and needs. Palliative care and hospice principles in recent years have helped 'humanise' the end-of-life within Western medical facilities by offering better pain and anxiety relief, more patient control and choices over the dying, and promoting a better understanding of the grieving process for both the patient and their families.

REFLECTION POINTS

10.1 Intention (motivation, message, meaning, emotion)

What was the intention of the nurse's tears? If 'being with' the patient in the moment produced tears for the nurse, do you think this was appropriate professional communication? Why or why not?

10.2 Reception (received message, response, feedback)

How did the patient respond to the non-verbal communication he was receiving, including avoidance and silence?

10.3 Perception (style, manner, impression, analysis)

Why do you think the patient had to be the initiator of the communication in his family's grieving process? What cultural or environmental factors may have influenced this?

QUESTIONS FOR REVIEW

1 Can you pick out the stages of loss and grieving for the patient, the wife and the nurse in this case study?
2 What would have been Erikson's age-stage related 'tasks' that needed to be resolved for each member of this family in this case study?
3 How might the wife and two young children have been affected had the family not discussed the father's dying?
4 What were some of the non-verbal emotional indicators and behaviours that communicated information in this case study?
5 What were the cultural and political factors that influenced the situation in this case study?
6 Can you think of a way the situation could have been handled differently?

REFERENCES

Arnold, E. & Boggs, K. (1989). *Interpersonal relationships: Professional communication skills for nurses* (2nd edn). Philadelphia, PA: W. B. Saunders Company.

Bailey, K. (1998). Communication issues. Patients' views on nurses' communication skills: A pilot study. *International Journal of Palliative Nursing, 4*(6), 300.

Berk, L. E. (2010). *Development through the lifespan* (international edn). Boston, MA: Pearson/Allyn & Bacon.

Durie, M. (1994). Māori perspectives on health and illness. In J. Spicer, A. Trlin & J. A. Walton (eds), *Social dimensions of health and disease: New Zealand perspectives* (pp. 194–203). Palmerston North, NZ: Dunmore Press Ltd.

Dyer, K. A. (2006). *Definition of a good death or an appropriate death*. Retrieved from http://dying.about.com/od/glossary/g/good_death.htm.

Foster, A. (2007). *Communicating at the end-of-life*. Mahwah, NJ: Lawrence Erlbaum.

Health and Disability Commissioner. (2009). *Other Reports*. Retrieved 14 February 2011 from www.hdc.org.nz.

Healthcare Commission. (2007). *Spotlight on complaints: A report on second-stage complaints about the NHS in England*. Retrieved from www.healthcarecommission.org.uk.

Hospice New Zealand. (2005). *Paediatric palliative care*. Retrieved 14 February 2011 from www.hospice.org.nz.

Hurtig, W. A. & Stewin, L. (1990). The effect of death education and experience on nursing students' attitudes towards death. *Journal of Advanced Nursing, 15*(1), 29–34.

Institute of Medicine. (1997). *Approaching death: Improving care at the end-of-life*. Washington, DC: National Academy Press.

Janssen, A. L. (2010). What can people approaching death teach us about how to care? *Patient Education and Counseling, 81*(2), 251–6.

Kaakinen, J. R. (1992). Living with silence. *The Gerontologist, 32*(2), 258.

Kübler-Ross, E. (2009). *On death and dying* (40th anniversary edn). New York, NY: Simon & Schuster.

Macdonald, J. & Park, J. (2007). The culture of health and illness. In D. Broom, B. Deed, K. Dew, M. Durie, J. Germov, A. Kirkman, J. Macdonald, P. Moon, J. Park, B. S. Turner & S. Walke (eds), *Health in the context of Aotearoa New Zealand* (pp. 155–67). Auckland, NZ: Oxford University Press.

Peterson, J., Johnson, G., Halvorsen, B., Apmann, L., Chang, P.-C., Kershek, S. et al. (2010). What is it so stressful about caring for a dying patient? A qualitative study of nurses' experiences. *International Journal of Palliative Nursing, 16*(4), 181–7.

Rogers, A., Karlsen, S. & Addington-Hall, J. (2000). 'All the services were excellent. It is when the human element comes in that things go wrong': Dissatisfaction with hospital care in the last year of life. *Journal of Advanced Nursing, 31*(4), 768–74.

Seno, V. L. (2010). Being-with dying: Authenticity in end-of-life encounters. *American Journal of Hospice, 27*(6), 377–86. DOI:10.1177/1049909109359628.

Taft, P. (2009). Breaking bad news. *Nursing Standard, 24*(10), 59.

Worden, J. W. (2002). *Grief counseling and grief therapy* (3rd edn). New York, NY: Springer.

WEBSITES

Hospice New Zealand: www.hospice.org.nz

Palliative Care in New Zealand: www.moh.govt.nz/palliativecare

Passing on: learning more about death and dying: www.tpk.govt.nz/en/in-print/kokiri/kokiri-20-2010/passing-on-learning-more-about-death-and-dying

{PART 2}

Communication and Human Engagement

Chapter 11 Communication and Survival ... 113

Chapter 12 Access and Communication ... 124

Chapter 13 Power Relations ... 140

Chapter 14 Culture ... 157

Chapter 15 Social and Interpersonal Dynamics ... 173

Chapter 16 Touch ... 187

Chapter 17 Media ... 197

Chapter 18 Types of Messages ... 212

Chapter 19 Language and Vocabulary ... 222

Chapter 20 Style and Manner ... 237

Chapter 21 Receiving the Message ... 247

Chapter 22 Written Communication ... 258

Chapter 23 The Electronic Message ... 269

Chapter 24 Creative Messages ... 283

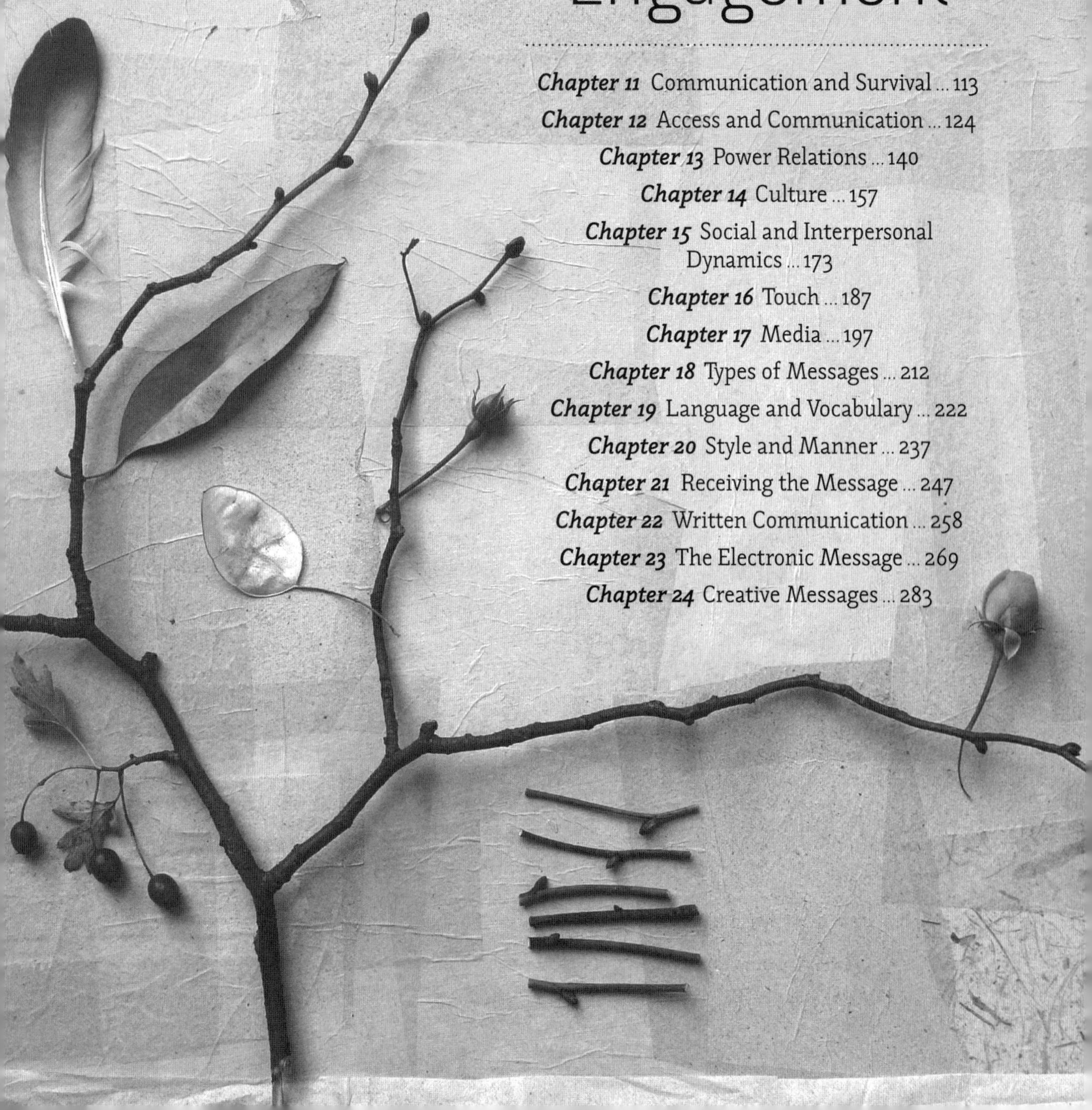

{11}

Communication and Survival

Chris Webb

CHAPTER OVERVIEW

This chapter covers the following topics:

+ Communication and survival
+ Situations of crisis and emergency
+ Truth and responsibility.

KEY TERMS

Base reactions
Social rules
Norms
Socialisation
Social networks
Body language
Congruence
Ethics

People react to many situations and their environment instinctively—such as sensing danger or experiencing severe pain, tiredness or hunger. These are known as **base reactions** or survival instincts. Often these reactions are learned reactions: a baby gets fed when they cry, therefore next time they are hungry they cry again. These become learned patterns of behaviour.

Base reaction The fundamental human drive to survive (survival instinct).

Social rules The accepted boundaries of behaviour within any particular group.

People learn **social rules** the same way. They learn to react with actions that are acceptable to the group of which they are a part. By reacting appropriately (for example, clapping when others clap or laughing when others laugh) individuals feel accepted by the group. Many animals live in social groups and learn how to behave within them. However, humans also have the ability to analyse their reactions and to learn to judge when or to what extent certain behaviour is acceptable or appropriate.

Learning these social expectations is complex compared with simply copying what others in the group are doing. As individuals, our communication is influenced by our attitudes, values and patterns of social behaviour. These are influenced by various sources such as home, school, social or peer groups. This is why families and schools are often blamed for their failure to socialise individuals who go on to transgress social **norms** or rules. Examples of these transgressions may include playing truant from school or having what people with different taste may consider inappropriate choices of music or clothes.

Norms That which is considered average or usual for a group of similar people.

Socialisation The process by which people learn to modify their behaviour to conform to the expectations of groups to which they belong.

Importantly, learning continues throughout life. The importance of the **socialisation** process is that it allows people to engage and interact with one another so that not only can they participate and function within their communities, but they can also ensure that these features will be carried on through subsequent generations. The way people participate and function within their communities are known as norms of behaviour. All communities have their own collection of shared norms, customs, values, traditions, social roles, symbols and languages.

With increasing globalisation and greater use of technology, communities are becoming more and more multicultural. This means that communities constantly face change as they accommodate new members with their own set of norms as well as developing social and cultural values of the wider society. People seek familiarity and interactions with activities and others that affirm their sense of self, identity, heritage and belonging. People are both individuals and members of numerous groups. Humanity can only survive if individuals survive. However, the individual needs the group to enhance their own odds of surviving—if people are accepted by the group then there is a far greater opportunity of them surviving. Thus survival is a tightly interwoven connection.

Communication and survival

The word 'survival' may conjure up visions of catastrophic events such as earthquakes, tsunamis, hurricanes, eruptions or avalanches. However, on a day-by-day basis the notion of survival may mean food and shelter or emotional fortitude to survive the pressures of life, depending on the context people find themselves in.

Communication is an essential component of human engagement and interaction. Through this process of engagement (understanding acceptable behaviours, social norms and the like) humans and their cultures survive. Because the way people communicate is very much influenced by the manner or culture in which they have been brought up, culture is highly relevant to communication. Communication is a complex effective survival tool, which is ever present in our lives. According to Beebe, Beebe and Ivy (2010), 'most people spend between 80 and 90 per cent of their waking hours communicating with others' (p. 24).

To engage with and communicate with others, and so heighten chances of survival, people create and maintain complex **social networks** or structures. These are made up of many cooperating and competing groups, from families to nations. Most people have a wide range of social networks, such as sports teams, study groups or housemates. Social networks change as people move between various roles and environments (such as the move from work or school to university) and these changes require adjustments to expectations, ways of interacting and shared goals and purposes.

Social networks Relationships between people as they interact within groups or organisations, which include virtual locations.

The ways people communicate with one another take many different forms and require frequent adaptations. In the course of a short period of time, people may find themselves chatting over coffee, texting and working out in the gym, all of which involve different communication styles and needs. In recent times, the possible ways of communicating have increased tremendously from face to face interaction and reading newspapers or magazines to engaging with the aid of technologies such as video conferencing, Skype, telephone, Facebook, Twitter, email and text messaging.

The emphasis on interpreting the meaning of an action means that at times people can wrongly interpret these actions; for example, mistaking a comment as a casual joke (and responding accordingly) when in fact the message was not casual and required a considered and formal response. Culture often determines how people interpret meaning. This leads to a very complicated social system, particularly as people become more aware and more sensitive to cultural differences. So it is that often the messages people receive are not necessarily the same as the messages sent.

This places real importance on effective communication. It also brings the realisation that the survival of organisations, relationships and people can be dependent on good communication, and negatively affected by ineffective interaction between people and groups. Human communication processes and systems are about engaging with others, and engagement is the connection that occurs between two or more people. However, people do not automatically engage with one another just because they have been told something or given a particular instruction. Effective communication occurs when someone is engaged with the person delivering the words or actions. People become engaged when they are involved. Face-to-face interaction is the most complete form of engagement because the receiver picks up messages from not only the words but also the tone of voice and **body language** of the person sending the message. Body language consists of facial expressions, gestures, body movements and stance, which all send signs and signals to the receiver. We never speak without sending out signals with our bodies. De Vito (2008) states that research has shown that we pick up over half of our messages from body language. This form of engagement, therefore, is possibly the most revealing because true feelings are likely to be communicated.

Body language
Communication conveyed through posture and other non-verbal expressions.

Situations of crisis and emergency

Every day there are situations of crisis and emergency that individuals, groups and whole communities face. A crisis is a crucial stage: a turning point that can lead to extreme trouble. While 'crisis' often refers to financial trouble within corporate organisations, it is also used synonymously with words like 'disaster' or 'emergency'. In situations of crisis and emergency, we find that the survival instinct is predominant. It is in times of crisis and emergency that humans, through their actions and behaviours, do all that they can to survive or assist others to survive.

The responses of people to emergency events provide examples where people have supported those affected by way of, for example, donations (through appeals), offers of volunteer labour (clearing away debris and rebuilding damaged houses), offers of temporary shelter and offers of replacement of lost items (donation of goods). Most human beings naturally want to help others to survive—it is a base reaction of how we interact with others in their time of need, believing that others value life and will do the same for us if we ever require assistance.

Immediately prior to or following a crisis or emergency, one or more people in authority communicate to try to restore calm and order so that widespread panic and confusion does not take over. Often the people in authority are those who are either appointed to such a position (for example, the chief executive officer of a company) or who have the power or expertise to act as an authority when an emergency occurs (for example, the ambulance service, fire service, police, civil defence emergency management and the defence forces). By communicating with the affected people, those controlling an emergency response try to ensure physical safety and well-being. Crises and emergencies require communication essentials in the form of warnings, risk messages, evacuation notices, messages of self-preservation and information on dealing with health issues, among many others. Different types of crisis and emergency require the communication of different messages. For example, communication issued prior to a hurricane may be different from those messages provided during a chemical spill or a flood. Further, the rise of bioterrorism (for example, anthrax scares) and large public health outbreaks (for example, SARS or avian flu H5N1) means the communication messages may need to be on a global scale.

In emergencies, authorities often rely on mass media and general public education campaigns to get the messages across not only to those affected by the emergency, but also to those not directly affected, who may be planning to travel to a region or who have family or friends living in the eye of the emergency. Recently, we have also seen examples where people have captured the immediate nature of the event and communicated it across the world via the internet well before the authorities have issued information. This puts a great deal of pressure on the authorities to communicate effectively in times of uncertainty. During these situations, messages must explain the nature of the event, identify possible consequences and provide specific information on how to reduce harm in a clear, honest, prompt and accurate way. These messages are more effective when they are matched to the audiences' needs, values, background, culture and experiences (Murray-Johnson et al., 2001). Whether emergency messages are conveyed in public buildings, public transport or newspapers, it is important that the format of these messages is consistent and clear. This means that people always see the same message and therefore their interpretation should be consistent. In times of crisis, people should know where to look for information and what actions to take.

In crisis and emergency situations, there are many ways that the messages between those affected and those in control are sent. Think of victims buried under a pile of rubble tapping to attract the attention of the rescuers, or flood victims writing 'save me' messages on the roof of their house.

Despite the best efforts of those authorities responsible for managing emergency and crisis events, many people ignore public warnings and other emergency messages. Warnings and emergency education campaigns are some of the ways that emergency agencies communicate with the public. People become engaged when they are involved—it is a two-way process of mutual understanding. However, people do not automatically engage just because they have been told something or given a particular instruction. When it becomes a one-way process of pushing information, it is no longer communication and, sadly, in situations like this severe damage and loss of life may occur.

CASE STUDY 11.1

Simeulue Island

On 26 December 2004, a magnitude 9.3 earthquake occurred in the Indian Ocean, close to Indonesia. This massive undersea earthquake created a tsunami that killed over 250,000 people in Indonesia, Sri Lanka, Thailand and India. However, on the island of Simeulue, the closest island to the earthquake's epicentre, only seven people from the island's population of 83,000 lost their lives. The reason for this minimal loss of life on Simeulue was communication. The people of this island were familiar with earthquakes and tsunamis, and they knew to leave the coast after the earthquake.

Reportedly a huge earthquake and tsunami hit Simeulue in 1907, killing many of its population. Many died when they rushed to the beach when they saw the sea going out and fish and coral exposed. Many went to collect the fish, not realising that the water would forcefully come back. Those who survived told the story of the 1907 tsunami to their children. It was largely because communication of this story, handed down verbally through the generations, that most of the island's inhabitants survived the 2004 tsunami.

The people of Simeulue say that because of this oral history they instinctively knew what to do when the 2004 earthquake and tsunami struck. Although village buildings were completely destroyed in parts of Simeulue when the 2m-high tsunami stuck, the loss of life was minimal (United Nations Information Management Service, 2005; McAdoo et al., 2006). Visit http://video.answers.com/how-the-simeulue-island-survived-a-tsunami-416308690 for a video link.

Truth and responsibility

Congruence When all messages that are conveyed (verbal, physical and emotional) agree.

Good communication engages people on an emotional level. The building of trust between those sending and receiving messages has the ability to turn negative emotions into positive ones. Trust is built when people can see **congruence** between the message, their experience and interpretation, and the person sending the message. Congruence occurs when what people are saying, thinking and feeling are all aligned. It is this consistency of behaviour that people pick up on and respond to. The effectiveness of good communication may be judged by the response of those receiving the message. If the response mirrors the message then it has been understood.

Much of the work needed to move from being a poor to an average to an excellent communicator is reliant on the individual conveying the message. The reality is that even the most proficient communicators have a bad day. When the beliefs, values and feelings line up with the message, then those receiving the message will sense congruence and trust the integrity of the sender; that is, body, mind, heart and words are aligned.

Credibility is evident when the people receiving the message perceive trustworthiness in the source of information. If the message is perceived by the listener or reader to be credible—in other words, if the deliverer of the message has taken responsibility to deliver the correct information—then the receiver of the information will engage with the information more readily and believe what is said or written. In this case, the engagement process has become more aligned or congruent.

Communication can be used to deliver positive or negative messages. A message that is clearly understood and achieves its intention—but happens to use false information, manipulates the message receiver or provides unfair choices—is not appropriate or ethical. According to Beebe et al. (2010), **ethics** are 'the beliefs, values and moral principles by which we determine what is right and wrong' (p. 8). Within all cultures, ethics and ethical behaviour have long been thought of as critical components of human behaviour. For centuries, philosophers have debated whether or not there is a universal moral or ethical code. Consider the religions of the world: they have a moral code that provides direction to their followers on how people should behave. Across most of the world's religions there is an underpinning ethic on how to treat others.

Ethics A system of values or principles, which outlines conduct.

However, philosophy and religion are not the only areas that have focused on ethical behaviour. Professions (such as medicine and law) all have codes of ethics that outline an ethical or moral framework for appropriate and inappropriate behaviour within that discipline. For most of the professions that have a code of ethics, key points include being sensitive to clients' or patients' needs, providing choices rather than forcing people to take a certain action, respecting clients' or patients' confidentiality, and being honest when presenting information.

The National Communication Association has developed a code for communication ethics that emphasises the importance of ethical communication:

> Ethical communication is fundamental to responsible thinking, decision making and the development of relationships and communities within and across contexts, cultures, channels and media. Moreover ethical communication enhances human worth and dignity by fostering truthfulness, fairness, responsibility, personal integrity and respect for self and others.
>
> *NCA Credo for Communication Ethics (1999, in Beebe et al., 2010, p. 9).*

Abiding with the truth is critical for ethical communication. If the sender knowingly withholds information, lies or distorts the truth then they are not communicating ethically or openly. Think of the 2010 BP oil spill in the Gulf of Mexico. What was the real situation and how was the information coming from the various stakeholders perceived? Who was delivering the truthful information?

CASE STUDY 11.2

Hindering message interpretation

A dietician is working with a morbidly obese patient explaining the need for a healthy diet and a regime of daily exercise. Consider the following scenarios and consider whether the obese patient, who may not want to be there in the first place, is likely to be engaged. What are the barriers that are preventing this engagement?

1 The dietician welcomes the patient into the clinic, but then proceeds to tell them that they are in a hurry as they have another appointment in a few minutes. Rather than find out about the patient from the patient himself or herself, the dietician says: 'I have read your notes and it appears that you need to lose 55 kilos. Take this pamphlet home and try what it says—it should work if you follow it closely. Come back to me in four weeks' time, but if you don't understand anything then ring my receptionist.'

2 The dietician welcomes the morbidly obese patient into the clinic and proceeds to provide facts and figures to the patient about the risks associated with obesity: World Health Organization figures on obesity and what this will mean for health services if this trend continues. The patient nods their head, but does not really understand what many of the words mean. The dietician then goes on to talk about the value of 'healthy' foods—which foods are better than others and why they are better. At the end of the appointment the dietician tells the patient that they need to be committed to losing weight and provides the patient with pamphlets about the facts and figures that were discussed during the appointment. The dietician's last words to the patient are: 'I look forward to working through this process with you, so please make another appointment for four weeks' time.'

3 The dietician welcomes the patient in to their office and immediately engages in a conversation with the patient about food in general—their likes and dislikes, how often they eat,

the type of job they are employed in and what they like to do in their spare time. The dialogue is continuing well and then the dietician tells the morbidly obese patient that although eating 'healthy' foods is important, they themselves eat fatty and processed foods, as they often do not have time to prepare meals. They will often get takeaways or snack on foods until they feel full. The conversation then turns to exercise and the importance of regular exercise. However, at this point the dietician is slouched in the chair and constantly looking at their watch. They excuse themselves to make a phone call and then admit that they do not have time to exercise regularly and that they would rather go and have a drink with friends than exercise: 'I'm lucky. I stay thin whatever I eat or do, so I don't need to exercise.' The dietician then asks the patient over the next two weeks to log the foods they eat and the times they are eating and to make a note of any exercise they do. The dietician says goodbye to the patient and suggests making an appointment in two weeks' time, adding that they really look forward to working with them to help resolve their obesity issues.

As you will have concluded, there are many barriers that are blocking the therapeutic relationship. These barriers include:

- providing information only and expecting the patient to be fully committed
- appearing to be enthusiastic about helping the patient, but then indicating that they are not committed themselves
- not using language that is understood by both parties
- not providing opportunity for questions from the patient
- not acknowledging that for the dietician this is the work they have been engaged in for years, while for the patient it is a new experience
- sending mixed messages: while the dietician may be enthusiastic their body language and tone of voice suggest otherwise.

The ways people communicate with one another are many and varied, and this requires constant interpretation and assimilation of meaning. The range of skills that are required to do this, and the speed with which they occur, can be a challenge in itself, especially for people unfamiliar with the culture or technologies involved.

{ SUMMARY }

Humans are naturally social beings and, as such, rely on social relationships for collective co-existence and help in times of duress. These social relationships include social rules that each of us learn so we can participate and function within our communities, as well as ensure that these features will be carried on through subsequent generations. Communication is an important part of this engagement and interaction process, and is a complex but effective survival tool. Effective communication requires a two-way process of mutual understanding. This process is enhanced when there is alignment between the message and the tone of voice and body language. This alignment and consistency of messages is critical in crisis and emergency situations. Communication that is clearly understood and does not provide false information or unfair choices is ethical communication. Ethical communication is often referred to within many professions as codes of ethics or codes of conduct.

REFLECTION POINTS

11.1 Intention (motivation, message, meaning, emotion)

What non-verbal behaviours will convey the message that you are interested in hearing what a person has to say?

11.2 Reception (received message, response, feedback)

Think about the statement: 'true communication is the response you get'. How do you know when a message has been received accurately?

11.3 Perception (style, manner, impression, analysis)

How is trustworthiness conveyed?

QUESTIONS FOR REVIEW

1 What are examples of the social rules that guide your communications with others?
2 How do these social rules change in regard to the age or gender of the person you are talking with?
3 How do emergency situations alter these social rules?

REFERENCES

Beebe, S. A., Beebe, S. J. & Ivy, D. K. (2010). *Communication: Principles for a lifetime* (4th edn). Boston, MA: Allyn & Bacon.

DeVito, J. A. (2008). *Essentials of human communication* (6th edn). Boston, MA: Allyn & Bacon.

McAdoo, B. G., Dengler, L., Prasetya., G. & Titov, V. (2006). Smong: How oral history saved thousands on Indonesia's Simeulue Island during the December 2004 and March 2005 tsunamis. *Earthquake Spectra, (22)*S3, 661–9.

Murray-Johnson, L., Witte, K., Liu, W. & Hubble, A. P. (2001). Addressing cultural orientations in fear appeals: Promoting AIDS-protection behaviours among Mexican immigrant and African American adolescents and American and Taiwanese college students. *Journal of Health Communication*, *6*, 335–58.

United Nations Information Management Service [UNIMS] (2005). *January10.SUM81012_Simeulue_Number_of_Deaths_Sub_district_HIC_2005-04-10_A4.pdf*. Retrieved from www.humanitarianinfo.org/sumatra.

WEBSITES

Emergency communication, Natural Hazards New Zealand: www.naturalhazards.co.nz/product.jsp?id=30

How the Simeulue Island survived a tsunami: http://video.answers.com/how-the-simeulue-island-survived-a-tsunami-416308690

Ministry of Civil Defence & Emergency Management: www.civildefence.govt.nz.Chris Webb

{12}

Access and Communication

Melissa Evans and Susan Shaw

CHAPTER OVERVIEW

This chapter covers the following topics:

+ Neurological impairment
+ Impact of neurological impairment on communication
+ Visual challenges
+ Impact of visual challenges on communication
+ Hearing impairments
+ Impact of hearing impairments on communication
+ Intellectual or learning disabilities.

KEY TERMS

Neuroplasticity
Aphasia
Apraxia of speech
Dysarthria
Cognitive communication disorders
Cataract
Uncorrected refractive error
Glaucoma
Macular degeneration
Conductive hearing loss
Sensorineural hearing loss

Disability is not attached to individual people. Individuals have impairments, while society constructs disability by making it difficult for people experiencing impairments to fully participate. Disability leads to discrimination, alienation and neglect, and as such has a lot in common with behaviours and attitudes associated with racism and sexism (New Zealand Disability Strategy, 2001). This chapter considers the needs of people with particular disabilities and the support that is available to assist with communication.

Neurological impairment

Interference with neurological function can occur for a number of reasons. For example, cerebral palsy, cerebral vascular accident (stroke) or a brain tumour can impact on both speech and understanding. Structures that may be affected include:

+ speech centres within the brain, as well as with the nerves that control parts of the body involved in speech, such as the lips and tongue
+ the motor planning part of the brain responsible for coordinating muscle contractions
+ the lungs that provide for air movement and therefore sound production
+ the use of the hand that enables us to hold a pen or use a keyboard.

While there is good evidence of how certain insults to the neurological system result in particular impairments, these should be considered within the context of emerging research about **neuroplasticity**, which explores the ability of the brain and nervous system to accommodate and adjust to change; for example, Doidge (2007).

Neuroplasticity
The ability of the nervous system to respond to insult or injury by building new pathways or connections (previously, it was believed that nerve tissue could not regenerate or modify its function).

Aphasia
Reduced ability to comprehend language or articulate ideas.

Apraxia of speech
Physical difficulty in speaking.

CASE STUDY 12.1

Neurological impairments

Aphasia is a language disorder that disrupts a person's ability to understand and use verbal, written or gesture symbols to produce verbal thought and/or communication. Aphasia can result in a reduced ability to speak and understand speech, read, write, use and understand gesture, and do arithmetic. The inability to understand speech, writing or gestures is termed Werniche's aphasia and the inability to express language via speech, writing or gesture is termed Broca's aphasia. Broca's aphasia has symbolic and motor aspects. The symbolic aspect relates to the ability to retrieve the correct word and place it in the correct order in a sentence. The motor aspect controls the actions for respiration, phonation articulation (voice), resonance and prosody (rhythm and melody of speech) (Tanner, 2009). Aphasia commonly occurs after a cerebral vascular accident or stroke to the left side of the brain.

Apraxia of speech occurs when there is damage to the motor planning area that is responsible for the sequence of actions that occur during a speech, writing or gesture. A person with speech apraxia may have difficulty speaking, have long pauses between words and will often use single words and incomplete sentences (Murdoch, 2010).

Dysarthria occurs when there is damage to the part of the brain that controls the muscle actions that produce speech. This includes any damage to nerve conduction for the lips, tongue, soft palate, pharynx, larynx and lungs. Impairments include loss of voluntary control of muscles, muscle weakness, difficulty controlling lips and swallowing problems. Generally, people with dysarthria have slow effortful speech that may be difficult to understand (Murdoch, 2010).

Cognitive communication disorders may occur when a person has had a traumatic brain injury. People with this condition are generally able to produce speech, but the content and structure of language may be affected by impaired memory and loss or reduction in abstract thinking, sequencing, monitoring self-performance and making appropriate social judgments. As a result, a person's speech may be disorganised, confused and disinhibited. Social behaviour rules of communication are disrupted and people may choose inappropriate topics, conversation may lose the art of turn taking, and the ability to express ideas fluently and concisely may be impaired (Murdoch, 2010).

How neurological speech and language impairments present is dependent on the exact location in the brain that is affected, as well as the extent of the injury (Tanner, 2009). As a result, a person may present with one or more speech and language impairments.

Dysarthria Difficulty with articulation of speech.

Cognitive communication disorders Impaired ability to transform thoughts into meaningful language or gestures.

Impact of neurological impairment on communication

When people lose the ability to express their needs and wants, and the ability to influence others, they also lose power. The self-concept of being an independent and competent person becomes compromised (Holland, 2006). A person's identity may develop negative characteristics; for example, from fluent to non-fluent or from independent to dependent (Shadden, 2005). Identity may be further eroded when communication attempts are met by rejection, ridicule, a lack of interest and miscommunication. These negative outcomes reduce the person's desire to communicate, and may isolate them from others. Reducing social interaction seems to have a further negative effect as remaining communication abilities deteriorate with disuse (Griffiths, 2009).

People with aphasia are restricted in many activities (Hilari, 2011). This lack of activity reduces the opportunity for conversation and the ability to take up meaningful roles. For example, people with post-stroke aphasia are reported as having less social contact with friends and attend fewer social activities than they did before the stroke (Brown et al., 2010). They are likely to rely on others for information support as they have limited ability to read and understand complex verbal information (Hilari & Northcott, 2006). Consequently, they may not make informed choices and others may take control over major decisions for them. Family members of the person with aphasia also experience stress. This may be a consequence of grieving the loss of a person's communication ability, and frustration from difficulties in communication. Family members are often seen as the person's translators and interpreters, and may feel incompetent as they struggle to assist the person to communicate in conversations with others (Shadden, 2005). A spouse may also become socially isolated as caring reduces their social contact and engagement in leisure activities (Michallet, Tetreault & Le Dorze, 2003).

Social isolation, loss of valued activities, and dependence on others may cause depression. One year after a stroke, the experiences of depression and emotional distress are higher in people with aphasia compared with people who do not experience aphasia (Kauhanen et al., 2000). Depression may also cause a change in the ability to process information, further compromising a person's ability to communicate.

Supporting people with neurological impairment to communicate

Given the severe social and quality of life concerns for people with speech impairment, support becomes hugely important and should acknowledge the competence and intelligence of the individual. Legg, Young and Bryer (2005) suggest maintaining conversations directly with the person (rather than with their caregiver), not avoiding complex topics and not 'talking down' to the person. Speaking louder is unhelpful and unnecessary. When communication breaks down, it is important to acknowledge confusion rather than pretending to understand. The problem in communications is a shared one: it does not reside with the person who has difficulty speaking. After two or three attempts at understanding, it may be helpful to try another way—using different words or visual cues—or to agree to come back to this part of the conversation again if it is not urgent. Increasing frustration tends to make speech impairments worse, so it is important to reduce any increasing distress.

Sustaining social communications fosters a sense of self-worth and identity (Shadden, 2005). Those involved with groups have been shown to have higher levels of social participation, less perceived social isolation and greater perceived social support, compared with those who did not attend groups (Vickers, 2010). The ability to have and do activities affects current and future quality of life (Cruice et al., 2010).

When a person has an acquired or congenital impairment that impacts on their ability to speak or write, communication may be enhanced with the use of technology. When a person has unclear speech, such a device may enhance, aid or supplement speech. An example of this type of equipment is a communication board made up of symbols representing topics or letters of the alphabet. There are various methods to select a word from a communication board, such as using a hand, foot, eye gaze or an aid such as a hand splint or electronic light pointer.

When the ability to produce speech is lost, a person can use a device that replaces speech. Some communication devices convert words or symbols into synthesised speech (Kangas & Lloyd, 2006). Technology can replace words or concepts with symbols, modify how the person selects the word and modify how the message is transmitted. When the person does not have sufficient motor ability to use these techniques, they can use a scanning technique. This strategy allows the person to scan a choice of words and then activate an electronic switch to select the word. Switches can be designed so that the smallest movements, such as wrinkling of an eyebrow, can activate the switch (Kangas & Lloyd, 2006). Following a full assessment, a device can be tailored to meet the individual's cognitive, sensory and motor abilities.

CASE STUDY 12.2

Support to talk

The TalkLink Trust is a nationwide organisation that assists people with disabilities to talk, write or control their environment using assistive devices and training. TalkLink provides an assessment of the person's communication and provides options for the person to trial. Once a communication method has been chosen, training is given to the person's communication partners; for example, health practitioners, family members, school teachers and caregivers.

Visual challenges

These include blindness and partial blindness. The most common vision impairments are cataract, uncorrected refractive error, glaucoma and age-related macular degeneration.

CASE STUDY 12.3

Examples of visual challenges

Cataracts occur when the lens of the eye becomes clouded, which prevents the light from being focused on the retina. A person with a cataract has difficulty seeing distinct shapes because the edges of objects blur with the background surroundings. The effect on vision is like 'looking at a mirror that has become fogged up with steam' (Global Blindness, 2008). A person's ability to perceive contrasts is further reduced if exposed to glare from direct or indirect light sources (Erber, 1996). This condition may be treated surgically by removing the lens and inserting a synthetic lens into the eye.

Uncorrected refractive error occurs when the lens of the eye loses the ability to change shape in order to focus light directly onto the retina, which results in reduced accuracy of vision. If the lens focuses light in front of the retina, it causes a loss of near vision (myopia or short-sightedness). Difficulty in seeing distant objects (hyperopia or long-sightedness) is caused by the lens focusing light behind the retina. With age, the lens begins to harden and is unable to change shape, which results in difficulty focusing on near objects (presbyopia).

Glaucoma occurs when there is damage to the optic nerve behind the eye. This damage may occur when the arteries in the eye become blocked, which prevents the fluid in the eye from draining correctly. The build-up of fluid damages the optic nerve and without treatment can cause permanent blindness in both eyes. There are two types of glaucoma: primary open angle glaucoma and acute angle closure glaucoma. Primary open angle glaucoma occurs gradually and results in a gradual loss of vision over time. The cause of this condition is uncertain, but known risk factors are family history, diabetes and damage to the eye. Acute angle closure glaucoma occurs quickly, can result in pain and sudden vision loss, and requires rapid medical attention. Early intervention can prevent further damage.

Macular degeneration is the primary cause of vision impairment in many countries. This occurs when cells in the macular area of the retina break down. Damage to these cells means that the retina is unable to transmit images between the retina and the brain. Macular degeneration results in blurred or absent central vision. People experiencing this degeneration may have difficulty reading, doing fine work, driving and seeing faces. Although the exact cause is unknown, the risk for macular degeneration increases if the following factors are present: being aged over 60 years, smoking, having a high fat diet, hypertension, family history, being female, exposure to the sun, and light skin and eye colour. Treatment consists of managing risk factors and adapting to the condition. For those with a particular type called wet AMD, treatment is available in the early stages of sight loss (Mitchell & Bradley, 2006).

Cataract Opaqueness of the eye causing impaired vision or blindness.

Uncorrected refractive error When the lens of the eye loses the ability to change shape in order to focus light directly onto the retina, which results in reduced accuracy of vision.

Glaucoma High pressure within the eye, which leads to damage and impaired vision.

Macular degeneration Progressive deterioration of the central visual field.

In the 2001 Household Disability Survey (Living with Disability in New Zealand, 2005), a visual impairment was defined as difficulty in seeing ordinary newspaper print or the face of someone across the room, even when wearing glasses or contact lenses. Using this definition, it found 2 per cent of all adults living in Aotearoa New Zealand households had such a disability. The highest rates for a visual impairment was in people 75 years and over, with one in every ten people in this age group experiencing some kind of vision limitation.

Impact of visual challenges on communication

Impaired vision limits the ability to perform daily activities, and reduces access to the environment and engagement in living and leisure activities (Laliberte-Rudman et al., 2010). In some cases, a lack of independence and increased personal safety risks may contribute to a person requiring care (Norwell & Hiles, 2005). Low vision may also limit an individual's access to social groups. The person may lose their ability to drive or feel unsafe when negotiating stairs and kerbs. They may not wish to engage socially due to the possible embarrassment of bumping into people or not recognising faces. Social opportunities may become reduced as the person may not have the necessary sight to gain pleasure from leisure activities (Laliberte-Rudman et al., 2010). Social situations may also be disrupted as the person with a visual impairment may not pick up on gestures, facial expressions and lip movements that contribute to our understanding of speech (Heine & Browning, 2004). People with visual impairments tend to reduce the number of hobbies they pursue, with reading, driving and crafts the most affected activities (Mitchell & Bradley, 2006). Visual impairment in people over 65 years has been identified as a consistent predictor of both the onset and persistence of depression (Chou, 2008; Hayman et al., 2007). In the elderly, vision impairment is associated with significantly reduced quality of life, reduced physical activity and social functioning, and poorer mental health (Fischer et al., 2009).

Supporting people with visual challenges to communicate

Low technology devices such as telescopic lenses may improve the ability to see distant objects, and magnifying lenses may assist with reading. Other low technology options include providing task lighting and light-absorbing lenses to regulate the amount of light transmitted to the eye. These lenses eliminate harmful sunrays, reduce glare, increase contrast and help with the transition between light and dark surroundings.

CASE STUDY 12.4

Electronic support for visual challenges

- Screen magnifiers enlarge a portion of the screen as the user moves the focus.
- Screen readers are software programs that present graphics and text as speech. A screen reader is used to verbalise, or 'speak', everything on the screen.
- Speech recognition (also called voice recognition) allows the person to convert speech to text without using a mouse or keyboard. Computerised speech synthesisers can 'speak out' the information on behalf of the person.
- Refreshable Braille displays convert the printed word or speech on the screen to tactile Braille display. Speech to Braille displays allow a person who is blind and deaf access to verbal communication in real time.

Talking books, magazines and newspapers enable access to print media. Communicating with others via the phone can be enhanced by having a phone with large print buttons and by using mobile phones that convert text to speech. Global positioning functions in mobile devices may also serve to improve orientation and mobility.

The Royal New Zealand Foundation for the Blind (RNZFB) serves people who are blind, partially blind and blind-deaf. To be eligible for RNZFB services, individuals must have severely limited vision.

Hearing impairments

A hearing impairment may be defined as having difficulty hearing a conversation with one person or when in a group of three people. Approximately 8 per cent of all adults living in households in Aotearoa New Zealand had some kind

Conductive hearing loss Hearing loss resulting from inability to conduct sound.

of hearing impairment. Hearing impairment is more common in people of 75 years of age and over, with 35 per cent of all males and 24 per cent of all females reporting a hearing impairment (Living with Disability in New Zealand, 2005).

CASE STUDY 12.5

Types of hearing impairments

Conductive hearing loss occurs when the structures of the outer and middle ear are damaged or blocked, causing poor transmission of sound waves to the inner ear. Conductive hearing loss results in reduced sensitivity to softer or weaker sounds (Martin & Noble, 2006). The outer ear includes the external ear canal and the tympanic membrane or ear drum. The middle ear consists of ossicles or small bones (commonly known as the hammer, anvil and stirrup), the middle ear space and the eustachian tube. Conductive hearing loss may occur when the external ear canal is blocked (for example, with hard wax) or when fluid builds up in the middle ear (for example, an ear infection—otitis media). Untreated infections may result in a perforated tympanic membrane, infection of nearby bone structures and a delay of language development in young children.

Sensorineural and auditory hearing loss occurs when there is damage to the hair cells in the inner ear or cochlear. As a result, the hair cells are unable to convert sound waves into nerve impulses that are recognised by the brain as sound. A specific cause of damage to this area is high levels of noise. People are at risk when they are exposed to noise; for example, from machinery, lawn mowers, loud music and stereo headphones (Martin & Noble, 2006). Auditory process hearing loss is due to damage to the auditory nerve and to the centres in the brain that process auditory information. These centres are responsible for our ability to localise and interpret sound. Sensorineural and auditory process hearing loss may result in a distortion of sound. People experiencing this may find it difficult to distinguish between sounds, recognise sound and hear sounds in a particular pitch. Consequently, a person may have difficulty understanding words and sentences (Erber, 1996).

Impact of hearing impairments on communication

Sensorineural hearing loss
Hearing loss resulting from damage to the inner ear or acoustic nerve.

A person with a hearing loss will find it more difficult to hear what is being said in noisy environments and when in a group conversation (Helvik, Jacobsen & Hallberg, 2006). A person with hearing loss may use lip reading, so understanding can be compromised if the conversation partner has their hands over their mouth or if they are not directly looking at the person while speaking.

Acquired hearing loss reduces a person's enjoyment in activities and pastimes. A person may not be able to hear television, films, music, theatre or natural sounds such as bird song, the wind and the sea. Hearing impairment significantly affects quality of life in the elderly (Fischer et al., 2009). A person may find they misunderstand words in a conversation; for example, hearing 'feel' rather than 'heel' and 'guess' rather than 'guest'. Such misunderstandings may lead the person to unintentionally change the topic, which can result in frustration for the communication partner. When people realise there has been a misunderstanding, attempts are made to 'repair' the conversation. This is desirable, but as a consequence the flow of conversation is disrupted (Erber, 1996). As conversation becomes more difficult, intimate or complex information may not be shared, conversation may be minimised to essential facts only, and people may pretend they understand the other person to avoid giving offence (Erber, 1996). In groups of elderly people with hearing difficulties, it was found women had greater psychological distress than men. However, being hearing impaired is less likely to result in psychological distress if a person is leading a life that meets their activity and participation needs (Helvik et al., 2006).

Supporting people with hearing impairments to communicate

New Zealand Sign Language is recognised as an official language and therefore has the same legal status as Māori and English. The Deaf Community has a strong cultural presence in Aotearoa New Zealand and while professionals may view deafness and hearing impairments as disabilities, this is not a perspective that is fully embraced within the Deaf Community. Hearing loss is an impairment, but the experience of being deaf or hearing impaired within society becomes disabling when institutions and decision-makers do not meet the needs of this group when planning and providing services.

The provision of captions for television programs is an example of an institution providing access to communication for deaf and hearing-impaired members of society. Television New Zealand (TVNZ) runs a 24-hour service, presenting news and information as text on screen.

CASE STUDY 12.6

Devices to enhance hearing

- Hearing loops are fitted into buildings. They work by converting sound waves from a microphone to an electrical current. The sound is then amplified and picked up by hearing aids. Loop systems take sound straight from the source and deliver it to the listener without background noise.
- Modified phones amplify sound transmitted via phone lines. To enable a person to hear the phone ring, the ring tone can be adjusted to a louder tone or changed to a different sound pitch that is easier to hear.
- Hearing aids are designed to amplify the sound frequencies the person has difficulty hearing (Holmes & Thomas, 2006).
- Cochlear implants are surgically implanted devices that provide hearing sensations for people with severe or profound hearing loss. Cochlear implants do not amplify sound but stimulate the auditory nerve with sound and speech information. The benefits of a cochlear implant vary from person to person. Some recipients may have improved awareness of sounds in the environment (such as being able to hear a knock on a door), some have improved lip reading ability and others have increased ability to understand speech. Cochlear implants are more likely to be successful if they implanted in early childhood and children are provided with ongoing rehabilitation from a hearing therapist (Holmes & Thomas, 2006).

Similarly, the New Zealand Relay service allows phone communication between people who are hearing impaired or deaf and those who are not. This service involves an operator being part of the call, who is able to convey either a typed message to speech or speech to a typed message. The typed message is displayed on a screen to the recipient.

CASE STUDY 12.7

Mr Portnuff

Colin Portnuff was a product development engineer who designed software and electronics. In 2004, he noticed that after physical exercise his speech became garbled and this became worse after long training runs. On visiting a neurologist he learnt that he had motor neurone disease (MND) or amyotrophic lateral sclerosis. This disease gradually causes loss of upper motor neurones, leading to progressive limb paralysis and swallowing difficulties. Patients with advanced MND may die as a result of respiratory failure. In some forms the disease causes cognitive deficits, but this was not a symptom in Mr Portnuff's case. In 2006, although not able to speak, he was able to give a 45-minute lecture to the Oregon Health Science University using a speech synthesiser. Using a laptop he was able to type his thoughts, which were then converted to spoken speech. This device enabled him to communicate with family and friends.

Although helpful, this device had several drawbacks. Mr Portnuff found people did not want to continue a phone conversation as they thought his 'voice' sounded like an automated marketing message. Delays in developing and conveying messages prevented him from engaging in group communication. In normal conversation we speak 150 words per minute, but Mr Portnuff could achieve only 30 words per minute. He wanted synthesised speech to be like his old voice and to have the ability to express emotion (changes in intonation). Most of all he wanted to be able to sing. Mr Portnuff's message to his listeners was communication devices need to be continually improved so that people can again find communication pleasurable and functional (Portnuff, 2006).

Intellectual or learning disabilities

A proportion of the population lives with disabilities that relate to the way they understand or process information (Ministry of Health, 2005). These challenges include developmental delays and are often referred to as intellectual or learning disabilities. There are many disorders or syndromes that are used to label specific intellectual disabilities, but the focus should be on providing support to enable people to participate in society. This field of disability support has changed dramatically in recent years, with the emphasis moving from sheltered support environments to assisting people to live and participate within the wider community. The phrase 'an ordinary life' (National Advisory Committee on Health and Disability, 2003) has been coined to explain the desire of people with intellectual disabilities to be part of the community rather than alienated from it.

Within Aotearoa New Zealand, the IHC is a national organisation that provides support and advocacy for people with intellectual disabilities. There are many smaller providers of services, and the Donald Beasley Institute in Dunedin supports research and development of services for people with intellectual disabilities and those around them.

CASE STUDY 12.8

Respecting support

One of the most contentious issues in the New Zealand disability support sector in recent years has been the payment for carers of people with intellectual disabilities to stay overnight in the community. There are a number of organisations that provide residential support for people with intellectual disabilities and the services often require that staff sleep overnight in community homes with residents. It is understood that the staff who are 'sleeping over' may need to be up during the night when residents need them. Whether or not staff should be paid for 'sleeping over' has been debated and it has been agreed that the staff should be paid for the hours they are at work. This has led to further discussions about the value society places on people with disabilities and those who support them.

Comprehension is difficult for people when communication includes technical or specialised language. It is made more difficult if the person has an intellectual or learning disability, which means that understanding requires special attention. Different ways of communicating need to be considered to support the understanding of people who do not easily comprehend detailed spoken or written information (Jahoda et al., 2009). It is equally important to consider that all people living with disabilities or impairments are individuals and that they need to be supported in ways that meet their unique needs.

{SUMMARY}

The ways in which we think about disability contribute to disabling conditions. In the past, professionals have tended to view disability as a personal problem to be 'fixed', but contemporary thinking is more socially inclusive, emphasising the reduction of social and environmental barriers to participation. Working alongside people with impairments requires emphasis on minimising the disabling effects of society. Neurological, visual and hearing impairments all have the potential to impact on communication, and there are various resources and tools to support people experiencing them to communicate and engage more fully with others.

REFLECTION POINTS

12.1 Intention (motivation, message, meaning, emotion)

How does working from a person-centred approach alter the way in which health practitioners work with people with disabilities?

12.2 Reception (received message, response, feedback)

How might you know if your communications are effective when working with people who have hearing or visual or neurological impairments? In what ways, if any, is this different from working with people without such impairments?

12.3 Perception (style, manner, impression, analysis)

'Disability is in society, not in me.' Do you think the society we are in is inclusive or disabling of people who relate differently?

QUESTIONS FOR REVIEW

Communication never involves only one person, so a problem with communication is necessarily a shared one. What strategies might you suggest for working with someone who has a:

+ problem in expressing themselves?
+ visual impairment?
+ hearing impairment?

REFERENCES

Brown, K., Worrall, L., Davidson, B. & Howe, T. (2010). Snapshots of success: An insider perspective on living successfully with aphasia. *Aphasiology, 24*(10), 1267–95.

Chou, K.-L. (2008). Combined effect of vision and hearing impairment on depression in older adults: Evidence from the English Longitudinal Study of Ageing. *Journal of Affective Disorders, 106*(1–2), 191–6. DOI: 10.1016/j.jad.2007.05.028.

Cruice, M., Hill, R., Worrall, L. & Hickson, L. (2010). Conceptualising quality of life for older people with aphasia. *Aphasiology, 24*(3), 327–47. DOI:10.1080/02687030802565849.

Doidge, N. (2007). *The brain that changes itself*. Melbourne, Vic: Scribe.

Erber, N. (1996). *Communication therapy* (2nd edn). Melbourne, Vic: Clavis Publishing.

Fischer, M. E., Cruickshanks, K. J., Klein, B. E. K., Klein, R., Schubert, C. R. & Wiley, T. L. (2009). Multiple sensory impairment and quality of life. *Ophthalmic Epidemiology, 16*(6), 346–53. DOI:10.3109/09286580903312236.

Global Blindness. (2008). Retrieved 25 February 2011 from http://webadmin.hollows.org/Assets/Files/Global Blindness[1].pdf.

Griffiths, C. (2009). The interface between communication and community living. In J. Goodman, J. Hurst & C. Locke (eds), *Occupational therapy for people with learning disabilities* (pp. 69–82). Edinburgh, UK: Churchill Livingstone Elsevier.

Hayman, K. J. M., Kerse, N. M. P. M., La Grow, S. J. E., Wouldes, T. P., Robertson, M. C. P. & Campbell, A. J. M. F. (2007). Depression in older people: Visual impairment and subjective ratings of health. *Optometry & Vision Science, 84*(11), 1024–30.

Heine, C. & Browning, C. J. (2004). The communication and psychosocial perceptions of older adults with sensory loss: A qualitative study. *Ageing and Society, 24*(1), 113–30.

Helvik, A.-S., Jacobsen, G. & Hallberg, L. (2006). Psychological well-being of adults with acquired hearing impairment. *Disability & Rehabilitation, 28*(9), 535–45.

Hilari, K. (2011). The impact of stroke: Are people with aphasia different to those without? *Disability and Rehabilitation, 33*(3), 211–18.

Hilari, K. & Northcott, S. (2006). Social support in people with chronic aphasia. *Aphasiology, 20*(1), 17–36.

Holland, L. (2006). Aphasia and related acquired language disorders. In N. Anderson & G. Shames (eds), *Human communication disorders* (7th edn) (pp. 409–35). Boston, MA: Pearson Education Ltd.

Holmes, A. & Thomas, C. (2006). Audiologic rehabilitation. In N. Anderson & G. Shames (eds), *Human communication disorders* (pp. 538–63). Boston, MA: Pearson Education Ltd.

Jahoda, A., Selkirk, M., Trower, P., Pert, C., Kroese, B. S., Dagnan, D. & Burford, B. (2009). The balance of power in therapeutic interactions with individuals who have intellectual disabilities. *British Journal of Clinical Psychology, 48*, 63–77.

Kangas, K. & Lloyd, L. (2006). Augmentative and alternative communication. In N. Anderson & G. Shames (eds), *Human communication disorders* (pp. 436–70). Boston, MA: Pearson Education Ltd.

Kauhanen, M., Korpelainen, J., Hiltunen, P., Maata, R., Mononen, H., Brusin, E. & Myllyla, V. (2000). Aphasia, depression, and non-verbal cognitive impairment in ischaemic stroke. *Cerebrovascular Diseases, 10*(6), 455–61. DOI:1015-9770/000/010-0455.

Laliberte-Rudman, D., Huot, S., Klinger, L., Leipert, B. D. & Spafford, M. M. (2010). Struggling to maintain occupation while dealing with risk: The experiences of older adults with low vision. *Occupation, Participation and Health, 30*(2), 87–96. DOI:10.3928/15394492-20100325-04.

Legg, C., Young, L. & Bryer, A. (2005). Training sixth-year medical students in obtaining case history information from adults with aphasia. *Aphasiology, 19*(6), 559–75.

Living with disability in New Zealand (2005). Retrieved 25 February 2011 from www.moh.govt.nz/moh.nsf/0/3679738AF457C693CC25701900788E31/$File/livingiwthdisability-summary.pdf.

Martin, F. & Noble, B. (2006). Hearing and hearing disorders. In N. Anderson & G. Shames (eds), *Human communication disorders* (7th edn) (pp. 504–37). Boston, MA: Pearson Education Inc.

Michallet, B., Tetreault, S. & Le Dorze, G. (2003). The consequences of severe aphasia on the spouses of aphasic people: A description of the adaptation process. *Aphasiology, 17*(9), 835. DOI:10.1080/02687030344000238.

Ministry of Health (2005). *Living with intellectual disability in New Zealand: Key results on intellectual disability from the 2001 household disability survey and the 2001 disability survey of residential facilities*. Wellington, NZ: Ministry of Health.

Mitchell, J. & Bradley, C. (2006). Quality of life in age-related macular degeneration: A review of the literature. *Health and Quality of Life Outcomes, 4*(1), 97.

Murdoch, B. (2010). *Acquired speech and language disorders* (2nd edn). Chichester, UK: John Wiley & Sons Ltd.

National Advisory Committee on Health and Disability (2003). *To have an ordinary life*. Wellington, NZ: National Advisory Committee on Health and Disability.

New Zealand Disability Strategy. (2001). *Making a world of difference: Whakanui oranga*. Wellington, NZ: Ministry of Health. www.odi.govt.nz/resources/publications/nzds/index.html.

Norwell, C. & Hiles, C. (eds). (2005). Why every hospital should have an eye clinic liaison officer. *International Congress Series, 1282*, 226–9.

Portnuff, C. (2006). *AAC—a user's perspective*. Retrieved 5 March 2011 from http://aac-rerc.psu.edu/index.php/webcasts/show/id/3.

Shadden, B. B. (2005). Aphasia as identity theft: Theory and practice. *Aphasiology, 19*(3–5), 211–23.

Tanner, D. (2009). *The psychology of neurogenic communication disorders*. New York, NY: iUniverse.

Vickers, C. P. (2010). Social networks after the onset of aphasia: The impact of aphasia group attendance. *Aphasiology, 24*(6–8), 902–13.

WEBSITES

Aphasia Association of New Zealand: www.aphasia.org.nz
Aphasia Institute, Canada: www.aphasia.ca
Connect UK: www.ukconnect.org
Donald Beasley Institute: www.donaldbeasley.org.nz
IHC New Zealand: www.ihc.org.nz
New Zealand Speech-Language Therapists' Association: www.speechtherapy.org.nz
TalkLink Trust: www.talklink.org.nz

{13}

Power Relations

Ruth DeSouza

CHAPTER OVERVIEW

This chapter covers the following topics:

+ Oppression
+ Power
+ Critical social theory
+ Organisational and management theories
+ Social psychological theories
+ Post-structural theories
+ Empowerment.

KEY TERMS

Power
'The state'
Surveillance
Oppression
Critique
Foucauldian
Consumerism

Many practitioners see themselves as apolitical and powerless, particularly with regard to their relationships with the structures of medicine and management. However, in reality practitioners are powerful both as individuals and as members of the groups with which they identify. The structures and cultures within which most health and disability practitioners exist and work are based on beliefs and practices that constrain autonomy. These constraints are at work through a number of mechanisms, such as the market, the infusion of targets and performance measures and quality programmes (Newman & Vidler, 2006). In addition, the changing role of consumers or service users from passive recipients of care in the past to people who may be informed, empowered, articulate and 'demanding' poses a threat to the 'knowledge–power knot' on which professional power rests.

When practitioners view themselves as people who are doing good, they tend to lack awareness of their complicity and embeddedness in relations of **power** that structure inequality. Yet, power is embedded in everyday practices and interactions (Bradbury Jones, Sambrook & Irvine, 2008). Practitioners within the wider health and disability support sector contribute to social regulation through their roles as employees of **the state**. They enact government policies for the benefit of the health of the citizens of the state; so they are both governed and governing. Members of recognised professional groups are provided with a moral authority by their capacity to define problems and pose solutions, and their role in defining and evaluating good or normal behaviour and health practices through **surveillance** of the population and the criteria for interventions on behalf of the state (Gilbert, 2001, p. 201).

Power The exercise of strength or control.

'The state' The politically organised leadership (or government) of groups of people or populations.

Surveillance The act of keeping watch over people and their actions.

These ambivalent relationships with power that are evident among health practitioners require exploration. This can be done by considering the various ways in which power is conceptualised and the micro and macro definitions of empowerment. Some shifts in power have occurred in the last few decades, largely influenced by various social movements. Maternity and mental health are two particular examples of professional practice and service delivery in which power can be recognised and ideas of empowerment can be translated into meaningful engagement between service delivery and those who engage with the service.

Oppression

It can be difficult to understand, but in the process of doing good, people can contribute to **oppression**. For example, medicine has historically dominated health care, but in recent times it has come to be thought about and understood in terms of power and relationships between institutions (and the practitioners

Oppression The unfair or unjust exercising of power over others.

Critique Critical comment, appraisal or evaluation.

within them) and those who seek care and support (Broom, Nicholls & Deed, 2010). This **critique** of power has significantly eroded the traditional position and role of medicine within our society. This desire to rebalance power has challenged assumptions within the professions in relation to personal and professional culture.

For example, there is an assumption that being a member of a group that provides health care and disability support services automatically means individuals are neutral and egalitarian. However, such assumptions have been challenged and the oppressive capacity of these services, systems, institutions and groups has been exposed.

Foucauldian In the spirit of French philosopher Michel Foucault and therefore with an interest in critique of institutions and power.

Young (1990) conceptualises oppression in the **Foucauldian** sense as 'the disadvantage and injustice some people suffer not because a tyrannical power coerces them but because of the everyday practices of a well-intentioned liberal society' (Henderson & Waterstone, 2008). The suggestion is that the actions of many people who are going about their lives contribute to the maintenance and reproduction of oppression, but few of those people (such as health practitioners) would see themselves as agents of oppression (Young, 1990). Oppression, therefore, goes beyond a few people's choices or policies. Its causes are embedded in unquestioned norms, habits and symbols, in the assumptions underlying institutional rules and the collective consequences of following those rules (Young, 1990). It is structural and woven throughout the system. Seeing oppression as the practices of a well-intentioned group removes the focus from individual acts that might repress the actions of others. Instead the focus is on acknowledging that 'powerful norms and hierarchies of both privilege and injustice are built into our everyday practices', which call for structural rather than individual remedies (Young, 1990).

Power

Many practitioners hold empowerment as a central concept to their work with clients, patients and consumers/tangata whai ora. However, in order to empower others, it is important to know what power is. The concept of power has three central themes:

1. Ability—the ability to do something or act in a particular way: capacity, capability, potential, faculty and competence.
2. Control—having the capacity or ability to direct or influence the behaviour of others or the course of events: authority, influence, dominance, mastery, domination, dominion, sway, weight, leverage, clout and teeth.
3. Strength—the physical strength and force exerted by something or someone: powerfulness, might, force, forcefulness, vigour, energy, brawn, muscle, informal punch.

It could be argued that practitioners have all these attributes and are enabled and constrained in their roles and behaviour by the institutions they work for. Practitioners are in positions of political or social authority or control, and have delegated authority (Gilbert, 2001). However, there are different ways of understanding power. Four main theories of power are explored here:

+ critical social theory
+ organisational and management theories
+ social psychological theories
+ post-structural theories.

Critical social theory

Within a critical social theory or liberational framework, power is viewed as a possession and hierarchies are central to the imbalance of power. The group with control has more power and status than other groups in society, which are in a subordinated position. Critical theory is concerned with helping disenfranchised groups in society to overcome this domination. Power is obtained through the surrender of another's power, and empowerment is equated with liberation. In order for this transfer of power to happen, a struggle must occur as powerful people will not readily transfer resources, information or responsibility (Bradbury Jones, Sambrook & Irvine, 2008). Empowerment is collective and is about increasing the power and influence of oppressed groups (Kuokkanen & Leino Kilpi, 2000). However, power is not always repressive and this is a limitation of critical social theory.

Organisational and management theories

Where critical social theory is concerned with oppressed groups, organisational and management theories are concerned with how power is distributed in organisations. Hierarchies also come into play, especially the idea of top-down power (Bradbury Jones, Sambrook & Irvine, 2008). Within this framework, there is an acknowledgement of structural factors and their capacity to empower and disempower, rather than focusing on the individual. According to Kanter (1993), four conditions are necessary for empowerment to occur within organisations, with the degree of empowerment related to how many of the four conditions are present: opportunity for advancement, access to information, access to support and access to resources. Power is then framed as the ability to get things done, and being empowered is having the opportunity to do things. However, the problem with this model and with critical social theory is that power is not only distributed in a top-down manner: it also operates from bottom to top and laterally (Foucault, 1977).

Social psychological theories

Social psychological theories contrast with organisational models of power in that they focus on the psychology or the point of view of the individual, rather than environmental factors. Power is framed as a personal attribute that can be nurtured, and personal growth leads to personal power and therefore empowerment (Bradbury Jones, Sambrook & Irvine, 2008; Masterson & Owen, 2006). However, it does not necessarily follow that individuals are empowered or able to assert their power in any given situation. It may be argued that individualistic empowerment deflects attention from socio-structural disempowerment, as well as social, cultural and structural factors that disempower (Masterson & Owen, 2006). Morrall (1996) challenges individual empowerment, saying that empowering the individual is like treating the symptoms of disempowerment rather than the cause. Other concerns are that an increase in self-confidence might result in an altered perception of power. This would then allow an individual to act or exert influence while power imbalances remain because there has not been an actual transfer of power.

Post-structuralist theories

A post-structural appreciation of power conceptualises it not as a thing (something that is possessed by individuals or organisations) but as a relation: something that is exercised (Foucault, 1977). Consequently, post-structuralism challenges the view that power can be relinquished in order to empower someone else (Bradbury Jones, Sambrook & Irvine, 2008). Michel Foucault (1926–1984) is a key theorist within post-structuralism. Foucault conceptualised power in a number of key ways that differ from the previous three theories: power is always shifting and moving; power is ubiquitous and omnipresent, coming from everywhere and moving in multiple directions and permeating like capillaries into every space and interaction; and power is productive. Within this framework, power is not a logical causal relationship where someone can take over or give up power. Power in this paradigm is about having an influence over thoughts, attitudes and social relationships (Kuokkanen & Leino Kilpi, 2000) and practitioners can be viewed as powerless in some circumstances, and powerful in others (Bradbury Jones, Sambrook & Irvine, 2008).

Empowerment

Empowerment is a central concept in recent approaches to health and health promotion, and acknowledges the importance of people having control or being able to participate in their own life and environment. Notions of 'patient empowerment' and participation in care can be identified throughout recent health-care policy and practice information and documents. Empowerment is almost universally viewed as a good thing. However, empowerment can be misapplied in such a way that a transfer of tasks away from formal care occurs without people and their families being resourced and supported. The risk is that traditional service providers and organisations can absolve themselves of the responsibility for supporting the health and well-being of the population by arguing that people should be taking care of themselves—without transferring the resources to the community for such support. The idea of empowerment can be operationalised in diverse ways in practice and differentially received by clients and families. There might be negative consequences for clients who do not value 'empowerment' as much as they trust professionals. For example, when someone does not want active involvement in certain decisions or tasks, promoting involvement can contribute to negative experiences, dissatisfaction, anxiety, fear and guilt.

CASE STUDY 13.1

Empowerment and recovery

Many people who have experiences of mental illness have been marginalised, experiencing social exclusion and the loss of their dignity, freedom, autonomy and rights. Collective action for empowerment by service users has produced many organisations in Aotearoa New Zealand, including Psychiatric Survivors and Mind and Body. These groups have been at the forefront of de-stigmatisation efforts, contesting negative perceptions of mental illness and exploring new ways of talking about mental health and illness (Masterson & Owen, 2006), particularly recovery. As a result of these efforts, the centrality of service users to New Zealand mental health services has been solidified through both legal and contractual frameworks and culture change, with service users employed within mental health services and playing a part operationally, strategically and nationally.

There is a growing expectation for service-user involvement at all levels of social service delivery, in part due to social and policy changes such as de-institutionalisation and community care.

These have led to a resistance to the supremacy of what has been considered the historically paternalist 'professional knows best' approach, a valuing of people's personal experiences of mental illness, and a growing ownership and pride among consumers. In New Zealand services, consumer participation has had impacts for consumers, health-care professionals and policymakers. Consumers are required to be involved in the planning, implementation and evaluation of service delivery at every level of mental health service provision. Transparent and clear processes that show this in service design and delivery are contractual requirements (Ministry of Health, 1995; Phillips, 2006).

Perhaps the most powerful impact has been on critiquing the normalising judgments of medico-psychiatric discourses that are also widespread in society, where labels of deviance such as 'psychiatric patient', 'schizophrenic' and 'mentally ill' have been accompanied by stigma and caused social exclusion and disadvantage (Masterson & Owen, 2006). The power of medico-psychiatric discourses has placed service users in a sick role, where they have been dependent on the knowledge and resources of professionals. Instead, advocacy, recognition of lay knowledge and personal experience of mental illness have resulted in the creation of alternative discourses, such as the recovery model, which have helped to reduce stigma and the power of health practitioners (Masterson & Owen, 2006).

The recovery model reconceptualises what has been typically called mental illness (Masterson & Owen, 2006), framing it as a natural phenomenon occurring along a spectrum of human experience, rather than long-term dysfunction. Prominent advocates of the recovery model include Deegan (1998), Copeland (1997), Jacobson and Curtis (2000) in the USA, and Campbell (1997), Barker and Buchanan-Barker (2005), and Repper and Perkins (2003) in the UK. In Aotearoa New Zealand, O'Hagan (2001) has developed recovery competencies for mental health workers.

The recovery model provides not only an alternative model but also a critique of professional dominance as seen in mental health policies and practices. Consumers charge that medico-psychiatric discourses obliterate hope, disempowering, stigmatising and removing choice from service users. By contrast, recovery advocates assert that regardless of claims about illness, chronicity and progress that are offered in medico-psychiatric discourses, all service users can achieve recovery. However, it is the individual—rather than services or practitioners—who drives the recovery process and what recovery means to them. Therefore, the recovery project provides a mechanism for empowered action and legitimates the rights of service users, supporting autonomy and self-direction as well the creation of user-run services and reformation of existing mainstream mental health services (Masterson & Owen, 2006). While societal and service 'buy in' is critical (without appropriation and professionalisation), this is not without its challenges. Embracing a recovery perspective requires challenging and transforming some taken-for-granted practices and developing new kinds of relationships with service users. Strategies might include redistributing power in tangible ways (for example, contractually); making professionals dependent on service users for training, education or performance assessment; and renegotiating the professional functions of therapy and carers.

Models and discourses of empowerment

Individual level or micro-level strategies of empowerment include the psychological model and the consumerist model. The psychological model involves developing power from within, by avoiding 'power-over'. Information giving is highly regarded as an essential step towards genuine empowerment (Masterson & Owen, 2006). It is thought that collaborative partnerships between practitioners and service users—founded upon relationships of trust, support, equality, respect, genuineness, empathy and positive regard—facilitate this. However, consumers/clients can be reluctant to challenge decisions made about their care for fear of consequences such as being labelled and experiencing the withdrawal of care or the imposition of punitive care (Masterson & Owen, 2006). Despite the presence of codes of patient rights within nations or organisations, users might be unable to exert them. Professionals might appear to facilitate service user decision-making, but still exert control over their decisions where power might be exercised in terms of limiting the range of decisions and maintaining 'expert' authority.

By contrast, **consumerism** involves delegating or sharing formal power through structural change and where there is a transfer of top-down power within services (Masterson & Owen, 2006). Increasingly in fields such as mental health, policy directives have centralised the role of the consumer and their whānau in terms of being able to shape, participate and evaluate health services. In Aotearoa New Zealand, service users have been taught leadership skills to facilitate their ability to assert themselves in organisations. However, while consumerism can mean service-user participation in decision-making (ostensibly giving them influence

Consumerism
Viewing human interaction with an emphasis on access to goods and services.

and allowing professionals and managers to appear empowering), power is still being retained by professionals and managers who set the terms of engagement, incorporating consumerist ideals into existing power structures without changing them (Masterson & Owen, 2006).

A social or macro perspective of empowerment assumes that large-scale action, to meet people's common needs, changes the social and material circumstances of society. There are two general approaches: socio-structural change and grassroots communal action. Socio-structural change encompasses such strategies as creating equal opportunities through structural change and through legislation, policy, financial and organisational means to ensure the social inclusion of all—regardless of ability, age, gender, race, income, social class, sexual orientation or any other form of difference. Power is evident through the unequal distribution of resources between those who are poor and socially excluded and those who are not. By devolving responsibility to patients and their families, the concept of empowerment achieves the goals of improving perceived control and self-efficacy—which are thought to enhance well-being—while fitting in with neo-liberal political and economic imperatives of efficiency and cost (Funk, Stajduhar & Purkis, 2011).

Consumer involvement in health-care decision-making, planning and policy making (as individual consumers, potential service users, citizens and organised groups) is a feature of the contemporary health-care scene (Coney, 2004). The growing centrality of the consumer is part of many efforts to change health systems so that they are more responsive. However, the advent of 'consumerism' has posed a set of challenges to professional, occupational and organisational power (Newman & Vidler, 2006), not least by threatening the hegemony of the medical model of health, whereby the replacement of the machine model of the body with more holistic models has required more personally tailored responses. This holism has been accompanied by challenges to professional judgment in favour of consumer 'choice' (Newman & Vidler, 2006). Critics of the term argue that 'choice' is inappropriate if a person is an unwilling or involuntary user, or if alternative services are scarce (Newman & Vidler, 2006).

CASE STUDY 13.2

Consumers and birth

The New Zealand midwifery profession has struggled for autonomy in the face of threats from medicine, hospitals and nursing (Stojanovic, 2008). It has shaped itself into an autonomous feminist profession founded on partnership with women (Surtees, 2003), creating a point of difference emphasising 'normal' and 'natural' births and the capability of women to 'naturally' carry and deliver a baby without the surveillance and interventions of physicians in a hospital setting (Macdonald, 2006). Mutually beneficial political lobbying by consumers and midwives in the late 1980s saw legislative changes occur that led to autonomous midwifery practice. Midwives wanted to differentiate their scope of practice from nurses and regain independent practice and autonomy, while maternity consumer activists viewed autonomous midwifery practice as a mechanism for gaining increased control over their own birthing (Pairman, 2006). The subsequent passing of the Nurses Amendment Act in 1990 heralded an era of choice in maternity care for Aotearoa New Zealand, allowing women to choose a caregiver (Lead Maternity Carer or LMC) who would either coordinate or personally provide the care they required from early pregnancy to six weeks post partum (Pairman, 2006). Direct access to government maternity funding means midwives can be self-employed, prescribe some pharmaceuticals, and access pathology and radiology services, hospitals and other birthing facilities. They can also consult with obstetricians or refer women to consultant obstetricians (Davis & Walker, 2010). In 2004, 75.3 per cent of New Zealand women were registered with a midwife to provide lead maternity care, demonstrating a high uptake of midwifery care (Ministry of Health, 2007).

Partnership

The concept of partnership between women and midwives in midwifery practice recognises the centrality of women as consumers in society and to the profession (Freeman, Timperley & Adair, 2004). Partnership was incorporated into the New Zealand College of Midwives' *Handbook for Practice* in 1993 (New Zealand College of Midwives Inc., 1993) and is named as the first of ten standards of midwifery practice: the midwife works in partnership with the woman and the twin forces of feminism and consumerism contributed to this ethic. The women's health movement in the 1970s and the Inquiry into the Treatment of Women for Cervical Cancer at National Women's Hospital (also known as the Cartwright inquiry) in the 1980s identified the omission of informed consent and choices in cervical cancer screening and treatment as evidence of the violation of women's rights (Surtees, 2003). This led to an emphasis on 'accountability, patient-centred care, self-determination and cultural sensitivity in the health service' (Surtees, 2003, p. 30). The centrality of the consumer role became instantiated in roles such as patient or consumer advocates in health services and consumer representation on committees.

The newly formed New Zealand College of Midwives, which had emerged from the New Zealand Nurses Association in August

1988, encouraged consumers as members and representatives in decision-making (Daellenbach & Thorpe, 2007). This partnership was a recognition of the value of the political and public support of midwifery, but also an acknowledgment that there was further collaborative work to be done. The midwifery autonomy regained in 1990 allowed for one-to-one working, and the partnership between the midwife and the woman came to underpin the midwifery model in New Zealand maternity services (Pairman, 2006). Partnership assumed equity between mother and midwife, and acknowledged that both parties were making equally valuable contributions. Midwives brought their knowledge, skills and experience, and the woman brought her knowledge of herself and her family, and her needs and wishes for her pregnancy and birth. Midwives argue that their point of difference from the more hierarchical professional models of medical, nursing and obstetric practice is the shift from authoritative models to partnership and collaboration, where women are empowered (Daellenbach & Thorpe, 2007). However, partnership rests on consumers who are informed and want to be informed (DeSouza, 2006).

Critics from within the midwifery profession challenge the model of partnership on two counts: first, because it assumes a white, middle-class subject; and second, because the relationship between midwives and clients is more akin to individualist contractualism, where individuals contract with each other but do not produce a participatory outcome (Skinner, 1999). Skinner's critique of contractualism contradicts the explicit claim by Guilliland and Pairman (1995) that the concept of partnership originates from their understanding of partnership as it is encapsulated in the Treaty of Waitangi. Instead, Skinnner argues that the Treaty is a contract that only has a contemporary reading of partnership and that the demands for tinorangatiratanga (self-determination), protection and equity remain absent in the midwifery partnership. Skinner (1999) concludes that partnership 'reflects a superficial analysis of society, neglecting to identify the dominant underlying right-wing philosophy of individualism, contractualism and patriarchy. It does not recognise inequalities in power or access to resources and is culturally elitist' (p. 16).

Choice

A second tenet of midwifery is the notion of choice and being an informed consumer. The assumption that choice is empowering is derived from the notion that women can be empowered by being consulted and actively involved in processes that affect them. Informed choice emerged as a women-centred, feminist mode of health-care communication, which provided a contrast to more hierarchical and paternalistic modes associated with biomedical obstetrical contexts (Spoel, 2007). Informed choice became both an ideological principle implicit in midwifery models of care and a rhetorical practice of midwives exchanging information with women in order to facilitate decision-making (Spoel, 2007). This led to the advancement of empowered and choice-making subjects who were no longer passively recipient 'patients' but active 'consumers' of health care (Tully, Daellenbach & Guilliland, 1998, p. 248). This notion of the choice-making subject is arranged around discourses of neo-liberal subjectivity and relies on an individual who is rational and responsible within the discursive culture of midwifery. Choice is also constrained by a tension within contemporary liberalism, where respect for the autonomy and privacy of individuals is posited against the concern for the regulation of social and economic life, and where expert knowledges are a mechanism for regulating the choices of individuals within the limits of government, thereby constraining the choices that are made (Murphy, 2003).

Liberal feminists view increasing choice in childbirth as a mechanism for enhancing women's perception of control, but radical and social feminists argue that choice has led to the illusion of freedom in an oppressive context where the status quo remains unchanged (Leap & Edwards, 2006). Leap and Edwards outline the limitations of the concept of informed choice. First, the person who is doing the informing has a powerful influence on the decisions that are made. Being given information about a limited range of choices is not a guarantee of involvement in decision-making. Ultimately, the health practitioner is a gatekeeper who decides what information is relevant. However, if the mother disagrees with the health practitioner, she needs to have either the resources to find alternative support or the attributes that will allow her to challenge the decision—such as being articulate, assertive and knowledgeable (Leap & Edwards, 2006).

Schmidt's (2008) example of breastfeeding information provided by the Ministry of Health is emblematic of the neo-liberal paradox. Schmidt contends that what appears to be the provision of scientific information about the benefits of breastfeeding and risks of formula feeding frames breastfeeding as the only rational option and appropriate choice for a good modern parent to make. Schmidt contextualises contemporary breastfeeding discourses in the new public health model, where neo-liberal ideals of individual informed choice are advanced in tandem with the narrowing of choices to those that advantage the state, such as those that reduce the costs of health care.

Natural childbirth

The legislative changes of 1990 that paved the way for greater midwifery autonomy in birthing also saw the advancement of natural childbirth as a philosophy that was strongly intertwined with partnership and informed choice. Central to this philosophy is the idea of being close to nature, and of returning women to the rewarding aspects of a labour.

However, natural childbirth discourses reflect class and race biases where control over birth and informed consumer choice are emphasised without the recognition that these require access to cultural and material resources that are available only to privileged women (Brubaker & Dillaway, 2009). The feminist notion of taking control of one's life and body is a very middle-class perspective (Lazarus, 1997). However, evidence is growing that alternative approaches to childbirth do not necessarily guarantee more fair or compassionate treatment, as seen by a growing body of work about the experiences of migrant and refugee birthing women (Bowler, 1993). Therefore, midwifery concepts of partnership, choice and natural childbirth derived from radical feminist critiques of medicalisation have been aligned to middle-class white subjectivity, but have not effectively changed the structures of biomedical dominance.

The emergence of the consumer movement in health occurred in the context of related social movements, including the civil rights, anti-racist and indigenous rights movements, the psychiatric survivors' movement and the women's movement. Groups coalesced around identity politics and demanded a larger say in health particularly in terms of policy, professional regulation and service planning (Coney, 2004). The women's health movement was the forerunner in challenging tenets of modern medicine and predated other consumer movements, such as patient's rights and disability movements. The emphasis on critiquing mainstream health care resulted in scrutiny of who held the power in the health sector: governments, health practitioners, health industries, the pharmaceutical industry, policymakers, researchers and funders.

Alongside these people-led developments came community development and public health approaches that advanced critiques of medical dominance and the desire for community-based primary health-care models. These developments were supported by the Alma Ata Declaration (WHO, 2008) and the Ottawa Charter (WHO, 1986). In particular, indigenous Māori and mental health consumers have articulated the need for community-controlled services.

Public health as a field has broadened its scope from communicable disease to the recognition of the role of social inequalities as determinants of health. With the medical model failing to substantively improve the health of deprived populations, the need for models that address the social determinants of health have led to greater involvement of communities in shaping such services. This has led to the development of new and innovative service delivery models by, for example, Māori, Pacific refugee and Asian communities.

{ SUMMARY}

Power is a complex phenomenon in health care and disability support where many professionals assume that because they are doing good that oppression does not exist. However, the rise of consumer movements demanding the redistribution of power in these contexts has foregrounded the empowerment agenda. Therefore, in order to provide services and support that are empowering, professionals must first understand the part they play in power relations. This chapter has outlined the ways in which power is conceptualised through four main theories: critical social theories, organisational and management theories, social psychology theories and post-structural theories. These theories range from viewing power as a possession to seeing power as a relation. In response to the professional dominance of human experiences, such as having a baby and experiencing mental illness, the empowerment agenda has been advanced in a range of ways. In mental health, the recovery model challenges the dominance of professional knowledge in mental health policy and practice, and demands that service user involvement occurs at all levels of care. Importantly, the consumer drives his or her own process of recovery. In the patriarchal area of maternity services, the use of partnership, choice and natural childbirth are viewed as ways of redistributing power back to women. However, empowerment through the redistribution of responsibility to the consumer and their family can be problematic if the corresponding resources are not made available.

REFLECTION POINTS

13.1 Intention (motivation, message, meaning, emotion)

What motivates the consumer movement in health care and disability support services?

13.2 Reception (received message, response, feedback)

Who has more power when practitioners are giving information to consumers?

13.3 Perception (style, manner, impression, analysis)

Do consumers always understand what practitioners say?

QUESTIONS FOR REVIEW

1 Outline the different models of power and empowerment. Which definitions appeal and why?
2 Is there a risk that practitioners and professions can absolve themselves of responsibility when they emphasise the empowerment of service users?
3 What does being empowered mean to you in a health context?

REFERENCES

Barker, P. J. & Buchanan-Barker, P. (2005). *The Tidal model: A guide for mental health professionals*. London: Routledge.

Bowler, I. (1993). They're not the same as us: Midwives' stereotypes of South Asian descent maternity patients. *Sociology of Health & Illness, 15*(2), 157–78.

Bradbury Jones, C., Sambrook, S. & Irvine, F. (2008). Power and empowerment in nursing: A fourth theoretical approach. *Journal of Advanced Nursing, 62*(2), 258–66.

Broom, B., Nicholls, D. A. & Deed, B. (2010). Approaches to healthcare provision. In S. Shaw & B. Deed (eds), *Health and Environment in Aotearoa/New Zealand* (pp. 60–76). Melbourne, Vic: Oxford University Press.

Brubaker, S. J. & Dillaway, H. E. (2009). Medicalization, natural childbirth and birthing experiences. *Sociology Compass, 3*(1), 31–48.

Campbell, J. (1997). How consumers/survivors are evaluating the quality of psychiatric care. *Evaluation Review, 21*(3), 357.

Coney, S. (2004). *Effective consumer voice and participation for New Zealand: A systematic review of the evidence*. Wellington: New Zealand Guidelines Group (NZGG).

Copeland, M. E. (1997). *WRAP: Wellness Recovery Action Plan*. Brattleboro, VT: Peach Press.

Daellenbach, R. & Thorpe, J. (2007). Independence in practice: A New Zealand case study of midwives in partnership. In L. Reid (ed.), *Midwifery: Freedom to practise? An international exploration of midwifery practice* (pp. 261–81). Philadelphia, PA: Elsevier.

Davis, D. L. & Walker, K. (2010). Case-loading midwifery in New Zealand: Making space for childbirth. *Midwifery, 26*(6), 603–8.

Deegan, P. E. (1988). Recovery: The lived experience of rehabilitation. *Psychosocial Rehabilitation Journal, 11*(4), 11–19.

DeSouza, R. (2006). *New spaces and possibilities: The adjustment to parenthood for new migrant mothers*. Wellington, NZ: Families Commission.

Foucault, M. (1977). *Discipline and punish: The birth of the prison*. London, UK: Allen Lane.

Freeman, L. M., Timperley, H. & Adair, V. (2004). Partnership in midwifery care in New Zealand. *Midwifery, 20*(1), 2–14.

Funk, L. M., Stajduhar, K. I. & Purkis, M. E. (2011). An exploration of empowerment discourse within home care nurses' accounts of practice. *Nursing Inquiry, 18*(1), 66–76.

Gilbert, T. (2001). Reflective practice and clinical supervision: Meticulous rituals of the confessional. *Journal of Advanced Nursing, 36*(2), 199–205.

Guilliland, K. & Pairman, S. (1995). *The midwifery partnership: A model for practice*. Wellington, NZ: Department of Nursing and Midwifery, Victoria University of Wellington.

Henderson, G. L. & Waterstone, M. (2008). *Geographic thought: A praxis perspective*. New York, NY: Routledge.

Jacobson, N. & Curtis, L. (2000). Recovery as policy in mental health services: Strategies emerging from the states. *Psychosocial Rehabilitation Journal, 23*(4), 333–41.

Kanter, R. M. (1993). *Men and women of the corporation*. New York, NY: Basic Books.

Kuokkanen, L. & Leino Kilpi, H. (2000). Power and empowerment in nursing: Three theoretical approaches. *Journal of Advanced Nursing, 31*(1), 235–41.

Lazarus, E. (1997). What do women want?: Issues of choice, control, and class in pregnancy and childbirth. In R. Davis-Floyd & C. F. Sargent (eds), *Childbirth and authoritative knowledge: Cross-cultural perspectives* (pp. 132–58). Berkeley, CA: University of California Press.

Leap, N. & Edwards, N. (2006). The politics of involving women in decision making. In L. Page & R. McCandlish (eds), *The new midwifery: Science and sensitivity in practice* (2nd edn) (pp. 97–121). Philadelphia, PA: Elsevier/Churchill Livingstone.

Macdonald, M. (2006). Gender expectations: Natural bodies and natural births in the new midwifery in Canada. *Medical Anthropology Quarterly, 20*(2), 235–56.

Masterson, S. & Owen, S. (2006). Mental health service user's social and individual empowerment: Using theories of power to elucidate far-reaching strategies. *Journal of Mental Health, 15*(1), 19–34.

Morrall, P. (1996). Clinical sociology and the empowerment of clients. *Mental Health Nursing, 16*, 24–7.

Ministry of Health (1995). *A guide to effective consumer participation in mental health services*. Wellington, NZ: Author.

Ministry of Health (2007). *Notice Pursuant to Section 88 of the New Zealand Public Health and Disability Act 2000*. Wellington, NZ: Author.

Murphy, E. (2003). Expertise and forms of knowledge in the government of families. *Sociological Review, 51*(4), 433–62.

New Zealand College of Midwives Inc. (1993). *Midwives handbook for practice*. Dunedin, NZ: Author.

Newman, J. & Vidler, E. (2006). Discriminating customers, responsible patients, empowered users: Consumerism and the modernisation of health care. *Journal of Social Policy, 35*(2), 193–209.

O'Hagan, M. (2001). *Recovery competencies for New Zealand mental health workers*. Wellington, NZ: Mental Health Commission.

Pairman, S. (2006). Midwifery partnership: Working with women. In L. Page & R. McCandlish (eds), *The new midwifery: Science and sensitivity in practice* (2nd edn) (pp. 73–97). Philadelphia, PA: Elsevier/Churchill Livingstone.

Phillips, R. (2006). Consumer participation in mental health research. *Social Policy Journal of New Zealand, 27*, 171–82.

Repper, J. & Perkins, R. (2003). *Social inclusion and recovery: A model for mental health practice*. London, UK: Bailliere-Tindale.

Schmidt, J. (2008). Gendering in infant feeding discourses: The good mother and the absent father. *New Zealand Sociology, 23*(2), 61–74.

Skinner, J. (1999). Midwifery partnership: Individualism contractualism or feminist praxis? *New Zealand College of Midwives Journal, 21*, 14–17.

Spoel, P. (2007). A feminist rhetorical perspective on informed choice in midwifery. *Rhetor: Journal of the Canadian Society for the Study of Rhetoric, 2*, 1–25.

Stojanovic, J. (2008). Midwifery in New Zealand 1904–1971. *Contemporary Nurse, 30*(2), 156–67.

Surtees, R. J. (2003). *Midwifery as feminist praxis in Aotearoa/New Zealand*. Christchurch, NZ: University of Canterbury.

Tully, L., Daellenbach, R. & Guilliland, K. (1998). Feminism, partnership and midwifery. In R. Du Plessis & L. Alice (eds), *Feminist thought in Aotearoa/New Zealand* (pp. 245–55). Auckland, NZ: OUP.

World Health Organization. (1986). *The Ottawa Charter for Health Promotion*. Retrieved from www.who .int/hpr/NPH/docs/ottawa_charter_hp.pdf.

World Health Organization. (2008). *International conference dedicated to the 30th anniversary of the Alma-Ata declaration on primary health care*. Retrieved from http://www.who.int/mediacentre/ events/meetings/alma_ata/en.

Young, I. M. (1990). *Justice and the politics of difference*. Princeton, NJ: Princeton University Press.

WEBSITES

About Mental Health Recovery and WRAP: www.mentalhealthrecovery.com/aboutus.php
Definition of Wellness: www.definitionofwellness.com/dictionary/empowerment-for-health.html
Maternity Services Consumer Council: www.maternity.org.nz

{14}

Culture

Denise Wilson, Ray Gates, Junior Sonny Samuela and Terry Weblemoe

CHAPTER OVERVIEW

This chapter covers the following topics:

+ Cultural difference
+ Cultural competence
+ Cultural safety.

KEY TERMS

Cultural difference
Culture
Ethnicity
Race
Colonisation
Assimilation
Cultural domination
Māori
Pacific People
Aboriginal and Torres Strait Islanders
Interpersonal racism
Linguists
Indigenous
Stereotypes
Cultural blindness
Cultural imposition
Institutional racism
Racism
Cultural competence
Cultural awareness
Cultural safety

Cultural difference The variations between groups that relate to their fundamental understandings about themselves, those around them and the communities of which they are a part.

Culture Beliefs, traditions and rituals originating within the family and community into which a person is born and raised, and transmitted from one generation to the next through a common language.

Ethnicity A group of people united by cultural or national heritage but residing in a place different from their place of origin.

Race A group of people who share distinctive characteristics.

Colonisation The movement to a new place by a group of people who maintain strong ties with their place of origin in the process of establishing a settlement.

Assimilation The process of attempting to make all people similar in terms of their beliefs and practices.

Before examining the concepts of **cultural difference**, cultural safety and cultural competence, it is important to understand what **culture** is and what it is not. Culture originates in the family and community in which a person is born and raised, where beliefs, traditions and rituals are transmitted from one generation to the next through a common language. Simply, culture provides a group of people with a shared identity based on beliefs, values and behaviours acceptable to that group, and influences the way its members see the world (Andrews & Boyle, 2007). Everyone has a culture of origin. Health practitioners also have a specific professional culture. Nonetheless, social, technological and global changes influence cultural beliefs, values and practices, which means that culture is dynamic, evolving over time as its members interact with cultural and social groups within and outside of their family or community of origin.

Often the concepts of culture, ethnicity and race are referred to interchangeably, even though they are different concepts. **Ethnicity**, while incorporating aspects of culture, develops within communities, where groups of people share common traits, loyalties and associations. Often people's nationality is used as a de facto term for ethnic identity (in Census polls, for example). It should be noted that this is a crude measure of ethnicity and cannot be used as a reliable indicator of culture, particularly in the case of Asian identity where a great number of nationalities are collapsed within an 'Asian' ethnicity descriptor. **Race**, on the other hand, broadly classifies people based on shared physical characteristics like skin pigmentation, facial features, body build and hair composition. Major race classifications in the Pacific include Polynesian, Melanesian, Micronesian and Caucasian, and are discernible by their physical characteristics. Defining people by race, ethnicity and culture, however, is problematic because identity, globalisation and inter-marriage contribute to identifiable features within the contemporary context.

Cultural difference

Effective communication with others from a different cultural background requires having a critical understanding of a country's history of **colonisation** and immigration. Countries like Australia and Aotearoa New Zealand were colonised by settlers from other countries, which resulted in their indigenous peoples being subjected to a loss of people, land, language and cultural practices through processes of **assimilation** and **cultural domination**. The colonising agenda was for indigenous peoples to conform to the dominant values, beliefs, behaviours and expectations of the settler culture, and the outcome was the cultures, social structures, roles, functions and traditions of the indigenous peoples were eroded. Not only have contemporary indigenous peoples—like **Māori**, **Pacific People**, **Aboriginal and Torres Strait Islanders**—suffered historical traumas, but most also live with significant contemporary socio-economic deprivation. They also experience inequalities in the access and use of health services, and in the quality of these services, which is generally perpetuated by institutional and **interpersonal racism**.

Cultural domination When one cultural group assumes superiority over others.

Māori The indigenous people of Aotearoa New Zealand.

Pacific People People indigenous to the islands of the Pacific region.

Aboriginal and Torres Strait Islanders The indigenous people of what is now known as Australia.

Interpersonal racism When individuals treat others in a prejudiced manner based on judgments about their race.

Professionals need to be aware of this in their practice and how it impacts on relationships and communication with indigenous peoples. Culturally determined and valued patterns of engagement and perspectives on communication style provide some insight into communication differences. Patterns of engagement differ in terms of the balances between individualism and collectivism. Pacific People tend to value the group needs, activities and identity (collectivism), whereas Europeans value individual achievement and recognition. In practical terms, this means that working in teams or emphasising the family as a whole may achieve more than emphasising individual efforts and rewards (Ting-Toomey & Chung, 2005). Other values in terms of engagement can be found in the different emphases placed on the roles people have within society. Western Europeans tend to value what a person does, can easily see a role as separate from the individual, and can understand interchangeable roles. For Pacific People, families and the relationships within groups are more important; they tend to define how the individual will work, who they are and how they will relate to each of a large number of people. While Western Europeans are more likely to introduce themselves to a new person by explaining what their role is or what job they do, Pacific People will generally want to know what the individual is like, what kind of person they are and how they are to relate to them (for example, their name, where they are from and who their parents are). Different appreciations of communicative style are also evident between cultural groups in terms of directness and indirectness. Europeans tend to emphasise the importance of verbal communication over non-verbal, the words over the context, and the content of the communication over the way the message makes the recipient feel, while at the same time using verbal softeners such as 'please' and 'thank you' for requests. For Pacific People, non-verbal communication, relationships and context are of greater importance.

Many communities are becoming increasingly culturally diverse due to globalisation and increasing migration. Minority and culturally and linguistically diverse groups are common in Australian and New Zealand communities, so health services and practitioners need to be aware of the challenges people belonging to these groups might face. Communication with those who belong to culturally and linguistically diverse communities requires professionals to work with others, such as interpreters, to ensure

Linguistics The study of language.

Indigenous The natural or native people of the land; the original inhabitants and carers of the place.

Stereotypes Beliefs held about a particular group that influence the way people respond to and treat people belonging to that group.

Cultural blindness The apparent inability to see cultural differences.

Cultural imposition The deliberate establishment of one set of cultural beliefs over those from other groups.

they provide safe and effective health care and disability support services. However, Mortensen (2010) reported that health practitioners lack the necessary cultural knowledge and skills of the culturally and **linguistically** diverse groups within their communities, which creates a major barrier to experiencing accessible, safe and equitable health services. Effective communication is important, and cultural safety and cultural competence can improve the practice of professionals working in communities that are culturally and linguistically diverse (DeSouza, 2008; Mortensen, 2010).

In situations where professionals lack critical analysis and understanding of contemporary **indigenous**, minority, and culturally and linguistically diverse groups, they risk acting on assumptions, **stereotypes** and faulty information. Often stereotypes are inaccurate, and negatively impact on the quality of health practitioners' communication with patients and service users. Acting on stereotypes or ignoring cultural differences contributes to **cultural blindness** (Johnstone, 2009). Cultural blindness facilitates a platform for **cultural imposition** (Andrews & Boyle, 2007), where professionals believe people should conform to beliefs and values of the dominant cultural group. Cultural imposition is evident in public health services in Aotearoa New Zealand, for example, whereby health practitioners impose the dominant biomedical view of health and illness on health service users.

Health is a socio-cultural construction formed in personal and professional lives (Wilson, 2008). Māori have an eco-spiritual holistic world view, which values collective responsibilities and obligations to whānau (extended family) members. Such a world view is at odds with the biomedical world view that is illness- and disease-oriented, valuing an individualistic perspective. Cultural difference becomes evident when a number of whānau members of a Māori patient in hospital want to visit or be present at a doctor's round, and the doctors and nurses focusing on the individual patient require visitors to adhere to visiting times and leave during the doctor's round. Whānau presence is important for the wairua (spiritual well-being) of a Māori patient.

In Australia and Aotearoa New Zealand there is awareness of cultural diversity, but it tends to be either poorly understood or insufficiently recognised and respected. For example, Aboriginal and Torres Strait Islander people are commonly grouped together and termed 'ATSI' or 'Indigenous'. It has been argued that neither of these terms is appropriate as they ignore unique tribal identities both between and within these groups (Gooda, 2010; Taylor & Guerin, 2010). By failing to recognise, appreciate and manage these differences, many individuals and services—albeit in some cases without intention—reinforce the harm that colonisation, assimilation and institutionalisation has inflicted on Aboriginal and Torres Strait Islander peoples (Ganguly, 2001; Taylor & Guerin, 2010) and Māori (Reid & Robson, 2007).

The continued ignorance of, or blindness to, cultural differences offers explanations for the persistent poor health status of Aboriginal and Torres Strait Islander peoples compared with the rest of the Australian population, and similarly for Māori and Pacific People in Aotearoa New Zealand. This is notably different from the experience of indigenous populations in other countries, where recognition and appreciation of cultural differences has led to improvements in the health of indigenous peoples (Couzos & Thiele, 2007; Ganguly, 2001). Couzos and Thiele (2007) have criticised the Australian Government as failing to meet its international obligations to improve the health of Aboriginal and Torres Strait Islander peoples, based on the belief that there is a continued practice of **institutional racism**.

Institutional racism Racism that is accepted and allowed within an organisational or powerful framework.

Racism Treating people in a discriminatory manner based on their heritage or race.

Institutional racism can be defined as 'the systematic disadvantaging of racial and ethnic minorities through systems or institutions' (Taylor & Guerin, 2010, p. 75). In terms of health, this could include potential barriers to accessing services or care (for example, transportation, service hours and staffing), failure to provide adequate services (for example, lack of interpreters for little- or non-English speaking patients) and failure to provide adequate care due to stereotyping. Jones (2000) identifies **racism** as occurring at three levels: institutional, personally mediated (whereby individuals display discriminatory behaviours or choose not

CASE STUDY 14.1

The dangers of stereotyping

A 56-year-old Aboriginal man presented to a regional hospital's emergency department, shouting, slurring his speech and staggering round the waiting area. Admissions staff had trouble understanding him due to his affected speech and, like many Aboriginal people in the district, his use of a pidgin form of English.

A triage nurse eventually guided him into a preliminary examination room. She knew the local community had a high level of alcohol abuse, and had frequently seen intoxicated community members present to hospital. Although she did not detect any alcohol on the man, she assumed he was drunk and believed all he needed was a couple of hours to 'sleep it off'. She instructed the man to rest on the examination table and said she would return shortly.

The nurse became busy with incoming patients, and was unable to return to the man until several hours later. The man was unresponsive, and on closer examination lacked any vital signs. The emergency was raised but the man was unable to be revived.

It was discovered that the man had been previously diagnosed with type I diabetes and had died from severe hypoglycaemia.

to acknowledge another person's culture) and internalised (when those subject to racist and discriminatory behaviours begin to believe the negative stereotypes imposed on them). Undoubtedly, racism has been linked to poor health outcomes and quality of care, at times resulting in adverse events (Davis et al., 2006; Harris et al., 2006). Blackman (2009) links the impact of racism on communication, stating: 'Perceived racism is a factor that can cripple the opportunity for honest and valuable communication between health care provider and the patient' (p. 213). Further, racism fuels mistrust and does little for the establishment of respectful relationships.

Institutional racism in the health-care system, whether intentional or not, at the very least places minority groups at a disadvantage, and at worst places them in jeopardy. It is important to understand that, in these circumstances, it is the culture of neither the patient nor the practitioner that leads to poor service provision (McMurray & Param, 2008). Rather, it is the failure to recognise and address these differences that leads to poor outcomes. As Fenwick (2006) states: 'If Western health care does not enhance Indigenous health due to the loss of emotional, social, spiritual and political support, it may be considered that the care delivered is culturally unsafe' (p. 220). Making services culturally safe remains an ongoing subject in both the Australian and New Zealand health-care systems.

CASE STUDY 14.2

Culturally appropriate support

It is common for Pacific People to be inaccurately thought of as one homogenous group. AUT University has developed an approach to supporting Pacific students based on the concept of a 'learning village'. The information below is directed at people from non-Pacific backgrounds to assist with interacting with Pacific students.

The setting is important—consider the environment in which information will be shared. Will everyone feel comfortable and culturally safe to speak their mind in that environment, or will they be overheard or feel foolish if they express themselves or their opinions in a way that is different from others? Do not assume how people experience or interpret information. Give them permission and facilitate their communication, especially within groups.

Make proper introductions—Pacific People want to know who they are speaking to, as a person, not just a job title or role. Be human and make an emotional connection with them. Try to put them at ease and spend some time to get the level right. Never trust stereotypes, but discover who they are as individuals.

Discover common ground—it helps if Pacific People can find common ground, such as someone or some place that both know, or even a common purpose. Aotearoa New Zealand and its various cultural groups are quite small. It is always a pleasant surprise to find out who you know in common. Gentle humour that includes them can often put people at ease.

Set the ground rules early—Pacific People need to know how to relate to strangers, what is likely to happen and who is in charge. There are many cultural expectations, in both the medical and the educational field, that Europeans have grown up with and internalised that are never articulated. Spell out what will happen, what is expected of them, what are the consequences and what kind of relationship they can expect.

Show that you truly care and meet them halfway—learn something about their culture and way of seeing the world. Do not just expect them to be culturally competent in your culture but reciprocate. Being interculturally competent does not necessarily mean that someone must know everything about their culture; rather, one should be open and flexible enough to build bridges and solutions between the cultures, and be willing to meet them halfway (Falconer, Watson & Hofner Saphiere, 2006).

Be persistent—keep checking understanding. In practical terms, this can mean such things as defining things as we go, repeatedly checking in with Pacific People that they are following our explanations or seeing if they have a question that we have not yet answered. They need to clearly understand what resources are available to them and exactly how to access them. This may require a step-by-step instruction or a visual demonstration. Do not assume that they necessarily know some of the things that are probably taken for granted in New Zealand culture, but equally do not assume that they do not know—always check, and give them credit for what they do know. Also do not assume that they see the world the same way that you do. Culture influences perception and the assumptions we make about what is going on, so check and check again.

Understand their background—learn something about their culture, their background and why they do what they do. Be interested and ask about their cultural understanding and their experiences, and what makes them comfortable or feel like they can fit in. Check in with Pacific People regularly, giving them permission to tell us when and how they see the world differently, and seeing if we can compromise or find a middle ground. Empower them to express themselves and to negotiate on equal footing.

Give examples they can relate to—the more that we know about their culture, the better we can use the examples and metaphors they already know to explain new concepts. We often forget how much of our illustrations are based on the history and technology of our culture, and therefore do not actually help to clarify meaning across culture. A good example that is culturally neutral, culturally shared or even culturally appropriate is much more facilitative to learning. Remember to be persistent. If one example does not trigger understanding, be willing to try something else or to demonstrate when possible.

Cultural competence

Cultural competence The concept that practitioners have the skills to interact in a culturally appropriate manner.

Cultural awareness A basic understanding that cultural difference exists and requires consideration and appropriate responses.

It has been argued that in order to help break down the barriers that cultural differences can place between patients and health-care practitioners and services, there is a need to establish a level of **cultural competence** (Gruen, Weeramanthri & Bailie, 2002; McMurray & Param, 2008). Many definitions exist regarding cultural 'competence' and it is often confused, or used interchangeably, with **cultural awareness**. In Australia, the provision of cultural awareness training has been incorporated into the curricula of many health and medical courses; however, there is little evidence about whether this translates into competence at the service-provision level. Authors such as Gruen and colleagues (2002), Henry, Houston and Mooney (2004) and Taylor and Guerin (2010) argue that it is not occurring.

Aotearoa New Zealand has adopted the concept of cultural safety, believing health practitioners need to be more than culturally aware. A clear history of this concept is obvious within nursing (Papps & Ramsden, 1996) and more information about it is presented later in this chapter. However, the Health Practitioners Competency Assurance Act 2003 in Aotearoa New Zealand has a focus on health practitioners being competent, and requires registered health practitioners to demonstrate cultural competence. Early versions of cultural competence required health practitioners to 'learn' the cultural practices of people they came into contact with. However, this is problematic as it is not possible to 'know' all cultural practices, given the culturally diverse people health practitioners come into contact with. Wilson (2008) defines cultural competence as the capability to 'articulate and demonstrate culturally appropriate and acceptable health services where clients feel culturally safe' and that these services reflect the professional's 'reflexivity, knowledge and skills, and an ability to work meaningfully with clients to meet their unique health and cultural needs during their health experience' (p. 185). Thus, cultural competence involves:

1 the knowledge, beliefs, attitudes and power dimensions of the professional
2 his or her actions contributing to improving health outcomes and health status of people from different cultural backgrounds
3 the ability to integrate the cultural values, beliefs and practices of clients into their plans of care (Wilson, 2008).

To do this requires a willingness and commitment to provide culturally competent care, and undergo ongoing education (Campinha-Bacote, 2002; Whaley, 2008).

Cultural competence is a progression from cultural awareness. It occurs when a given system (for example, a hospital, health service or collection of health practitioners) is able to identify and use behaviours, attitudes and policies to work effectively despite cultural differences (Nguyen, 2008). The questions in Table 14.1 can be used to guide self-reflection to determine the level of knowledge and skills a practitioner currently possesses, and the further development needed to attain cultural competence.

TABLE 14.1 *A self-reflection activity on cultural competence*

Self-reflection activity
What do I feel about people from other ethnic and cultural groups in my community?
What do I know about the cultural and ethnic world views of the range of people in my community?
What do I think about people from other ethnic and cultural groups in my community?
What interactions have I had with people from different cultural groups?
What stereotypes, prejudices and racism do I have about those from cultural groups different from mine?
What knowledge and skills do I possess to undertake appropriate and safe cultural assessments? What knowledge and skills do I need?
What aspirations do I have to be culturally aware, safe or competent?

A practitioner must not only have a level of awareness of the cultural diversity of their patients, but must also understand how their own cultural background and beliefs can impact upon the practitioner–patient relationship; they should also consider the ways in which they can approach that relationship to achieve a positive outcome for the patient (Nguyen, 2008; Williams, 1999). The aim is not to make the practitioner an 'expert' on the culture of a given patient, but rather to enable the practitioner to recognise and overcome potential barriers to effective service provision. Translating this understanding into the clinical, educational and policy-development systems can facilitate the development of culturally safe services.

Cultural safety

Cultural safety
A concept, closely associated with health practitioners in Aotearoa New Zealand, relating to the expectation that people receiving services should experience security and respect in terms of their cultural identity.

Cultural safety originated from the concerns of Māori nurses (and also Māori students in nursing programmes) about the quality of care patients received and the differences in outcomes compared with others (Ramsden, 2002). Over time, cultural safety has evolved to include cultural groups beyond ethnic groups, such as age, gender, occupation and sexual orientation. While cultural safety is determined by the patient about their experiences of interactions with health practitioners and a health service, there is an onus on health practitioners to undergo a process of critical reflection on their own cultural values, beliefs and traditions, and how this impacts on others. It is also useful to identify and reflect on the power a health practitioner has, which may or not be used to benefit patients. In situations where professionals lack this analysis, they risk acting on stereotypes and faulty information, and inadvertently using their power to disrupt access, use and quality of health services. In the absence of cultural safety, patients have their cultural identity diminished and demeaned, and as a consequence are disempowered during their health experience.

CASE STUDY 14.3

Compromising cultural safety

Matiu is a 40-year-old Māori man who lives with his whānau (his wife, Mihinui, and three school-aged children) in rented accommodation near the local marae. He has not worked for some time as he has serious health conditions associated with having rheumatic fever as a child, including obesity and sleep apnoea. He survives on the sickness benefit and relies on others for transport as he cannot afford the costs associated with having a car. Their home does not have a telephone.

Matiu finds it difficult to keep his health clinic appointments at the hospital, which is a one-hour drive away from his home. This is affecting his wairua (spiritual well-being) as he would really like to get better control of his health, but does not really understand his conditions and the treatments associated with them. When he has tried to ask questions in the past, the health practitioners he has come into contact with either ignore him or use language he cannot understand. In fact, he believes health practitioners only care about his illnesses and not about other things affecting his health. He also believes they trample on his mana, leaving him feeling inferior and worthless by the time he leaves. Matiu would really like to take his wife with him to his appointments to help him understand, but he really does not want to expose her to the disrespectful way in which he gets treated. He has received letters from Mary, the nurse at the health clinic, but he does not understand some of the words used and has decided to ignore them, as the money it costs to pay for petrol for someone to take him to the hospital is better spent on food for his children.

Mary, the registered nurse at the local health services, has given up on Matiu as he consistently does not attend clinic appointments. She has concluded Matiu does not care about himself, and has heard that the whānau are known for not conforming. For example, his tamariki (children) often do not attend school, according to Mary's friend who is a school teacher. Matiu's actions confirm all the things Mary knows about working with Māori—they are lazy, difficult and always late for (or miss) appointments. If they would just do what everyone else does, everything would be fine. To date, Mary has only communicated with Matiu in writing.

This is a situation where Matiu's cultural safety is being compromised as Mary has imposed her own cultural beliefs and values (such as the importance of time-keeping and conforming to expectations) onto Matiu. She has also acted on unvalidated assumptions (such as the hearsay about the school attendance of Matiu's tamariki) and stereotypes. In this situation, Mary would benefit from reflection on her own and her professional cultural beliefs, values and practices, and how this may impact on others she works with from a different culture.

From a cultural perspective, Matiu's whānau are important and a priority, and in his situation of limited resources he has prioritised feeding his children over the costs of transport. He has also decided not to expose his wife to the poor treatment he receives. Having health practitioners who can communicate in a respectful manner—providing Matiu with time to understand the information he is receiving and to ask questions—and acknowledging important cultural beliefs and practices related to his health would pave the way for a different outcome from the one described here.

In addition, cultural safety was grounded in the Treaty of Waitangi, the agreement Māori made with the Crown in 1840. The Treaty of Waitangi outlines the nature of the relationship Māori have with Crown agents, including health practitioners working in publicly funded health services. The Treaty guaranteed Māori the right to self-determination, to equality with other citizens living in Aotearoa New Zealand, and to protection. The principles of the Treaty are translated into health practitioners' practice in three ways: partnership (formation of a meaningful relationship for working *with* the patient and his or her family), participation (involvement of the patient and family in their care) and protection (determining key cultural and spiritual values, beliefs and practices that need to be included into plans of care). A fourth 'P'—power—also should be considered; that is, the power health practitioners possess and the manner in which they use it.

The need to provide culturally safe environments in all services to Aboriginal and Torres Strait Islander peoples has been identified by Australian governments since the late 1960s, and has been recommended in almost every report on Aboriginal and Torres Strait Islander health since the National Aboriginal Health Strategy in 1989 (NATSIHC, 2004). A generally accepted definition of cultural safety, as it applies to Aboriginal and Torres Strait Islander peoples, is 'an environment which is safe for people: where there is no assault, challenge or denial of their identity, of who they are and what they need. It is about shared respect, shared meaning, shared knowledge and experience, of learning together with dignity, and truly listening' (Eckermann et al., 2010, p. 174). Inherent in this definition are elements that can be attributed to basic human rights: identity, recognition, acceptance (or, at the very least, tolerance) and respect.

In the scope of providing health services, cultural safety equates to empowering patients from diverse cultural backgrounds to determine for themselves what sort of care is most appropriate for them (Nguyen, 2008; Peiris, Brown & Cass, 2008). In particular, the power imbalance that commonly exists between practitioner and patient needs to be equalised, so the practitioner can be seen as a resource that the patient can access—or, in broader terms, that health services can be seen as a resource for the community (McMurray & Param, 2008; Peiris et al., 2008).

An example of this has been described by Abbott, Gordon and Davison (2007), where Aboriginal Health Workers (AHWs) are utilised as a means of balancing the relationship between non-Indigenous nurses or doctors and Aboriginal patients. Within this arrangement, the practitioner, AHW and patient are seen as equals who work in partnership to achieve an identified outcome. AHWs often take the role of a 'cultural mentor' for the non-Indigenous practitioner, providing advice and understanding on cultural and other barriers that may limit the implementation of a care plan, and working with both the practitioner and the patient to effectively address and overcome these barriers (Abbott, Gordon & Davison, 2007). Similarly, Māori Community Health Workers are also a useful cultural resource for those working with Māori communities.

CASE STUDY 14.4

Aboriginal Health Workers as cultural mentors

During a 6-month placement at an Aboriginal Community Controlled Health Service in western Sydney, a GP registrar has a patient walk out of the consultation without discussing further details of her complex medical and social problems. He is concerned because the patient is potentially very ill, and confused because he felt that his communication skills were quite good.

He consults the service's AHW about the incident and the issues he encountered during the consultation. They agree that he should videotape some consultations, with full consent from the patients, with the aim of reviewing them together to discuss cross-cultural communication skills in an Aboriginal setting. In the meantime, the AHW contacts the patient involved to ensure appropriate health management can be initiated.

Adapted from Abbott et al. (2007, p. 71)

Facilitating cultural safety in the health service setting requires examination of service provision, not just in terms of what services are available but more importantly in terms of how services are delivered. This has implications at all levels of the organisation, from direct-contact staff (practitioners and administrators) to managers, internal policies and programmes, and even the organisation's infrastructure (Williams, 1999). Many authors, including Wepa (2005), Williams (1999), Nguyen (2008) and, most recently, Taylor and Guerin (2010), have suggested a set of minimum requirements for developing cultural safety principles (see Table 14.2).

TABLE 14.2 *Suggested minimum requirements for cultural safety guidelines*

Individual level
• Undertake a process of critical reflection on personal and professional cultural backgrounds and how these impact on those from differing cultural backgrounds. • Demonstrate a readiness to be culturally safe. • Have a willingness to listen and communicate appropriately with those who belong to indigenous, culturally and linguistically diverse, and minority groups. • Have an understanding and respect for different cultures, knowledge, experiences and obligations. • Avoid practices or attitudes that may diminish or demean an individual's identity or dignity, or disempower an individual. • Minimise the power differential between self and individuals.

(Continued)

TABLE 14.2 *Suggested minimum requirements for cultural safety guidelines (cont.)*

Organisational level
• Make a commitment to the practice of cultural safety throughout the organisation that is evident in its organisational policies. • Actively engage with individuals and the community to address appropriate issues. • Provide access to interpreters. • Identify groups and resources within the community to assist. • Recognise and empower community control and ownership. • Achieve clarity and consistency in decision-making.

Health services need to become accountable to the communities within which they provide services, and in so doing facilitate the development of a mutual level of trust and respect (Gruen, Weeramanthri & Bailie, 2002; Vicary & Andrews, 2001). This means recognising the impact that colonisation has had upon the health and well-being of indigenous peoples, and working towards 'decolonising' our health institutions, with the aim of developing reconciliation between indigenous and non-indigenous peoples (Edwards & Taylor, 2008; McMurray & Param, 2008; Sherwood & Edwards, 2006).

{ SUMMARY }

Cultural differences can present barriers to the effective and safe provision of health-care services to indigenous, culturally and linguistically diverse, and minority groups. There is a professional onus on those working in health services to develop the ability to provide safe and effective services to those who belong to these groups. Developing cultural competence can assist individual practitioners to develop their capability to work effectively with those from another culture, and overcome these barriers. Cultural safety occurs when patients and service users feel their cultural identity is recognised and respected, and their rights to equal health care are observed. Cultural competence facilitates cultural safety when it is practised at both individual and organisational or systemic levels.

REFLECTION POINTS

14.1 Intention (motivation, message, meaning, emotion)

What are some examples of how culture shapes the beginning stages in a therapeutic relationship?

14.2 Reception (received message, response, feedback)

When working with a person from a different cultural background, what cues would indicate how accurately the information you shared was received? How could you ensure the person understood what you were talking about?

14.3 Perception (style, manner, impression, analysis)

Reflect on occasions when communicating with someone from a different cultural background. Knowing what you now know about cultural safety and cultural competence, reflect on the way in which you communicated (that is, your communication style, manner and body language you adopted). How could you check out your communication style, manner and body language?

QUESTIONS FOR REVIEW

1 Consider the outcome in Case study 14.1. What changes would you suggest need to be implemented on the part of both the triage nurse and hospital management to avoid this happening in the future?
2 How would you describe the differences between cultural awareness and cultural safety?
3 How do you evaluate your own cultural competence and cultural safety?
4 Do you think cultural safety is a journey or a destination?

REFERENCES

Abbott, P., Gordon, E. & Davison, J. (2007). Expanding roles of Aboriginal health workers in the primary care setting: Seeking recognition. *Contemporary Nurse*, *26*(1), 66–73.

Andrews, M. M. & Boyle, J. S. (2007). *Transcultural concepts in nursing care* (5th edn). Philadelphia, PA: Lippincott Williams & Wilkins.

Blackman, R. (2009). Knowledge for practice: Challenges in culturally safe nursing practice. *Contemporary Nurse, 32*(1–2), 211–14.

Campinha-Bacote, J. (2002). The process of cultural competence in the delivery of healthcare services: A model of care. *Journal of Transcultural Nursing, 13*(3), 181–4. DOI: 10.1177/10459602013003003.

Couzos, S. & Thiele, D. D. (2007). The international covenant on economic, social and cultural rights and the right to health: Is Australia meeting its obligations to Aboriginal peoples? *Medical Journal of Australia*, *186*(10), 522–4.

Davis, P., Lay-Yee, R., Dyall, L., Briant, R., Sporle, A., Brunt, D. et al. (2006). Quality of hospital care for Māori patients in New Zealand: Retrospective cross-sectional assessment. *The Lancet, 367*(9526), 1920–5.

DeSouza, R. (2008). Wellness for all: The possibilities of cultural safety and cultural competence in New Zealand. *Journal of Research in Nursing, 13*(2), 125–35. DOI: 10.1177/1744987108088637.

Eckermann, A., Dowd, T., Chong, E., Nixon, L., Gray, R. & Johnson, S. (2010). *Binaŋ Goonj: Bridging cultures in Aboriginal health* (3rd edn). Sydney, NSW: Elsevier Australia.

Edwards, T. & Taylor, K. (2008). Decolonising cultural awareness. *Australian Nursing Journal*, *15*(10), 31–3.

Falconer, T., Watson, B. & Hofner Saphiere, D. (2006). *Cultural detective (NZ): Series facilitator guide* [Registered Training Package]. Retrieved from www.culturaldetective.com.

Fenwick, C. (2006). Assessing pain across the cultural gap: Central Australian Indigenous peoples' pain assessment. *Contemporary Nurse, 22*(2), 218–27.

Ganguly, I. (2001). The third dimension: Cultural awareness for non-English speaking background health professionals. *Australian and New Zealand Journal of Public Health*, *25*(2), 109–10.

Gooda, M. (2010). *Social justice report 2010*. Canberra, ACT: Australian Human Right Commission.

Gruen, R. L., Weeramanthri, T. S. & Bailie, R. S. (2002). Outreach and improved access to specialist services for indigenous people in remote Australia: The requirements for sustainability. *Journal of Epidemiology and Community Health*, *56*(7), 517–21.

Harris, R., Tobias, M., Jeffreys, M., Waldegrave, K., Karlsen, S. & Nazroo, J. (2006). Racism and health: The relationship between experience of racial discrimination and health in New Zealand. *Social Science & Medicine, 63*(6), 1428–41.

Henry, B. R., Houston, S. & Mooney, G. H. (2004). Institutional racism in Australian healthcare: A plea for decency. *Medical Journal of Australia, 180*, 517–20.

Johnstone, M.-J. (2009). *Bioethics: A nursing perspective*. Sydney, NSW: Elsevier Churchill Livingstone.

Jones, C. P. (2000). Levels of racism: A theoretic framework and a gardener's tale. *American Journal of Public Health, 90*, 1212–15.

McMurray, A. & Param, R. (2008). Culture-specific care for Indigenous people: A primary health care perspective. *Contemporary Nurse, 28*(1–2), 165–72.

Mortensen, A. (2010). Cultural safety: Does the theory work in practice for culturally and linguistically diverse groups? *Nursing Praxis in New Zealand, 26*(3), 6–16.

NATSIHC. (2004). *National Strategic Framework for Aboriginal and Torres Strait Islander Health: Context*. Canberra, ACT: Office for Aboriginal and Torres Strait Islander Health.

Nguyen, H. T. (2008). Patient centred care: Cultural safety in indigenous health. *Australian Family Physician, 31*(12), 990–4.

Papps, E. & Ramsden, I. (1996). Cultural safety in nursing: The New Zealand experience. *International Journal for Quality in Health Care, 8*(5), 491–7.

Peiris, D., Brown, A. & Cass, A. (2008). Addressing inequities in access to quality health care for indigenous people. *Canadian Medical Association Journal, 179*(10), 985–6.

Ramsden, I. M. (2002). *Cultural safety and nursing education in Aotearoa and Te Waipounamu* (PhD thesis). Wellington, NZ: Victoria University of Wellington. Retrieved from http://culturalsafety.massey.ac.nz/thesis.htm.

Reid, P. & Robson, B. (2007). Understanding health inequities. In B. Robson & R. Harris (eds), *Hauora: Māori health standards IV. A study of the years 2000–2005* (pp. 3–10). Wellington, NZ: Te Ropu Rangahau Hauora a Eru Pomare. Retrieved from www.hauora.māori.nz.

Sherwood, J. & Edwards, T. (2006). Decolonisation: A critical step for improving Aboriginal health. *Contemporary Nurse, 22*(2), 178–90.

Taylor, K. & Guerin, P. (2010). *Health care and Indigenous Australians: Cultural safety in practice*. Sydney, NSW: Palgrave MacMillan.

Ting-Toomey, S. & Chung, L. C. (2005). *Understanding intercultural communication*. Los Angeles, CA: Roxbury Publishing.

Vicary, D. & Andrews, H. (2001). A model of therapeutic intervention with Indigenous Australians. *Australian and New Zealand Journal of Public Health, 25*(4), 349–51.

Wepa, D. (2005). *Cultural safety in Aotearoa New Zealand*. Auckland, NZ: Pearson Education New Zealand.

Whaley, A. (2008). Cultural sensitivity and cultural competence: Toward clarity of definitions of cross-cultural counselling and psychotherapy. *Counselling Psychology Quarterly, 21*(3), 215–22.

Williams, R. (1999). Cultural safety—What does it mean for our work practice? *Australian and New Zealand Journal of Public Health, 23*(2), 213–18.

Wilson, D. (2008). The significance of a culturally appropriate health service for indigenous Māori women. *Contemporary Nurse, 28*, 173–88.

WEBSITES

Australian Indigenous HealthInfoNet: www.healthinfonet.ecu.edu.au

Hauora: Māori health standards of health: www.hauora.maori.nz

Tataū Kahukura: Māori Health Chart Book: www.moh.govt.nz/moh.nsf/indexmh/tatau-kahukura-māri-health-chart-book-2010

{15}

Social and Interpersonal Dynamics

Louise Miller

CHAPTER OVERVIEW

This chapter covers the following topics:

+ Boundaries and appropriateness
+ Zone of helpfulness
+ Dual relationships
+ Breaking bad news
+ Truth telling
+ Reassurance
+ Communicating with peers.

KEY TERMS

Boundaries
'Being with'

Each person brings their own social, cultural, gender and personal experiences to relationships, and effective practitioners recognise the influence of the social, political and cultural contexts that their relationships occur within. Stein-Parbury (2009) maintains that communication strategies cannot be adopted in the same way that one selects a recipe from a cookbook, because interactions are never free of context. Thus, communication requires thinking skills in order to make choices that support rather than oppress the self and others. Decisions and actions in a personal relationship are often based on emotions, whereas cognition and knowledge form the basis for decision-making in a professional relationship (Anewalt, 2009).

Undeniably, relationship skills involve the self, and among the most challenging are the issues of self-awareness and self-discipline.

Boundaries and appropriateness

Wright (2006) discusses the setting and maintenance of limits when involved with patients to provide safe, therapeutic care. Distinctions between personal and professional roles provide **boundaries** that ensure patient safety and help to offset the patient's vulnerability, protecting the space between the professional's power and the patient's availability (Anewalt, 2009). Becoming personally involved in a patient's world makes it almost impossible to return to a therapeutic framework (Holder & Schenthal, 2007).

Boundary The area between territories that marks the difference between them.

Appropriate boundaries are linked to professional roles and ideas of good practice, and should not be confused with boundary disputes between different professional groups. Boundaries identify what is considered acceptable or unacceptable in one's scope of practice and behaviour, both at work and outside it (Doel et al., 2010).

Holder and Schenthal (2007) assert that the majority of boundary violations are deliberate exploitation because professional boundaries are related to concepts of power differentials. Although boundary crossings may occur in a therapeutic context, all crossings run a risk of harm and collapsing the distance separating the powerful practitioner from a dependent vulnerable patient (Anewalt, 2009; Holder & Schenthal, 2007). Boundary violations range from acts of cruelty and dehumanising of patients to accepting gifts. Sexual violations are the most commonly reported boundary violation (Doel et al., 2010).

Boundaries may also be perceived as changing or negotiable, relative to the context. From this perspective, boundary crossings are not violations or transgressions since they may be fluid, and indeed practitioners might cross boundaries when trying to be helpful (Doel et al., 2010). Practitioners need to beware of multiple therapeutic boundary crossings (Wright, 2006). Once a boundary has been crossed, self-awareness and insight are needed to avoid further potential boundary violations.

Zone of helpfulness

The concept of the 'zone of helpfulness' (National Council of State Boards of Nursing, 1996; Peternelj-Taylor & Yonge, 2003) identifies the elements of appropriate and supportive relationships between practitioners and patients. This is consistent with the principles of the Treaty of Waitangi: protection, participation and partnership. The practitioner is involved enough to participate emotionally, spiritually and intellectually in interactions with patients, and at the same time remain distant enough to maintain control and use the situation to assist patients (Stein-Parbury, 2009). This tension between under-involvement and over-involvement is depicted in Figure 15.1.

FIGURE 15.1 *Zone of helpfulness*

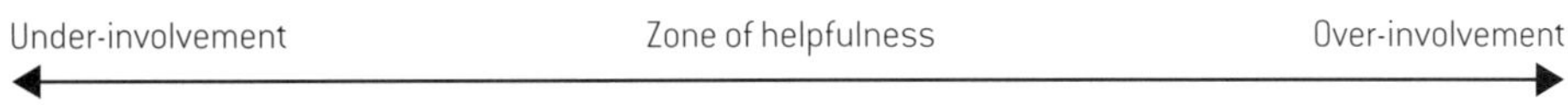

Under-involvement

Many practitioners are skilful conversationalists; however, if they refrain from going beyond this superficial level they risk becoming under-involved and providing less than adequate care or support. By distancing themselves from a situation, the practitioner is shielded from the emotional burden of caring. Practitioners need to develop their own coping strategies so that they can listen and be empathic with patients. In some situations there is not a requirement for emotional involvement, and if the practitioner is technically competent, the patient's needs may be satisfied. However, remaining distant and not recognising or responding to patients' need for support demonstrates being under-involved.

Over-involvement

With or without conscious thought, practitioners can become over-involved with patients who appeal to them on a personal or emotional level (Anewalt, 2009) and thus run the risk of becoming over-involved. One of the challenges of health care is to avoid shifting the focus to the self and to acknowledge feelings of discomfort and powerlessness (Stein-Parbury, 2009). Holder and Schenthal (2007) believe that boundary violations are often committed by well-educated, ethical, law-abiding health practitioners during periods of stress or personal trauma. The risk of over-involvement can develop when an individual believes they are the only one who can help (or rescue) a patient, when they cannot imagine the relationship with a patient ending, or when they themselves are over-extended or overwhelmed by the situation (Wright, 2006). Another example of over-involvement is when a practitioner does not see any separation between how personally important faith or religion is to them and their role as a practitioner (Anewalt, 2009). This is why the use of prayer (karakia) or reference to religious beliefs regarding health and illness must always be initiated by the patient or whānau.

CASE STUDY 15.1

Recognising boundary crossing

Boundary-crossing behaviours can lead to violations of the boundaries between patients and practitioners. These situations are always risky and potentially harmful. Examples of such behaviours include:

- providing or exchanging personal contacts with a patient, such as home telephone numbers, mobile phone numbers or email addresses
- spending more time with a favourite patient
- working extra hours as a favour to patients and families, which might include making personal visits or phone calls either outside of normal working hours or additional to the care plan
- doing personal favours; for example, minor house repairs or babysitting
- performing postal, banking or any other financial transactions for the patient
- providing gifts, clothes, toys or meals
- inviting a patient or their family members to social events or accepting the invitation to such functions
- maintaining personal relationships after professional contact has ended
- imposing one's personal or religious belief or initiating unsolicited discussions related to religious matters
- discussing personal problems with the patient
- keeping secrets with the patient, such as excluding other practitioners or the patient's family from decisions and information
- believing that no one else can meet the patient's needs; that is, assuming that a special rapport exists and that no one else could do everything for the patient
- having a patient pay excessive attention to you, such as commenting on your own physical appearance.

Professional judgment and common sense is needed to distinguish between boundary violations and helpful strategies. Doel et al. (2010) consider that boundaries should not always be seen as problematic, as service users can appreciate professionals who can cross boundaries, but that such practices must be transparent and undertaken in a considered manner. In other words, it is the context that determines if the boundary crossing is harmful (Holder & Schenthal, 2007).

Certain contexts have a higher risk of boundary crossing than others. Practitioners who work in isolated environments, lack direct supervision and provide home care are more at risk of boundary violations (Anewalt, 2009; Holder & Schenthal, 2007). Practitioners also may be resistant to looking at their behaviour, or lack the insight and maturity to understand their own vulnerability to boundary crossing (Holder & Schenthal, 2007). Practitioner vulnerability can stem from unresolved personal issues such as childhood trauma, stress, low self-esteem or professional and personal identity issues. New graduate practitioners often tend to want to be friends with their patients, and are more vulnerable to boundary crossing and boundary violations (Stein-Parbury, 2009).

Dual relationships

In small towns and rural communities, it is common for practitioners to know their patients in another capacity and thus have a dual relationship with that person (Doel et al., 2010). Anewalt (2009) found that many patients do not understand why it is important to keep health-care relationships distinct from other contexts.

It is essential that practitioners deliberately and thoughtfully establish and maintain clear boundaries. Boundary setting is a skill that requires self-awareness, fluent use of immediacy and assertiveness, and the ability to refocus conversations on patient concerns. The use of immediacy involves openly discussing what is going on in the immediate relationship between people, and overlaps with the skill of assertiveness. For example:

> I don't like it when you shout and swear at me. I would be more than happy to talk about what is upsetting you if you are willing to sit down and talk about it with me, without raising your voice or swearing.

Successful resolution of boundary issues depends on achieving balance between personal privacy, the safety of vulnerable patients and the protection of the wider public (Doel et al., 2010). Establishing and maintaining appropriate boundaries is vital to ensure the safety of patients and practitioners. While not an easy skill, practitioners must use judgment and critical thinking skills to determine reasonable and appropriate boundaries that are based on the patient's need (Wright, 2006).

CASE STUDY 15.2

Communicating complaints

Even though the need for good communication skills is clear, poor communication ranks as one of the most frequent complaints made in the health-care sector (Health and Disability Commissioner, 2010). Examples of poor communication include practitioners not listening, information being withheld and a lack of concern or respect (Health and Disability Commissioner, 2010; Lloyd et al., 2009). Not attending to a patient's psychological or spiritual needs that are largely reliant on communication means practitioners fail to fulfil a duty of care.

Many believe the time required to understand a person's experience is a luxury (Stein-Parbury, 2009); however, communication can occur alongside other health interventions. If practitioners can use their skills positively in everyday practice, then the challenges of breaking bad news, truth telling and providing comfort and reassurance are less of a problem.

Breaking bad news

The communication of bad news is never a pleasant task. Bad news marks an unwelcome transition in life for patients and their family, and can imply the loss of well-being, youth, hope, health or relationships (Lloyd et al., 2009). The range of circumstances and attitudes that have a bearing on the context in which information is delivered is huge (Bryant, 2008). Not all bad news concerns terminal illness; for example, explaining the implications of test results or the details of a recent diagnosis. Harrahill (2005) notes that the way in which news is delivered can be as important as the actual news itself. Bad news given in a clumsy manner hampers the patient's ability to cope (Chauhan & Long, 2000a). Regardless of what the bad news entails, patients and families need information to make appropriate choices to allow them to initiate strategies that will manage health and/or lifestyle changes. Beyond just communicating bad news, practitioners must also provide technical competence and knowledge of how to manage psychological and spiritual distress (Schmidt Rio-Valle et al., 2009).

While there are many reasons why delivering bad news is a challenge, most are related to practitioner discomfort and distress. Concern about the negative impact on the patient—such as dashing hope or showing sensitivity to the wishes of the family—may appear to be empathic, but these justifications are often red flags of over-involvement and boundary violations. Sometimes practitioners try to protect themselves from the pain of facing difficult questions, and possibly blame, as the bearer of bad news (Chauhan & Long, 2000b). Schmidt Rio-Valle et al. (2009) found in Spain and other Mediterranean countries that the tendency to conceal the diagnosis and prognosis from the patient is contextual and related to a fatalistic belief in the lack of control over one's own destiny, which is reinforced by the Catholic faith. They also discovered that most practitioners were convinced that even if the patients did not ask questions, they knew or suspected what was happening. Schmidt Rio-Valle et al. (2009) concluded that there are no benefits to concealing bad news, but practitioner's attitudes depend on their sense of personal responsibility and commitment to patient's rights, as well as the cultural context. While no similar study has been reported in Australasia, current health legislature in the New Zealand context requires patients to be given all the information they need to make informed decisions.

Taft (2009) considers that discomfort when communicating bad news is normal and a facet of empathy. However, it can be empowering if the practitioner adopts the attitude that, even though the situation is difficult and uncomfortable, there's an obligation to engage in it, so it should done as well as possible.

Truth telling

In challenging communication scenarios, there is always the potential for practitioners to censor or manipulate the information they choose to impart. Challenges exist between practitioners and patients, and between practitioners and relatives, in relation to giving information. To tell a prognosis to relatives before the patient is questionable, but to engage in a conspiracy of silence and tell relatives not to tell a patient cannot be justified (Parker, citied in Chauhan & Long, 2000b; Schmidt Rio-Valle et al., 2009).

In some situations, the truth is avoided when practitioners are silent, use jargon or take the conversation off on a tangent, and attempts are made to justify this as avoiding patient harm (Chauhan & Long, 2000b). Another common practice is where false hope is given, and the impact of illness is minimised or not fully explained. Both of these responses are inappropriate as people have a right to know about what is affecting them. Self-awareness is vital as it is difficult to see one's own avoidance of questions, along with deceptions and fabrications, as the lies they really are (Chauhan & Long, 2000b). Whatever the context or the reasons given, if a practitioner fails to share what they know, or if they dodge the issue, then the truth has not been told: such behaviour is an abuse of power and a violation of boundaries. Once trust or rapport has been broken, the practitioner is responsible for preventing further harm—a simple apology is a good place to start.

If known information is not shared, then basic communication skills of congruency and trust are compromised. Practitioners are accountable to actively assess preferences and to act in the patients' best interest. When patients are going for investigations, it is important to find out what they would like to know about the results, and what the impact of the results might be. Be open and discuss the potential for bad news, and ask who they would like to be there for support and whether they want anyone else informed of the findings. Listen to the client and respond to cues, as questions that may appear superficial can mask deeper issues. For example, 'Will I be able to finish my degree?' might actually mean 'How long have I got?' or 'Will this cancer kill me?' During times of stress, such as life-changing health events or hearing bad news, patients may need comforting and reassurance that is grounded in truth.

Reassurance

Reassurance can be defined as a planned, purposeful skill to help manage anxiety (Teasdale, 1995). Unfortunately, literature is sparse and most often this skill is developed by experience alone (Cooper, 1996). When someone is given reassurance, it is assumed that comfort is restored and the person is free from pain and more able to cope with whatever was causing their anxiety. Many coping strategies are viewed as inappropriate and maladaptive; for example, wishful thinking, self-blame, denial and avoidance. Nevertheless, coping is dependent on the situation and the strategy used is often adaptive, especially in extreme situations. To get through a traumatic situation, a patient will do whatever they have to. Reassurance must be a purposeful strategy that promotes a sense of safety and control, and supports whatever coping the person is using at that time. Most importantly, reassurance does not make everything all right—as often this is simply not possible—but establishes and/or maintains the patient's sense of hope, control over the situation and courage to cope with the adverse health event.

Unfortunately, reassurance is frequently offered in the form of trivial clichés that have no specific meaning, such as 'Everything will work out' or 'Don't worry—it will be all right'. These responses, which are often uttered in an almost automatic or stereotypical way, avoid underlying concerns and are examples of false reassurance (Stein-Parbury, 2009; Chauhan & Long, 2000a). They signal the inability of the practitioner to help and a failure to ease discomfort (Stein-Parbury, 2009). Such reassurance in reality means reassuring the practitioner (Chauhan & Long, 2000a). Optimistic assertions are promises or guarantees made with the intention of reassuring a person; for example, 'You will sleep after this pain medication'. The response appears to provide information, but in reality identifies an expected outcome that may or may not be related to the current event. Pain medication may reduce pain and encourage sleep, but if the patient is anxious, this in itself can preclude sleep and even heighten the perception of pain.

Appropriate and effective reassurance is reliant on first establishing what the patient is concerned about and why (Chauhan & Long, 2000a; Cooper, 1996). Practitioners must refrain from assuming control and attempting to fix the situation, and communicate with the patient to explore the meaning of the situation and the essence of the patient's discomfort. Reassurance must be directly related to the patient's situation and the meaning they attach to it. Receiving information and knowledge of facts eliminates the fear of the known and unknown. Accurate information that is readily understood—such as details of treatment and the nature of the condition—enables patients to make informed decisions and have a sense of control. In some situations, when it is not clear what the future might hold, practitioners can be reassuring by being open and by detailing what they are doing and why. In extreme situations, a small amount of information provided regularly is vital, and may also include information regarding the totality of the event, such as what is happening elsewhere.

Reassurance can also be conveyed through non-verbal means. '**Being with**' implies empathy or being in tune with the person who needs reassurance. The connection between practitioner and patient is the sense of sharing an experience to some degree. Communication skills of empathy and self-disclosure are useful here. 'Being there' is more physical. It is time with the person; a sense of the practitioner being there for the person and not for any other reason. To convey a sense of security, one does not have to be next to the person but rather accessible and available.

'Being with'
The process of supporting (being present with and for) people, which is not dependent on physical tasks or being busy.

Automatic, unthinking responses can meet the patient's need for reassurance if the practitioner is aware and then follows up with a more helpful response. This might be immediate or later in the day. For example, if you responded automatically with 'Don't worry', you could follow up with 'Let me sort out a few things and then I can sit with you'. Or the practitioner could acknowledge their own reality and apologise: 'Sorry, but earlier today I realised I did not give you my full attention when I said "Things will be all right".'

CASE STUDY 15.3

Reassurance techniques

- Answer specific anxieties.
- Provide an explanation of symptoms that directly relates to the patient's current experience.
- Fit the reassurance to the patient, as appropriate reassurance is dependent on contextual factors such as culture, age and gender.
- Put things into perspective.
- Emphasise the positive.
- Identify the plan for ongoing support.

Adapted from Cooper (1996)

In conclusion, communication with patients requires practitioners to be cognitively alert and to have dual awareness in order to hear and respond to patients in ways that are helpful. Good communication requires preparation and a willingness to bear one's own discomfort to ease the patient's.

Communicating with peers

Because health care brings people into close proximity with human vulnerability, suffering, pain, fragility and anxiety, internal coping resources of practitioners are often stretched. The communication skills used with patients are also part of the toolbox a practitioner can draw on to support or receive support from peers. Supportive relationships with colleagues are not automatic; they require active effort in order to develop and grow (Leever et al., 2010). Time constraints are very real and there is often a perception of never having any time to support each other, even though time might be found to complain about situations such as working conditions, which could be equally well utilised in peer support (Leever et al., 2010).

Peer relationships in the workplace are often also social as well as professional in nature. A key question to consider is: what are appropriate boundaries between peers? Instances of bullying are clear violations and inevitably reflect power differentials. As with appropriate boundaries between practitioner and patient, the same rule of thumb can be applied. If there is harm, there is boundary violation. Issues related to dual relationships and dual awareness also exist within the context of peer support and colleague relationships.

Sound professional communication and mutual respect improves collaboration between practitioners, which then can improve morale, as well as patient satisfaction and quality of care (Leever et al., 2010; Wackerhausen, 2009). Rapid development in health care has caused a growth in the number of clinical specialties, and has altered health and disease profiles. No single profession can manage patients who frequently have complex and time-consuming problems (Leever et al., 2010). Communication failure is commonly identified as a root cause during reviews of sentinel events (Dunsford, 2009).

Barriers to interprofessional collaboration are located within and external to professionals. Dunsford (2009) identifies external barriers to collaboration as high practitioner:patient ratios (resulting in heavy workloads and acuity), staff shortages and few experienced staff. Nancarrow and Borthwick (2005) note that the need for flexible working practices and more unskilled workers (such as health-care assistants taking on tasks previously only performed by professionals) has placed pressure on boundaries of practitioners.

Barriers that exist within the profession relate predominantly to boundary disputes and 'turf wars' (Reeves et al., 2009). Medical dominance of established professions protects and maintains boundaries (Harris, 2007). Wackerhausen (2009) states that while practitioners share the same basic goal—to do what is best for the patient—barriers to professional collaboration exist from the habitual ways of talking, explaining, perceiving, valuing, doing and assuming within practice. Differences in communication styles lead to misunderstandings, frustration, errors and poor patient outcomes (Pope, Rodzen & Spross, 2008).

Full collaboration requires that practitioners communicate with each other and constructively explore their differences in search of solutions that go beyond each practitioner's own limited vision of what is possible (Leever et al., 2010). Adopting a structured communication tool such as SBAR (see Case study 15.4) can reduce the risk of errors from communication misinterpretation and improve patient safety (Anderson, 2008). Practitioners with different communication styles have a consistent means of communication that's clear, concise and easy to use (Pope et al., 2008).

CASE STUDY 15.4

Applying SBAR

SBAR (which stands for Situation, Background, Assessment and Recommendation) is a method for interacting with fellow professionals. You can use SBAR any time to pass on patient information. It can enable handovers between staff to be orderly, ensuring all essential aspects of the patient's needs are covered. Before you use SBAR, be prepared to answer any questions. Assess the patient, have all the information you need and review the patient's health record, recent progress and handover notes.

Situation—the first step is to describe the situation. Identify yourself, your unit, the patient's name and room number (or address if in the community). Briefly state the problem, including when it happened or started and how severe it is. The situation is ideally described succinctly in less than 10 seconds.

Background—provide information pertinent to the situation; for example, the admitting diagnosis and date of admission. Avoid giving a full history of events; state only what is relevant to the current situation such as recent mental status, vital signs and successful or unsuccessful interventions.

Assessment—state how severe the problem is, such as whether the situation is life-threatening or not. Identify what you think might be going on, use phrases like 'might be' or 'could be helpful'. If unsure of causes, determine the broad body system that is involved. Provide objective assessment details to substantiate your assessment.

LOUISE MILLER

Recommendation—propose a recommendation for resolving the situation or what you need from the practitioner you have contacted. For example, do you want them to see the patient, transfer them to a high level of care or to chart medication? Clarify how the client will be assessed or monitored and under what circumstances you are to recontact the person with whom you have consulted. Get a time frame for actions to be completed by, or when the desired effects of a treatment should be visible.

{ SUMMARY }

Practitioner interactions with patients and with peers are influenced by a multitude of social and interpersonal factors. Professional relationship boundaries are reliant on practitioners making thoughtful choices based on insight into their professional identity and personal life. Use of communication skills without self-awareness and considered intent may cause more harm than good. The patients' need for comfort and reassurance, truthful sharing of information and imparting of bad news requires constant attention to the contextual factors that exist in the situation. While such moments are challenging for practitioners, they are often remembered as key moments in patients' lives. Collaborative and supportive communication with peers is reliant on individuals using the same skills with thoughtful purpose.

REFLECTION POINTS

15.1 Intention (motivation, message, meaning, emotion)

Professional boundaries are concerned with issues of power and exploitation. What factors are inherent in the health practitioner and client relationship that makes for unequal power dynamics?

15.2 Reception (received message, response, feedback)

A useful strategy for setting limits or professional boundaries is to use assertiveness and immediacy. This involves talking about what is going on right now in the relationship between yourself and the person you are speaking with as well as speaking assertively. Reflect on a conversation you have been involved in where limit setting might have been useful. Using the skills of immediacy and assertiveness, how might you have handled this differently?

15.3 Perception (style, manner, impression, analysis)

In the management of any dispute, fair treatment involves taking up the concern (assuming there is no threat of violence or abuse) directly with the person concerned in the first instance. If this is unsuccessful, what do you think should be the next step to take?

QUESTIONS FOR REVIEW

1 When referring a client to another health practitioner for treatment or assessment, what are the key elements that should be included in this handover?

2 What challenges may arise for practitioners who are breaking bad news?

3 What are the indicators that colleagues may not be functioning within the zone of helpfulness and how may this be addressed?

REFERENCES

Anderson, D. E. (2008). Bridging the professional chasm: Tools for collaborative communication. *MedSurg Matters, 17*(1), 8–9.

Anewalt, P. (2009). Fired up or burned out? Understanding the importance of professional boundaries in home health care and hospice. *Home Healthcare Nurse, 27*(10), 590–7.

Bryant, L. (2008). Breaking bad news. *Practice Nurse, 35*(5), 37.

Chauhan, G. & Long, A. (2000a). Communication is the essence of nursing care 1: Breaking bad news. *British Journal of Nursing*, *9*(14), 931–8.

Chauhan, G. & Long, A. (2000b). Communication is the essence of nursing care 2: Ethical foundations. *British Journal of Nursing*, *9*(15), 979–84.

Cooper, C. (1996). The art of reassurance. *Australian Family Physician*, *25*(5), 695, 697–8.

Doel, M,. Allmark, P., Conway, P., Cowburn, M., Flynn, M., Nelson, P. & Tod, A. (2010). Professional boundaries: Crossing a line or entering the shadows? *British Journal of Social Work, 40*, 1866–89. DOI: 10,1093/bjsw/bcp106.

Dunsford, J. (2009). Structured communication: Improving patient safety with SBAR. *Nursing for Women's Health, 13*(5), 385–90. DOI:10.1111/j.1751-486X.2009.01456.x.

Harrahill, M. (2005). Giving bad news gracefully. *Journal of Emergency Nursing*, *31*(3), 312–14. DOI: 10.1016/j.jen.2005.01.006.

Harris, L. (2007). Professional boundaries and competence. *Practice Nurse, 33*(7), 26, 30.

Health and Disability Commissioner. (2010). *Annual report for the year ending 30 June 2010*. Retrieved 10 January 2011 from www.hdc.org.nz/publications/other-publications-from-hdc/annual-reports/annual-report-for-the-year-ending-30-june-2010.

Holder, K. V. & Schenthal, S. J. (2007). Watch your step: Nursing and professional boundaries. *Nursing Management, 38*(2), 25–30.

Leever, A. M., Hulst, M. V. D., Berendsen, A. J., Boendemaker, P. M., Roodenburg, J. L. N. & Pols, J. (2010). Conflicts and conflict management in the collaboration between nurses and physicians—A qualitative study. *Journal of Interprofessional Care*, *24* (6), 610–24. DOI: 10.3109/13561820903550762.

Lloyd, M., Bor, R., Blache, G. & Eleftheriadou, Z. (2009). *Communication skills for medicine* (3rd edn). New York, NY: Churchill Livingstone.

Nancarrow, S. A. & Borthwick, A. M. (2005). Dynamic professional boundaries in the healthcare workforce. *Sociology of Health and Illness, 27*(7), 897–919. DOI: 10.1111/j.1467-9566.2005.00463.x.

National Council of State Boards of Nursing. (1996). *Quick reference for professional boundaries and sexual misconduct cases*. Chicago, IL: Author.

Peternelj-Taylor, C. A. & Yonge, O. (2003). Exploring boundaries in the nurse-client relationship: Professional roles and responsibilities. *Perspectives in Psychiatric Care, 39*(2), 55–66.

Pope, B. B., Rodzen, L. & Spross, G. (2008). Raising the SBAR: How better communication improves patient outcomes. *Nursing, 38*(3), 41–3.

Reeves, S., Rice, K., Conn, L. G., Miller, K., Kenaszchuk, C. & Zwarenstein, M. (2009). Interprofessional interaction, negotiation and non-negotiation on general internal medicine wards. *Journal of Interprofessional Care, 23*(6), 633–45. DOI: 10.3109/13561820902886295.

Schmidt Rio-Valle, J., Caro, M. P. G., Juarez, R. M., Pena, D. P., Vinuesa, A. M., Pappous, A. & Quintana, F. C. (2009). Bad news for the patient and the family? The worst part of being a health care professional. *Journal of Palliative Care, 25*(3), 191–6.

Stein-Parbury, J. (2009). Patient and person: Developing interpersonal skills in nursing (2nd edn). Sydney, NSW: Churchill Livingstone.

Taft, P. (2009). Breaking bad news. *Nursing Standard, 24*(10), 59.

Teasdale, K. (1995). Theoretical and practical considerations on the use of reassurance in the nursing management of anxious patients. *Journal of Advanced Nursing, 22*(1), 79–86.

Wackerhausen, S. (2009). Collaboration, professional identity and reflection across boundaries. *Journal of Interprofessional Care, 23*(5), 455–73. DOI: 10.1080/13561820902921720.

Wright, L. D. (2006). Violating professional boundaries. *Nursing 2006, 36*(3), 52–3.

WEBSITES

Breaking Bad News: www.dhsspsni.gov.uk/breaking_bad_news.pdf
Health and Disability Commissioner: www.hdc.org.nz
Institute for Healthcare Improvement: www.ihi.org
Overcoming Communication Barriers in Emergency Situations: Some Basic Tools: www.patientprovidercommunication.org/index.cfm/useful_information.htm

{16}

Touch

David Nicholls

CHAPTER OVERVIEW

This chapter covers the following topics:

+ The culture of touch
+ Touch through the lifespan
+ Touch and communication
+ Touch and professional practice
+ Touch and human well-being.

KEY TERMS

Haptic
Integumentary system
Therapeutic touch
Purposeful touch
Inappropriate touch

> ***When we honestly ask ourselves which person in our lives means the most to us, we often find that it is those who, instead of giving advice, solutions, or cures, have chosen rather to share our pain and touch our wounds with a warm and tender hand.***
>
> *Henri Nouwen (1990)*

Of all the senses, touch is probably the most valuable to other people. While hearing, sight, smell and taste provide vital information that enables human function, it is the ability to touch that makes people social. Combine touch with the ability to communicate with words and it is clear how humans developed as higher order beings. Touch allowed people to feel their way out of the dark cave and into the sunlight; to rub sticks together to make fire; to wield tools to provide and prepare food; to build machines and tall buildings; to plough fields; and, importantly, to heal other people's suffering. Touch is the most practical and the noblest of the senses, and is an essential component of modern life.

Touch means much more to us than merely what we can feel with our hands. This is apparent in common references to touch, such as people saying they 'feel for you' when showing sympathy, or that someone 'touched a nerve' in relation to something being painfully true. To 'catch your breath', 'grasp at straws', 'hold that thought' and 'grab a drink' are other examples of touch in everyday language. It is also common to refer to the working of the human mind in terms of tactile language—how people 'feel'.

Touch, therefore, is far more complex than it would first appear, but it is a vital subject for those who aspire to work with others, and particularly those in the professions that use touch as a regular part of their work. Novice practitioners often make the mistake of thinking that tactile, or **haptic**, communication is innate and cannot be taught; that it is a skill that some people are simply born with. While this might be true to some extent, expertise is achieved through months and years of practice, along with the application of skills that certainly can be acquired. Touch is so powerful, rich and complex that students of health must have at least a rudimentary appreciation for its ability to bring relief to people, and they must grasp some of its subtlety and complexity.

Haptic Relating to the sense of touch.

There are several social and theoretical aspects of touch. Culture and history indicate the importance of touch for humans. Across the lifespan, tactile forms of communication take various forms. The complexity inherent in the language of touch is important to understand; its place in professional practice also requires attention.

The culture of touch

People have used touch to hurt and to heal for as long as we have recorded history. From earliest fumblings in the dark world of prehistoric peoples, through the manual labour of the pre-industrial age, to the computer-aided technologies of the twenty-first century, touch has been vital to the identity of humans and has served as a marker of evolution. Touch is now so pervasive and necessary for our civilisation that it is easy to overlook how important it is to human existence, ways of life and standards of living (Calvert, 2002).

Prior to the Industrial Revolution, most Western cultures relied on small-scale manufacture of goods and agriculture for income. By necessity, work was local, with things being made as they were needed and food being harvested in season. With the advent of machinery in factories and on farms, mass-produced commodities began to appear in homes, and food began to be gathered in vast quantities and shipped as refrigerated cargo around the world. Populations subsequently grew in number, size and affluence; birth rates increased and death rates declined.

But while the marvels of modern technology were celebrated, people also began to yearn for a simpler time. As far back as two hundred years ago, writers like Charles Dickens and Thomas Hardy, and painters like John Constable and Jean-François Millet, mourned the loss of a pastoral way of life. Concerns that people were 'out of touch' with nature began to pervade aspects of Victorian culture and led to some seeing technology as the cause of much illness and suffering. In many ways, today's environmental campaigners and advocates for locally grown, organic food are repeating many of the same arguments: expressing a yearning for a simpler time when people made things by hand.

Touch has played a complex and multidimensional role in modern culture, and it is simplistic to say that touch, or touch technologies, are simply good or bad. Take, for example, the current fascination with smartphones and touch technology. It is difficult to imagine the appeal of an iPad or iPhone without the touch-screen, or a computer without a mouse or keyboard. Touch is ubiquitous in modern technology and for many years science writers have written about a future in which haptic technology or haptics play an increasingly important part in our methods of communication. From touch-screens (such as the screens used in the films *Minority Report* and *Quantum of Solace*) to touch-activated communication systems, haptics will offer assistive technologies for people, whether they have difficulties with speech, want to reach a mass audience or simply want to communicate with someone on the other side of the globe.

One of the most interesting aspects of touch in our culture is not the technological innovation coming in the next few years, but the way that touch has influenced our various social histories. Many of the social tensions that now define human civilisation have, in some way or other, involved touch. The sexual revolution in the 1960s broke down traditional stigmas around touch, for example, but these new-found freedoms were soon cut short by epidemics of AIDS, avian flu and SARS that made people more fearful of touching others (this cultural shift is illustrated in the Austin Powers films). HIV/AIDS was such a frightful thing in the 1980s that Princess Diana caused controversy when, in 1987, she publicly touched the hand of an AIDS victim, commenting that people need hugs and that she believed everyone needs to be touched. More confusion and ambivalence in relation to touch are apparent in the ubiquitous nature of cleaning products, in terms of the debate that children's immune systems may not be able to properly develop in sanitised environments.

The sophistication of human society is built on some rather basic physiological functions, not least the prehensile ability, which in anthropological terms means to be able to grasp objects. Many other species 'feel' through their hands and paws, and some have adapted tails (monkeys), claws (cats), noses (elephants) and even lips (horses) that allow them to grasp objects in the absence of human-like hands. But few outside the primates have the ability to move the thumb across the palm to touch the other digits (a function called 'opposition'). The prehensile ability of early humans allowed them to grasp objects, fashion weapons and wield tools, and this vital evolutionary advantage may have even led directly to us walking erect (because animals cannot wield tools in their hands if they rely on four legs to stand and walk). This, in turn, allowed humans to grow in size and brain power, adapt their diet and evolve rapidly. Touch is a tool that has brought us to civilisation.

Touch through the lifespan

The experience of touch (both given and received) is vital for normal child development. A newborn baby first relies on their other senses to find out about the world beyond their grasp. Only when they begin to crawl then walk do they really experience the world of surfaces, materials, textures and temperatures, and then parents and others around them spend inordinate amounts of time teaching them to discriminate between those that are safe and those that are not.

Children learn that not all tactile experiences are good or pleasant. Accidents occur: some will trip and hurt their hands on the gravel, touch a hot pan or trap their fingers in doors. Some will experience physical abuse at the hands of others. Much is learnt and remembered from early tactile experiences and some of it will stay with a person for their whole life.

Adults, too, rely on touch for growth and maturation. Much of our sexuality is inherently derived from touch. The sensuality of the world around us is appreciated in large part from our sense of touch. Indeed, the experience of pain so common in adulthood is thought by many philosophers to be vital to our very existence as humans (see, for example, the work of Friedrich Nietzsche or the writings of Marcel Proust). Touch is also a major form of social engagement for adults who use handshakes, kisses, hand-holding, slaps and punches to communicate to others what words sometimes cannot say.

Integumentary system Skin and related structures.

For the elderly, who are prone to frail skin and illnesses that compromise their **integumentary system**, touch takes on new meaning. An inability to move as freely and as comfortably as when they were younger often means long periods sitting or lying, and a reliance on others for help with movement. Fragile skin can easily break down and ulcerate, and poor circulation results in very slow healing. A cerebro-vascular accident (or 'stroke') may affect the sensation over half of the body, and heart disease may cause the limbs to swell and the skin stretch until it splits. Arthritis may deform the joints of the hands and make using even simple tools like knives and forks, garden trowels and knitting needles impossible. Touch, therefore, accompanies people through the various stages of life, helping to define their experiences and engagement with the world. This is most clearly seen in the way people use touch to communicate.

Touch and communication

Touch is incredibly complex and multifaceted. Touch cannot be understood simply by knowing the anatomy of the hand, or the cultural history of tools, or the pathology of arthritis. It is not possible to know how important touch is by thinking only of one aspect of its role for individuals and societies. Its role in communication is immeasurably more complex.

While technical skill is hugely important in health-care practice, it is people's ability to communicate that truly makes the difference to people's experience of health care and disability support, and may also determine whether a treatment is effective or not. Given that the vast majority of communication is non-verbal (through gestures, body language and expressions), it is reasonable to assume that touch plays a large part in determining the outcome for those receiving care and support.

However, touch in health care is, in some ways, made more complex by social taboos about what can be touched, when and by whom. Each culture reflects its history and cultural identity in the way that touch is used. In English culture, for example, it is normal to shake hands on meeting someone, while in French culture people exchange kisses. In Māori culture the hongi carries enormous significance as a gesture of welcome. Simple though they are, these gestures betray deep roots that relate directly to collective histories, beliefs and values.

In Western cultures touch has been a problematic issue for many centuries, since certain forms of touch associated with pleasure and sensuality were considered sinful by the early Christian church. The Christian attitude towards 'sins of the flesh' led to a purge against early forms of massage in Western Europe. All forms of **therapeutic touch** were considered blasphemous and many of the handwritten texts of Greek and Roman physicians and healers were burned. Had it not been for the intervention of Persian scholars like Ibn Sīnā (or more fully, Abū Alī al-usayn ibn Abd Allāh ibn Sīnā, 980–1037), who translated these texts into Arabic, the works

Therapeutic touch Touch that is deliberate and intended to help and heal, and is understood accordingly.

of Celsus and Galen would almost certainly have been lost, along with much of what is now known about these therapies.

The height of our Western society's anxieties about touch came in Victorian England towards the end of the nineteenth century. This period coincided with the birth of modern medicine, nursing, midwifery and physiotherapy, and these professions (and others that have followed) had to negotiate how society could give them licence to touch people while not causing offence. One of the ways this was achieved was through clearly defined ethical codes of conduct and the technical teaching of **purposeful touch**.

Purposeful touch
Touch that has a meaningful and honourable intent.

Purposeful touch defines the intent of the giver, and says less about the experience of the receiver. It is not the casual contact between two friends or the unintentional brush against another person on a bus, but the deliberate, thoughtful and often highly technical contact between a skilled practitioner and a client or patient. Importantly, it may require one of the parties to touch the other in a way that would not normally be socially acceptable. Taking blood, inserting urinary catheters, bathing people in bed and replacing hip joints, for example, all require forms of intimate contact that would be totally unacceptable were they to take place in the cinema or at the mall. But in hospital or at the local clinic, under the care of a qualified health practitioner, it is possible to encroach upon people's personal space in the most intimate manner. Given this ability, it is vital that consideration be given not only to the technical aspects of touch, but also to how that touch will be perceived.

Touch is an intimate connection between two people who in all probability have different histories, beliefs and values. Each experience of touch is unique, because the second after being touched change may take place, and the touch no longer exists. There is an aphorism that states: 'You cannot dip your toe in the same place in the river twice.' It means that every encounter in life is specific to that exact moment in time, and this is true of those occasions when people touch others.

Not surprisingly, the power of touch to harm and to heal intimidates some people, but people are surrounded by touch. The difference in the health-care setting is that the poser of touch is harnessed with the goal of improving the well-being of others. This requires the learning and careful development of skills that others may not have. The ability to touch people purposively costs nothing, but it has the ability to profoundly impact on those who receive it.

For all its mystical virtues, however, touch is obviously not always good. The harsh reality is that if the intent of the person is to be cruel, to hurt or to abuse, touch can be a profoundly harmful experience for the recipient. It is no surprise that centuries-old forms of torture involve the use of extreme physical punishment. However, not all forms of abuse involve the use of violence against the body. People can also experience trauma by being denied loving or healing touch as much as through the use of excessive force. To complicate matters further, there are occasions in health care where it is necessary to cause a person pain to bring about healing; for example, performing surgery, administering medications via injections or stretching limbs and scar tissue. Once again, in these situations it is the intent implied in the touch that defines whether the work is ethically justifiable.

Touch and professional practice

The ability to touch people, as a necessary part of health-care practice, is often taken for granted. For example, a primary care practitioner uses touch to take blood pressure and examine ailments, while a visit to a dental professional is obviously going to involve touching the face and mouth. But not all practitioners are allowed to touch people freely, and there are strict social codes around how, where and when the touch can take place (Lawler, 1991).

Society has traditionally allowed some practitioners to touch only when they have demonstrated competence, completed extended training and gained registration with a licensing authority. For their part, these practitioners have restricted their forms of touch to purposeful or intentional touch. This form of touch is different from the kinds of touch that happen in everyday personal and public life. Often it is touch that requires training, skill, purpose and the acceptance of the person receiving it. Surgeons, for instance, can touch the body in areas physically inaccessible to others (like the hip joint or the heart) while the person is anaesthetised. Nurses often perform very intimate procedures involving touch that would be unacceptable in any social location other than a hospital ward or clinic. Other practitioners use touch in the form of therapeutic manipulation (Oerton, 2004).

In recent years, the stranglehold that orthodox professionals had over the licensing of therapeutic touch has started to relax, and now a wider range of alternative and complementary practitioners use touch. The need for formal training and strict registration for practitioners has dissipated, and yet there remain some social conventions about where and when touch should take place. This increasing comfort with forms of therapeutic touch exists alongside an acute sensitivity to forms of **inappropriate touch**. Domestic violence and child abuse are widely acknowledged and condemned, although people young and old still experience physical and sexual violence, harassment and persecution. Physical violence need not involve another person: self-harm occurs when people inflict pain or injury upon themselves and may be considered a form of inappropriate touch.

Inappropriate touch Touch that is unwanted or of questionable intent.

Those who are given licence to touch in the course of their work have complex responsibilities. Not only are there shifting boundaries around who can and who cannot touch, but there are also considerations of the context, necessity and technical application of touch by the practitioner. Add to this the history and prior experiences of the giver and receiver, and the difficulties of navigating this complex social interaction are apparent. In the past, orthodox practitioners created rituals and cultural practices (like wearing white coats, working within hospitals and using special language that was reserved for those with special training) to sidestep many of these complex social tensions around touch. Latterly, however, society has shown an eagerness to dispense with these traditional practices, and has encouraged practitioners to look, talk and behave more like the people they serve, as well as leave their hospital wards and move out into the community.

With this change in the power dynamic between professionals and the lay public, a greater uncertainty has emerged about who can touch, when and where it can happen, and, indeed, when it is good or bad. Touch, like other aspects of the interactions between practitioners and patients or clients, requires consent and an appreciation of the appropriateness and potential interpretation of it.

Touch and human well-being

To be human and to be alive is to be in touch. We might well ask: 'Would we be able to survive without a sense of touch?' Clearly, people who have had neurological impairments—like spinal cord injuries and strokes—lack some ability to sense touch, but they survive regardless and often prosper. Equally, there are many that shy away from touch because it is hurtful or destructive, but they still come into contact with surfaces (chairs, beds, floors etc.) at every moment of their lives, and so have no choice but to move through a world of touch. All humans exist in a world of touch and navigate their way through it. In many ways, touch is the most dynamic sense, in that it brings people—literally and figuratively—into contact with the world and one another. It is vital that people engaging with the public in the provision of health care and disability support services grasp the complexity and importance of touch for others.

There are many issues to consider in relation to touch, including culture, touch through the lifespan, communication and professional practice. An understanding, curiosity and respect for the complexity of touch and its remarkable power to hurt and to heal is essential to good communication.

CASE STUDY 16.1

Touch in practice

Think of a situation in your own practice where you would need to touch another person physically. Now, follow this exercise as a way to show just how much the success of that experience depends on the context you find yourself in.

1 Keep the 'encounter' as it is, but imagine it takes place in a village in sub-Saharan Africa. You no longer have the white clinic room, or the technical equipment, but a dirt floor and a mud hut.

2 Now, remove the protection you carry as a health practitioner (your uniform, training and discipline). You are now just a neighbour.

3 Now ask yourself how your touch would be different.

Try to list at least five changes you would have to make given the new situation you find yourself in.

The purpose of such a task (and it is one you can simulate for any number of aspects of your practice) is to make you think the elements of touch that you might otherwise dismiss.

Touch is—on the one hand—so obvious and everyday it is easy to ignore its complexity and power. Practitioners need to be mindful of the value of it.

{ SUMMARY }

This chapter has considered the cultural significance of touch, the role of touch in technology and touch throughout the lifespan, and its role in defining professional practice. Touch is an essential component in practice and also plays a key role in communication. It is critical to have a broad appreciation of the power of touch—regardless of whether it is used as a primary mode of healing, or incidentally in the routine act of their everyday practice. Touch has profound significance for people, culture and society, and is able to profoundly impact on health and well-being. It is imperative that people working in the health care and disability support sector have a sound appreciation of the power and importance of touch, and equally that they are able to reflect on their practice and interactions in terms of appropriateness.

REFLECTION POINTS

16.1 Intention (motivation, message, meaning, emotion)

How does purposeful touch differ from other forms of casual touch?

16.2 Reception (received message, response, feedback)

How would you gain feedback in regard to whether touch is perceived as welcome or unwelcome?

16.3 Perception (style, manner, impression, analysis)

How does our use of touch help to define us as professionals?

QUESTIONS FOR REVIEW

1 How has touch influenced our culture as humans?
2 What role does touch play in modern technology?
3 How do children, adults and the elderly experience touch differently?
4 How can the language of touch help us express our feelings?

REFERENCES

Calvert, R. N. (2002). *The history of massage: An illustrated survey from around the world*. Rochester, NY: Inner Traditions/Bear & Company.

Lawler, J. (1991). *Behind the screens: Nursing, somology, and the problem of the body*. London, UK: Churchill Livingstone.

Nouwen, H. J. M. (1990). The *road to daybreak: A spiritual journey*. New York, NY: Doubleday.

Oerton, S. (2004). Bodywork boundaries: Power, politics and professionalism in therapeutic massage. *Gender, Work and Organization, 11*(5), 544–65.

WEBSITES

DePauw University Touch and Emotion Lab: www.depauw.edu/learn/lab
General Council for Massage Therapies (UK): www.gcmt.org.uk
Massage New Zealand: www.massagenewzealand.org
University of Miami Touch Research Institute: www6.miami.edu/touch-research

{17}

Media

Greg Treadwell

CHAPTER OVERVIEW

This chapter covers the following topics:

+ Principles of openness
+ Types of media
+ The business model
+ The effect on news
+ Censorship
+ Access, citizen journalism and the digital divide.

KEY TERMS

Mainstream media
Democracy
Freedom
Convergence
Multimedia
Broadcast
Digital revolution
Narrowcast
Internet
Business model
Censorship
Propaganda
News values
Citizen journalism
Agenda setting
Digital divide

> ***Were it left to me to decide whether we should have a government without newspapers, or newspapers without a government, I should not hesitate a moment to prefer the latter.***
>
> *Thomas Jefferson*

> ***From Gutenberg to Twitter, mankind has been chronicling itself for posterity.***
>
> *US journalist Christina Guerrero*

Anyone considering the media in the world's liberal democracies today has to do so against the background of fundamental and rapid change that the communications industry is experiencing. It is hard to provide cosy, reliable analysis of the media's role in contemporary society because the changes taking place before our eyes are so rapid and significant, and may well fundamentally affect that role. To generalise, the numbers of journalists employed in traditional newsrooms are shrinking as the **mainstream media**'s income from selling advertising decreases and the growth of digital media continues exponentially. Both advertisers and readers/viewers are heading online where the action is, leaving traditional media behind. More qualitative evidence, perhaps, tells us that a relatively sudden decline in the fortunes of 'old media' markets across the world, after decades of strong growth, is threatening democratically significant journalism (Ellis, 2010; McChesney & Nicholls, 2010; Hirst, 2010). Global media companies are cutting the resources they put into producing journalism, and this must, to some degree, imperil the expected norms of social and political life. In ironic counterpoint, many so-called developing countries, including some in Aotearoa New Zealand's own backyard, have a media crisis of their own as ideologies of access and **democracy** fail for multiple reasons, and political regimes hostile to openness reject transparency as a prerequisite for government.

Mainstream media The prevailing information sources that are available to and accessed by the public, including network television and large-circulation newspapers.

Democracy A system of government in which the majority of the people hold the power to decide.

Principles of openness

Key to having a safe place in the world today is knowing what is going on. The media, for all its sins, is the network that gives us that knowledge and helps to create that safe place. It is a semi-amorphous zone in which those societies with the necessary constitutional, political and legislative structures in place to guarantee **freedom** of speech enjoy a free exchange of ideas. The media are where communications and politics meet in any open society. Free speech is so fundamental to our idea of freedom that in post-world-war 1948, the United Nations enshrined the principle in Article 19 of its Universal Declaration of Human Rights: 'Everyone has the right to freedom of opinion and expression; this right includes freedom to hold opinions

Freedom Living with choice and without fear, coercion or restraint on beliefs or behaviour.

without interference and to seek, receive and impart information and ideas through any media and regardless of frontiers' (United Nations, 1948).

Indeed, the first amendment to the US constitution, contained in the Bill of Rights, had done very much the same thing generations before. Among other things, such as the right to peaceful assembly, it guaranteed the all-important freedoms of speech and of the press. In early colonial days in Aotearoa New Zealand, the press was a feisty force but subject, nevertheless, to laws of libel and contempt of court.

CASE STUDY 17.1

Official information

As the colony of New Zealand modelled itself on the Westminster (British) system of government, it also employed the prerogatives given to, and the restrictions placed on, the mother country's media.

It was not until 1982 that a fundamental shift took place in New Zealanders' expectations of government accountability, with the introduction of the Official Information Act, which gave reporters and other citizens a mechanism by which they could expect and demand access to the vast majority of information held by the government. This represented a hugely significant change in philosophy away from its predecessor, the Official Secrets Act, which was an act enabling secrecy by the government and limited access to official information by the public.

By comparison, the new Act's purposes were radical:

(a) to increase progressively the availability of official information to the people of New Zealand in order

- **(i)** to enable their more effective participation in the making and administration of laws and policies; and
- **(ii)** to promote the accountability of Ministers of the Crown and officials,

and thereby to enhance respect for the law and to promote the good government of New Zealand:

(b) to provide for proper access by each person to official information relating to that person:

(c) to protect official information to the extent consistent with the public interest and the preservation of personal privacy.

New Zealand Legislation (2011)

While these so-called rights to information and free speech may be fundamental in theory, globally they are not very widespread in practice. Reporters Without Borders, an active advocate for press freedom, regularly publishes a map outlining how well each country matches up to its expectations of the provision of such liberties. A quick glance at the 2011 version confirms that real freedom of the press is a precious and rare thing. Aotearoa New Zealand is among a small number of countries to be coloured white and accorded the highest status of 'Good Situation' (see Figure 17.1).

FIGURE 17.1 *Freedom of the press worldwide, 2011*

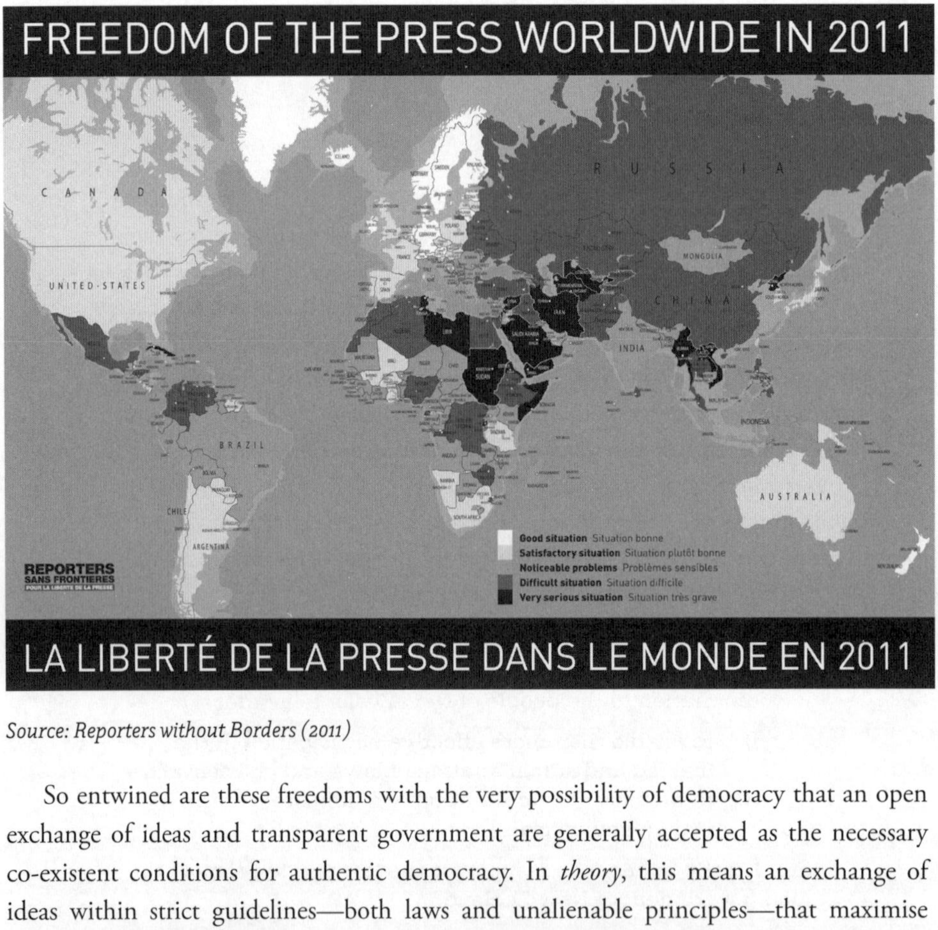

Source: Reporters without Borders (2011)

So entwined are these freedoms with the very possibility of democracy that an open exchange of ideas and transparent government are generally accepted as the necessary co-existent conditions for authentic democracy. In *theory*, this means an exchange of ideas within strict guidelines—both laws and unalienable principles—that maximise the likelihood of positive outcomes for those involved or otherwise scrutinised in the media's daily furore. In New Zealand media, practitioners operate according to industry-developed codes of ethical practice and have watchdogs, such as the Press Council and the Broadcasting Standards Authority, to censure them when necessary. As well, defamation and contempt of court laws are there to protect against poor behaviour by media. In *reality*, however, the news media are subjected to often damning scrutiny from many quarters for having breached standards of independence, impartiality, quality and good taste. These charges come from politicians, from media studies academics and former journalists, from its own increasingly involved audience and from its own practitioners, all of whom question the way it goes about its business. Journalistic ethics are famous for rating little better with the public than those of used-car salesmen. Those seeking power usually cry foul at their treatment, while academics condemn the media for its multiple failings, including its inherent function of legitimising power imbalances, in all their varied forms, between people. As for the quality of the news these days, it seems almost every day that discussion of this issue takes place somewhere. On nz.herald.co.nz, a reader commented under a column about the media: 'Sure, you can get up at 9 o'clock on a Sunday morning in an atempt [sic] to get the answers to some of the important political and economic issues of the day, but the timeslot is itself symbolic of where journalism is at and what the modern media's priorities are' (Drinnan, 2010). At the top, the introduction by the columnist (in news-story format) read: 'An academic critic of New Zealand media says journalism is "heading for hell in a handbasket"' (Drinnan, 2010).

The criticism just keeps coming, which is good—the relationship between media consumers and their suppliers needs to be a strongly critical one, for there must also be checks and balances on the power and influence of the media. Increasingly, people seem to be asking who is watching the watcher; in many ways, the media has never been under so much scrutiny. Freedom of speech and freedom of information are the ideologies of democracy and if the very things considered prerequisites for any notion of self-government are threatened by the failure of the commercial model delivering them, then trouble would most certainly be afoot.

Types of media

The term 'media' these days covers a **convergence** of multiple platforms, myriad types of message with innumerable purposes, and an array of media professionals and non-professionals producing content in often quite dissimilar working environments. Radio stations also use the web to stream content, newspapers have ever-more dynamic and interactive online presences complementing their hard-copy editions, and television stations now provide content post-broadcast on demand via the web. Journalists are increasingly expected to be able to produce and edit news content for more than one platform: reporters who plan to have a long career writing solely for newspapers like their dear old dad did are going to be disappointed. Already, newsrooms around the world are producing content for multiple platforms and have significantly advanced news selection processes to take advantage of the variety of formats. For example, editorial executives in large newsrooms will now decide, perhaps in consultation with reporters, which platform each story is best suited to. Dramatic news, for example, is surely heading for publication on the internet and as quickly as possible. Even then, after an initial newsbreak, editors will need to decide how best to create a package for

Convergence The point at which ideas meet or come together.

its expansion. Their aim is to produce a whole from complementary (or *interlocking*) parts. These parts include an ever-increasing array of display mechanisms for delivery and discussion of digital news content:

+ headlines and text—both rich with hyperlinking possibilities
+ audio—both raw tracks and packaged soundscapes
+ video—both raw footage and packaged items
+ still photography—enhanced by slide-show technologies and audio enhancement
+ information graphics—usually highly dynamic
+ various levels of reader contribution—comment, interaction and feedback.

The online editor of today looks at their resources (the content submitted by journalists and readers/viewers) and the mix of avenues they have at their disposal for its dissemination and discussion (technologies). The decisions they make are of a new and developing class in the world of journalism. Sub-editors on newspapers make similar packaging decisions concerning the use of text blocks, pictures, graphics and so on as they lay out the pages of tomorrow's paper. But the **multimedia** package under development by news sites is often viewed as three-dimensional, compared with the two-dimensional, one-way narratives of old media like newspapers. It is three-dimensional both because it is delivered in multiple formats—a combination of text, audio and video—and because a reader is not necessarily limited to starting the story at its text component's beginning. Hyperlinking makes it perfectly possible that the reader/viewer has arrived in the middle of a story, or even in the comments generated by readers at the end, rather than at the reporter's carefully crafted introduction. These concepts are challenging the old ways of storytelling across society.

Multimedia The combined use of various types of media (text, graphics and animation) in any given context or situation.

Indeed, not so long ago, the term 'media' pretty much meant radio, newspapers and television to New Zealanders. Today, the internet, fast-growing social networking and an ever-growing array of mobile and handheld touch-screen devices cannot be excluded. Until recently, those who produced news for the media could (fairly) safely be called journalists—based in print or **broadcast** delivery on a one-to-many model, which was supported successfully for much of the twentieth century by healthy growth in advertising sales. Now the broader definition of media also encompasses an array of new media professionals, bloggers and commentators who contribute in other ways, and amateur photographers and videographers who have taken to uploading content to social and other media. Some argue it also includes those who sort through online content, rating it on social media sites, ordering it, aggregating it and, in a sense, republishing it—or at least creating innumerable ways to access it. Somewhere, amid this still-emerging morass of communicators who have widely varying intentions and communication skills, sits the media that those aged over 25 grew up with: the mainstream media, now dubbed the MSM by commentators on digital media.

Broadcast Transmission to the general population, as in television or radio.

The MSM became quite used to its privileged, authoritative position—given to it by the unilateral direction of its communication and reinforced through the repetition of cultural norms—but for some time now, the MSM has had to adapt to survive the onslaught of the **digital revolution**.

Digital revolution
The radical change to digital technology enabling widespread access to information and technology.

The business model

It can be argued that the development of the mass media over the twentieth century (the one-to-many model of communication) came with the failures inherent in the commodification of news; for example, sensationalism, a focus on what sells rather than what is important, and ultimately a corporatisation of the power associated with knowledge and its dissemination. However, the current shift we are experiencing to so-called **narrowcast** publishing (the many-to-one and peer-to-peer models of communication) brings with it its own thorny set of issues. Consider, for example, the credibility of the information that flows through our constantly active social and media networks, now the digital revolution has arrived. It may not be reasonable in this context to expect accuracy from daily news media, or even to identify who was responsible for errors. The speed with which reporters now have to file their stories for online publication—and the shrinking resources for copy editing, fact-checking and other quality-assurance mechanisms—are often blamed for inevitable accuracies in online journalism. In the digital world, information flows in countless directions at the same time and it is often impossible to trace the origin of any particular message. Add to that the potential for the message to be moderated any number of times along the chain, and the lack of accountability for its veracity becomes clear. Should they want to be a responsible citizen, the onus increasingly is on the news consumer to find the reliable news brands—which are not always the tried and true—among the increasingly kaleidoscopic information markets.

Narrowcast
Transmission to an identified or limited group within the general public, as in digital platforms.

But perhaps the biggest issue facing this new type of journalism is just how media companies are going to pay for it. Budget cuts and staff layoffs have characterised newspaper and other media workplaces across many developed nations, including Australasia, in 2011. A period of soaring profits in worldwide media conglomerates has come sharply to an end and long-established newspapers across the USA are being closed down. New Zealand journalist and researcher Gavin Ellis (2010) predicts some short-term recovery, but adds that news media will now 'return very average profit margins that will not make them particularly attractive to investors'. In 2008, the share value of Australian media companies, which own most of New Zealand's media, fell by 50 per cent. In response to a declining revenue stream, thanks in part to the mass migration of classified advertising to the web, media corporations reached for the scalpel:

> The cost cutting saw many editorial budgets slashed to the bone. Newsrooms found that company accountants, who had been making their presence felt for more than a decade, had become sabre-wielding hussars. The picture was the same wherever one looked. In the United States, total newspaper employment has dropped to 1949 levels. The 2010 American *State of the News Media* report … estimated that the number of reporting and editing positions on American papers dropped by 27 per cent between 2007 and 2009. In Britain one group alone shed 2500 staff. In New Zealand, Fairfax, APN, TVNZ and MediaWorks cut staff including journalists. In Australia the number of fulltime journalists is estimated to have declined by 13 per cent between 2001 and 2008. The effect on journalism has become obvious.
>
> *Ellis (2010)*

Internet The electronic means (and protocols) to connect computer users to information from a vast array of sources.

Associated with, and perhaps inseparable from, this accelerating decline is the migration of readers to the **internet**, where news is fast and free but does not in any way attract enough advertising to support fundamentally sound journalism. How, then, did newspapers end up putting much of their news online for no financial reward? In the late 1990s, when they first moved content online, it was pretty much yesterday's news. After all, their main business was publishing newspapers—and if people read it first online, well, they might not buy the newspaper. However, pressure quickly built to take advantage of the immediacy of the web. It was becoming increasingly ridiculous to not publish information immediately; in fact, it was verging on anti-journalism. It was also becoming increasingly dangerous to hold a story because competitors were likely to take the scoop.

In 2006, the *Guardian*, in Britain, announced it would publish first to the web and not hold important news for the following day's paper (Fletcher, 2006). It was a defining moment because the *Guardian* was a leader in the world of online news and it signalled a clear shift in direction. There were protests (Greenslade, 2006b), but other newspapers followed. The move to publishing much, if not all, of a newsroom's hard-won content on the internet without charge was soon complete. Newspapers had done their best, if belatedly, to cut their internet-only rivals off at the pass—but in so doing had committed to online provision of content before they had a **business model** to support it. The mood seemed to be: get online and work out how to pay for it later. Some attribute much of the difficult situation now faced by newspapers to this 'mistake'; that there is still no proven business model some five years later may well give them confidence in this view. However, more astute commentators have pointed out that newspapers were in trouble before this: circulations have been in decline for various reasons for years.

Business model The concepts that underpin the ideals to make money.

Strong demand for advertising that returned healthy profits eventually meant that multinationals came to own media companies all over the world. In Aotearoa New Zealand, two Australian companies, Fairfax and Australian Provincial Press (APN), own most newspapers and many radio stations. Advertising sustained the increasingly corporate model for providing journalism during the twentieth century—at least until the current so-called media crisis and global economic recession. Now questions are being asked about its sustainability and just where the replacement business model that will sustain the online journalism of the future might be. News online simply does not provide enough income. Moves are afoot, most visibly by Rupert Murdoch's News Corp, to try to change that with the introduction of paywalls on key sites. These block access to content the publisher believes people will be prepared to pay for and enable micropayments (or similar) to access that content. Critics have pointed out that locking out willing readers through the establishment of paywalls will just drive them to the many other sites that offer free online content—including news in all its guises. Most people will be satisfied with what they can access for nothing, even if some websites are claiming to have content worth paying for.

The effect on news

The economic model that gave life to news in the twentieth century has faltered across the starting line of the twenty-first century, and looks like asphyxiating. The future of journalism is placed in very real doubt by this development and people from all walks are saying it. Christopher Warren (2010), Federal Secretary of the Media, Entertainment & Arts Alliance in Australia, viewed an initiative by Australian media companies to roll out iPad applications for their newspapers as a positive step. But he said the real question was not one of business models, but journalism:

> How can we ensure that journalism's core functions will be maintained: holding the powerful accountable for their actions, providing a voice for those who otherwise have no power and ensuring that our political servants fulfil the pledges they make to us when we elect them to office? These are the key jobs that journalism performs. If those jobs can no longer be performed, Australian democracy is in trouble.
>
> *Warren (2010, p. 3)*

And it is not just union leaders and academics who have come to this conclusion. A report called *The Evolution of News and the Internet* concluded that newspapers in OECD countries 'face increased competition (free dailies, internet, multiple television and radio sources) and often declining advertising revenues, titles and circulation, as well as declining readership' (OECD 2009, p. 7) and that the global economic meltdown has accelerated the trend: 'While the newspaper industry is experimenting with new distribution models, the economic crisis and related fall in advertising revenues have accentuated the downward spiral of many forms of printed news. The economic foundations of journalism have to be rethought' (OECD 2009, p. 12).

In 2006, Professor Roy Greenslade, from London's City University, said the following at a conference at the Auckland University of Technology:

> Overall, what I want to make abundantly clear is that the key issue for all of us—citizen and journalist, politician and academic, young and old—is not so much the future of newspapers as the future of journalism. We must not allow ourselves to be blinded by technology and the variety of delivery platforms from the continuing need to carry out our essential task: holding the people in power to account. We must engage with the enhanced democracy of the digital age to ensure that the journalism of 2050 is more vibrant, more penetrating, more questioning and, ultimately, more beneficial for the citizens of the world than it is today.
>
> *Greenslade (2006a)*

There is no doubt about the seriousness of the issues facing the mainstream media: the so-called public forum on which the health of any democracy is utterly dependent.

Censorship

Censorship
Judgments about the suitability of, and access to, information and media content.

Censorship is the antithesis of free speech. Political regimes that deny their peoples the right to free speech have to resort to some level of censorship to ensure the media are not propagating anti-government sentiments. Examples of autocratic censorship litter human history and are still widespread. In Fiji, for example, leaders of the military government that took power in a 2006 coup installed government censors in the newsrooms of the islands' media to make sure anti-government opinion was not published. In other countries around the world, including the Pacific, censorship may not be that explicit—it may simply be that journalists have accepted the informal message that anti-government stories will not be tolerated. Of course, this is still censorship. According to Reporters Without Borders (2011), in 2010 there were fifty-seven journalists killed and 153 imprisoned for their journalistic work around the world.

But there are other types of censorship that are even less explicit and that operate in democracies that are supposedly alive and well. These forms of determining what is and is not published in our news media are tied up in the structures that form the media and its corporate owners, and the nature of news work itself. According to theorists working in this area, journalists constantly 'self-censor' their work to make sure it fits with the expectations of their editorial managers and, indeed, the owners of the media organisation that employs them. In theory, there should be no connection between the publisher and the reporters in any news organisation, so that readers or viewers can be confident the news agenda is not being shaped by the self-interest of the company that publishes it. However, in reality this is not so simple. Reporters, argue the theorists, work within the expected norms of their practice and these very boundaries limit the type of news that is produced. A story that either does not support the ideological orientation of the news organisation or hurts its attempt at profit-making for its owners or shareholders is far less likely to be published than other stories. Other so-called 'norms' of the profession—from the constant use of official sources for news to the shape of the daily news cycle (what do we have time and resources to cover?)—help to shape decisions on what can and cannot be published.

In a still wider circle of theory, the media are seen as an inherent part of keeping in place society's existing structures and the powerful people who sit on top of them, even if reporters working on the ground say their job is to question everything. Most famous in this area are Herman and Chomsky (1994), who borrow a term from journalist and intellectual Walter Lippmann when they describe the media as 'manufacturing consent' for the dominant ideologies and social structures within which they work:

> Leaders of the media claim that their news choices rest on unbiased professional and objective criteria and they have support for this contention in the intellectual community. If, however, the powerful are able to fix the premises of discourse, to decide what the general populace is allowed to see, hear and think about, and to 'manage' public opinion by regular **propaganda** campaigns, the standard view of how the system works is at serious odds with reality.
>
> *Herman and Chomsky (1994, p. xi)*

Propaganda Information designed to further a cause, while damaging another one.

To put it another way: 'Although journalists do not set out to report the news so that the existing politico-economic system is maintained, their professional norms end up producing stories that implicitly support the existing order' (Soloski, 1997, p. 152).

According to such sociological perspectives, what generally constitutes news is to some degree predetermined by the mutually agreed work procedures journalists must undertake to work in the media; for example, covering today's court cases or meeting tomorrow's deadline. So-called **news values** like proximity (nearness), novelty (newness) and negativity (bad news), which reporters use to evaluate their stories, also come under scrutiny in such an approach to the media. Berkowitz (1997, p. xi) points out such values are constructed through an informal consensus between journalists over time and, in fact, do not exist at all in their stories outside that context.

News values The criteria used to identify the merit of a story (for example, proximity, novelty and negativity).

Access, citizen journalism and the digital divide

Digital-savvy citizens thriving on broadband speeds now enjoyed in the developed world are engaged in our communications storm in ways that simply were not possible in the now-defunct analogue era. They are not just reading the paper or rushing home to catch the news; they are reading, watching and commenting on pretty much whatever they like, wherever they like and at whatever time of day suits them. At work, at home, at the airport, outside the library (even when it is closed), on the bus or ferry—access to the media has never be so easy and publishing never so cheap. At the turn of the millennium, there were almost 361 million users of the internet worldwide (Internet usage statistics, 2011). At the time of writing the same source declared there were more than 1.96 billion internet users on the planet in 2010, a growth rate over a decade of more than 444 per cent. Another source (Pingdom, 2011) provides data for 2010 that reveals 152 million blogs being published (up 26 million from 2009), 25 million tweets (microblogging messages) sent every day and more than three billion photos uploaded to Facebook each month. YouTube now serves up two billion videos a day.

Citizen journalism The involvement of members of the public (rather than journalists) in the process of reporting and presenting information to others.

People who feel disenchanted with, or disenfranchised by, the mainstream media—such as Dan Gillmor, author of *We the Media: Grassroots Journalism by the People for the People* (2006)—celebrate the development of this so-called **citizen journalism** for its perceived ability to challenge the corporate-based status quo of the media, or at least to provide an alternative to it. Digital technologies are turning the once-passive consumer of news and information into an active, responding, contributing and, ultimately, publishing member of a new, interactive media landscape. Through ever-active social networks, microblogging, blogging, postings to other websites, eyewitness accounts and amateur footage—and through the ranking, rating and hyperlinking of news and information—people are contributing media content in numbers and ways that were impossible just a few years ago. The argument goes that if access to the technologies of the media is much more universal, then the freedom of information at the heart of democracy must be invigorated. News corporations, with their self-interest as an unavoidable given, have skewed the news agenda when its own interests conflict with the wider interests of community. Now citizens who perceive this to be the case can comment directly and even influence that news agenda:

Agenda-setting The process of managing information to achieve political impact.

> The citizen journalism movement does not signal the end of **agenda-setting** by professional or elite media organizations. Such institutions still break *and* frame a large proportion of the news stories circulating through the online sphere and this is unlikely to change in the foreseeable future. But those

> institutions must now vie for attention in competition with a diverse range of alternative news sources, from hyperlocal sites to unofficial and untamed celebrity gossip sites (news media dealing in scandal and salacious rumor-mongering can now be beaten at their own game by online sites more free of ethical and even legal constraints than they).
>
> *Goode (2009, p. 1293)*

In terms of communicating in the public sphere, it is certainly true that never before has the ordinary citizen had such access to the seat of power, but that access does not in any way guarantee a homogeneity of response. The term 'citizen journalism' encompasses an array of enterprises from journalism that is a real alternative to the mainstream media to the 30 seconds of fame available to the public that masquerades as important user-generated content on mainstream sites like CNN's iReport. At one end of a different scale sits OhMyNews, the world-famous Korean site for motivated and productive citizen journalism that now has 30,000 contributors (Hirst, 2010, p. 109), while at the other end is 'Ms Solo Citizen of Anytown', faithfully publishing her weekly blog on community issues. Citizen journalism takes many forms, and each makes its own quite different contribution to the mediascape. The term is so widely used for a range of different media enterprises that it is dangerous not to be more specific when talking about the public interest role of the media. And it is foolhardy to celebrate such access as universally beneficial to democracy when it is often provided by untrained reporters with little understanding of the requisite detachment for professional journalism. Indeed, goes the counter-argument, if legions of so-called citizen reporters are doing the work that paid, trained and experienced journalists once did under scrutiny and professional standards, then that can hardly be good for democracy.

Of course, issues of access can be approached from a completely different angle, and here, no matter how citizen journalism is viewed, access to contemporary digital and global communication technologies are restricted to less than 30 per cent of the world's population (Internet usage statistics, 2011). Internet 'penetration' stands at 77.4 per cent in North America but just 10.9 per cent in Africa. In between are Europe (58.4 per cent), Oceania and Australia (61.3 per cent), the Middle East (29.8 per cent) and Asia (21.5 per cent). This **digital divide** remains hauntingly in the background as digital utopians in the West celebrate citizen journalism: 'The concept of the digital divide provides a reality check when considered against the "techno-enthusiasm" of those who over-sell the democratic potential of online participation and Web 2.0 technologies' (Hirst, 2010, p. 45).

Digital divide The gap between people with electronic (internet) access and those that do not have it.

Returning to the Reporters Without Borders map of media freedom (Figure 17.1), it is clear that the state of open media in much of the world is in horrific contrast to that with which the intellectuals of the developed world are dissatisfied.

{ SUMMARY }

The media performs a role critical to the functioning of any open society. In its absence, or if it is performing that role poorly through under-resourcing or intimidation by authorities, the heart of that democracy will be missing. Progressive freedom of information mechanisms in Aotearoa New Zealand have ensured a society that values and supports openness and the right to free speech, though such 'rights' are extremely limited within a global context. While we can be pleased with the freedom of New Zealand's media, in another context sociologists point to the very nature of our corporate media—and the roles and routines its reporters carry out—as evidence for journalism's implicit support of existing social organisation and power structures and its inability to authentically challenge them.

Western media are in such a state of change as they deal with fundamental threats to the advertising-supported business model that has delivered journalism for more than a century, plus the exponential growth of online media that is drawing readers but not advertisers. Some argue journalism must be reinvented and new ways found to deliver it. Whatever the outcome, we can be sure change is already under way.

REFLECTION POINTS

17.1 Intention (motivation, message, meaning, emotion)

How might freedom of information be both a 'good' and 'bad' thing when related to dissemination of information on health?

17.2 Reception (received message, response, feedback)

Given open access to information via the internet, what are the implications of this for practitioners?

17.3 Perception (style, manner, impression, analysis)

Should health information on the internet be relegated? If so, how might this occur? Alternatively, could people be taught to be more 'digitally literate' and what might this involve?

QUESTIONS FOR REVIEW

1 What does living in a free society really mean in the early part of the twenty-first-century society?

2 In terms of communication, how better off are those living in liberal democracies than those living in developing countries? What challenges does the media in each 'type' of society face?

3 Can the media ever really question the fundamentals of a society that provides the economic base for journalism?
4 What might the business model for journalism look like at the end of the twenty-first century?

REFERENCES

Berkowitz, D. (ed.) (1997). *Social meanings of news*. Thousand Oaks, CA: Sage Publications Inc.

Drinnan, J. (2010). *Good journalism versus evil market*. Retrieved 21 February 2011 from www.nzherald.co.nz/nz/news/article.cfm?c_id=1&objectid=10655864.

Ellis, G. (2010 August). *Paying the Piper*. Paper presented as part of the series: The end(s) of journalism? Seminar conducted at the University of Auckland, New Zealand.

Fletcher, K. (2006) Web trail. *Guardian*. Retrieved 1 October 2006 from www.guardian.co.uk/technology/2006/jun/12/news.mondaymediasection?INTCMP=SRCH.

Gillmor, D. (2006). *We the media: Grassroots journalism by the people for the people*. Sebastopol, CA: O'Reilly Media.

Goode, L. (2009). Social News, citizen journalism and democracy. *New Media and Society, 11*, 1287–305.

Greenslade, R. (2006a). Untitled. Keynote address presented at Journalism Downunder: The future of the media in the digital age. Auckland, New Zealand.

Greenslade, R. (2006b). Print first, web second, says Independent's Kelner. *Guardian*. Retrieved 24 February 2011 from www.guardian.co.uk/media/greenslade/2006/jul/20/printfirstwebsecondsaysin?INTCMP=SRCH.

Herman, E. & Chomsky, N. (1994). *Manufacturing consent—The political economy of the mass media*. London, UK: Vintage.

Hirst, M. (2010). *News 2.0—Can journalism survive the internet?* Sydney, NSW: Allen & Unwin.

Internet usage statistics. (2011). *Internet world stats: Usage and population stats*. Retrieved 27 February 2011 from www.internetworldstats.com/stats.htm.

McChesney, R. & Nicholls, J. (2010). *The death and life of American journalism—The media revolution that will begin the world again*. New York, NY: Nation Books.

New Zealand Legislation. (2011). *Official Information Act 1982*. Retrieved from www.legislation.govt.nz/act/public/1982/0156/latest/DLM65364.html#DLM65364.

OECD (2009). *The evolution of news and the internet: The Organisation for Economic Co-operation and Development's Working Party on the Information Economy*. Retrieved from www.oecd.org/dataoecd/30/24/45559596.pdf.

Pingdom (2011). *Internet 2010 in numbers*. Retrieved 28 February 2011 from http://royal.pingdom.com/2011/01/12/internet-2010-in-numbers.

Reporters Without Borders. (2011). *Press freedom barometer—Journalists killed*. Retrieved 28 February 2011 from http://en.rsf.org/press-freedom-barometer-journalists-killed.html?annee=2010.

Soloski, J. (1997). News reporting and professionalism: Some constraints on reporting the news. In D. Berkowitz (ed.), *Social meanings of news* (pp. 138–54). Thousand Oaks, CA: Sage Publications Inc.

United Nations (1948). *Universal Declaration of Human Rights*. Retrieved from www.un.org/en/documents/udhr/index.shtml.

Warren, C. (2010). *Life in the clickstream II—The future of journalism*. Sydney, NSW: Media, Entertainment & Arts Alliance.

WEBSITES

Citizen Journalism: Global Perspectives: http://citizenjournalism.me

List of Citizen Journalism Websites: www.sourcewatch.org/index.php?title=List_of_citizen_journalism_websites

The Pros and Pros of 'Citizen Journalism', the Online Journalism Review: www.ojr.org/ojr/people/stverak/201003/1830

{18}

Types of Messages

Brenda Costa-Scorse

CHAPTER OVERVIEW

This chapter covers the following topics:

+ Conversation
+ Chat
+ Gossip
+ Delivering information
+ Nice to know versus need to know
+ Difficult messages.

KEY TERMS

In-depth
Light-hearted
Candid
Continuum of care
Systematic
Patient handover

Individuals communicate with ease when messages are received or delivered without ambiguity. It is impossible to separate the delivery of information or types of messages completely from personalities, the various roles of an individual, the dynamics of the group, where the interaction is taking place, and the context or circumstances of the communication. This chapter explores the types of messages that individuals utilise to make their way in the world. Some of the types of messages may help inform, educate or enhance people's life journey, while other delivery styles and message content may hinder, frustrate, anger or hurt an individual's equilibrium. By understanding the benefits, limitations and traps of various types of messages, you will be able to develop further expertise with these communication tools.

Conversation

A conversation is informal talk between two or more people. Good conversation is the glue between people that can be described by some people as intellectually stimulating, **in-depth** or **light-hearted.** Conversation weaves people into groups. Depending on a person's status in an informal conversation, the interaction can also be associated with power dynamics.

In-depth Detailed and thorough.

Light-hearted Relaxed, happy and without fear.

The degree to which a person engages in in-depth conversation may be associated with issues of trust and confidence. Social norms generally dictate that in-depth conversation is appropriate in the context of a trusting relationship that has developed over time. On meeting a person for the first time, health practitioners have the privilege of jumping from first base to conversations that involve personal vulnerabilities. However, health practitioners sometimes miss the 'getting to know a person' preamble before the in-depth conversation. With jumps from pleasantries to in-depth communication in a short space of time, practitioners need to be mindful of how in-depth they actually need to go. For example, when assessing a person that has overdosed on prescription medications and alcohol, the paramedic or the triage nurse in an emergency department will ask, 'Have you done this before?' This direct closed question lends itself to an affirmative or a negative response. If a person responds 'Yes', this may lead to disclosure of intimate information that the person has not disclosed to those close to them. In-depth conversations have boundary issues where the conversation moves from gathering information for a diagnosis to therapeutic communications that constitute counselling.

When formalising conversation, the interaction may occur in a meeting structure. The different status of individuals in conversation may become more obvious in a meeting room where the hierarchy and social norms within a group might limit open **candid** conversation. To ensure specific topics are covered by the group, an

Candid Honest and without affectation.

agenda is often used in meetings. To make sure that a meeting was not merely a convivial conversation, meeting notes are transcribed. Often the meeting notes record action points to make sure that there are specific outputs. When you are called to attend a meeting, do you make sure that you are au fait with the topics on the agenda? To make a constructive contribution to group conversation in a meeting, it is important to strive for purposeful, well-informed conversation that ends with a clear understanding of the actions required before the next meeting.

Chat

Chat is a friendly conversation that is often brief and light-hearted. When seeking to understand another individual's point of view, the quick chat may not necessarily suit the situation. Conversely, if a person is delivering a 'need to know' message, a long explanatory conversation would not be appropriate. For example, if a dental therapist only has a brief light-hearted chat with a client about cleaning their teeth and flossing, but omits to include information on the risks associated with early gum disease, the person may be very casual about their dental hygiene. The light-hearted way the conversation was constructed may result in the message not being heard or being deemed unimportant.

Chat also may change tempo. Another example of chat is when a colleague has been pulled aside by their boss for a quick chat. The descriptor 'quick' paints a scenario that possibly this is not a friendly interaction and that the person may be reprimanded. Conversely, hearing laughter when people are chatting conveys a light-hearted picture. Have you ever sat in a public space and tried to guess what people are chatting about by looking at their body language? People are unique and communication is fascinating.

Gossip

Different types of conversations conjure up a kaleidoscope of scenes in life. Conversations that focus on the affairs of others are variously termed gossip, hearsay, idle banter, rumour, tittle-tattle and half truths. There is a long tradition within some media genres of publishing personal information that can be sensationalised and may or not be true (Deuze, 2005). The burgeoning popularity of social networking may also contribute to this type of communication as personal information and messages are passed on to wider audiences with or without consent or censure. There is possibly a constructive element to gossip where people are attempting to make sense of the nonsensical; however, the motives of people are not always kind, ethical or honourable, and gossipy messages lend themselves to mixed interpretation. The opening line of a gossipy conversation or chat may begin: 'Did you hear about …?' This type of question potentially could be associated with half truths, where one part of the discussion is factual and the rest of the information has been twisted to suit the personal needs of the person delivering the information. Some people are manipulative, so it is always worthwhile maintaining a healthy scepticism in social interactions that include idle gossip. There are two sides to every story and it is important to establish the facts and gain a balanced view.

In workplace settings, family relationships, social groups of friends or sports teams, the dynamics between people can be undermined by baseless rumour. Individuals can become disenfranchised by gossip and the power of words can derail an individual's equilibrium. When messages are passed on to others, the deliverer may abbreviate the message and take a small sound bite from the original conversation. The original content may then become distorted as it is translated by others. It is important to choose your words carefully as all words in all situations convey meaning. People often convey what they really mean (their intention) in the choice of the words they use. Cultural and social contexts provide people with the cues to interpret these word messages. When words are poorly selected, the message may be more easily misinterpreted. It is important to remember that the very fact that people can choose from a wide range of terms to convey any message means that individuals are responsible for the messages they convey; in other words, they personally decide how they construct the message. The tone of the delivery also adds different layers of meaning.

Delivering information

Communication that utilises appropriate language delivered in an appropriate format is a powerful tool. All professional groups, cultures and organisations have particular understandings of unique words that define their particular groups. Part of the process of joining any group involves developing an understanding of the language used by the group, including the history of the group and the intention of the communication style.

The environment in which people communicate always impacts on the messages and how they are sent and received (Holmes, 2000) and this is particularly important to appreciate within the context of health care and disability support (Holmes & Major, 2003). Struggling to articulate a point of view or talking past each other may thwart understanding and lead to stress. The purpose and the potential pitfalls of various types of messages that individuals can select from need to be fully understood to enhance communication.

Poor communication has been identified as a key factor in serious adverse events in the health sector in general (Lawrence, 2004) and is a feature of many cases published by

Continuum of care The provision of appropriate services over a period of time, which is relevant to the needs of individuals.

Systematic Following a planned and accepted pathway.

Patient handover The process of health practitioners giving information and giving or taking responsibility for the care of patients.

the Health and Disability Commissioner. Many investigations into adverse events highlight the importance of good delivery of information. In health care, the number of professionals involved in a person's **continuum of care** is often mind-boggling. Ensuring that continuity of care actually occurs requires accuracy in the delivery of information and also requires that the full message does not get lost when passed from person to person.

Memory joggers, mnemonics or acronyms are used to instil a **systematic** approach to communication about the patient during handover between practitioners. For example, when a paramedic is handing over a patient who has been injured in a motor vehicle accident, it is important that the emergency department triage nurse has a clear understanding of the mechanics and severity of the injury, and the working diagnosis on which pre-hospital treatment was based. How fast was the vehicle travelling? What was the point of impact? Was there any vehicle intrusion? Was the person restrained by a seatbelt? Establishing answers to these questions will provide an index of suspicion of underlying pathology and determine the next set of assessment and treatment requirements. MIST, DeMIST, SOAP and SAMPLE are memory joggers that are used to create ordered systematic communication at **patient handover** (Talbot & Bleetman, 2007):

+ MIST: Mechanisms–Injuries–Signs–Treatment
+ DeMIST: Demographic–Mechanisms–Injuries–Signs–Treatment
+ SOAP: Subjective–Objective–Assessment–Plan
+ SAMPLE: Symptoms–Allergies–Medications–Past history–Last meal–Events.

These prompts ensure that the person handing the patient over to another health practitioner covers all of the pertinent information, and that the receiving health practitioner is fully cognisant of the patient history and can build on the original patient management plan. When practitioners use the same handover system there are clear expectations of what constitutes complete communication. These systematic approaches to the patient handover reduce the risk of important information being omitted, such as severe allergic reactions to medications. Missing such important information such as allergies may clearly compromise the well-being of the injured or ill person.

Nice to know versus need to know

Communicating 'nice to know' and 'need to know' information to patients or fellow health practitioners is a balancing act. When practitioners communicate the facts to patients, they may do little to allay people's fears: the succinct delivery of 'need to know' facts may escalate anxiety in the recipient. Conversely, cutting to the chase and establishing the pertinent need to know information is essential when there are time-critical elements to the communication. A rambling long-winded conversation may switch the listener off, while in an emergency situation, overly verbose conversation may compromise patient care. A monotone delivery is another way of switching off the receiver. Ensuring sufficient 'nice to know' and 'need to know' information is passed on is a skill that needs to be fostered. Insufficient communication can be risky, as important messages may get lost. Patients rely on all members of the health-care team to communicate effectively, both with them and with others who are involved in their care. Similarly, other work places rely on clear, unambiguous communication to be productive and to foster job satisfaction.

When practitioners are communicating in life-threatening situations, communication is brief and to the point. For example, when treating a person that has lost blood from stab wounds, the key information (or 'need to know') is on the risk of volume-related shock (hypovolaemic shock). It is important that paramedics pass on information of the estimated volume of blood lost and the amount of intravenous fluids that the person has received in transit to hospital. In other words, the 'need to know' information related to fluid loss and fluid replacement informs ongoing treatment decisions. If there was no communication, an injured person might become overloaded with fluid. The impact of overload of fluids could lead to the dilution of circulating red blood cells (haemoglobin) and a reduction in the person's oxygen carrying capacity—and oxygen is essential for cell life and organ function.

There is a cause-and-effect chain in communication. If there are missing links in the chain, these communication failures could have grievous effects on the patient and prevent the practitioners entrusted with their care from doing their best.

The treatment details and the mechanism of the assault are initially the 'need to knows'. The 'nice to knows' move to 'need to knows' when the patient is stabilised and discharge decisions are being made. The circumstances in which the injuries occurred (the 'nice to knows') will clearly be very important for future holistic family-centred care. In the case of the person who had lost blood from stab wounds, descriptive information from the hysterical scene—with dogs barking and children screaming—and the reason for the assault should prompt planning for short- and medium-term health and social care. Are the children that were left at the house safe? When visiting the house, will the social worker find the dog tied up? Is it safe for the assault victim to return to their home? Are social interventions needed? What are the pressures on this family? The psychological scars might be greater than the physical wounds. If so, what other referrals are required? Understanding whether there is a history of domestic violence, and what prompted these traumatic events, will be very important to help to ensure that both the patient and their family thrive in the future.

Difficult messages

One of the most common challenges for both people receiving health services and those delivering care is the breaking of bad news. Recently diagnosed conditions that are life altering—such as diabetes or multiple sclerosis, babies born with disabilities, renal failure, terminal cancer, Alzheimer's and a myriad of other conditions—recalibrate people's perceptions of the way their future looks. These types of situations contain many difficult messages in conversations where people are constantly seeking to understand their situation. The suddenness of news of a disaster, acute injury or an illness that may be chronic or terminal generally derails people: the capacity to absorb volumes of information is not possible. Difficult messages need to be brief, informative and consistent. Messages may need to be repeated more than once, as many of the details may be lost due to an individual's emotional state. After communicating the first difficult message, it is absolutely appropriate to give people the space of silence—there is no need to fill the silences with a lot of chatter. It is important to let people recover their bearings as sad or complex news sinks in. More detailed information can be provided in the days ahead.

The final writing on this chapter took place during the tragic events of the earthquake that devastated Christchurch on 22 February 2011. This was New Zealand's second worst natural disaster (after the 1931 Napier earthquake) and the first weeks after the quake were tremendously difficult times, with the death toll climbing each day. The messages of grief were mixed with accounts of incredible fortitude, inspirational tales of survival, and stories of the generosity of the human spirit as help arrived from across Aotearoa New Zealand and the world. Hope galvanised a community and the country. As a senior lecturer who has been privileged to teach paramedics for over 20 years, 22 February was a day of difficult messages as working ambulance staff studying at the university scrambled to make contact with family and were coordinated to fly home to Christchurch with the air force and the paramedic multi-casualty response team. Of the eight Cantabrians in Auckland attending lectures that week, all were on different places of the disbelief continuum. These calamitous events encourage one to acknowledge the fortitude of emergency service colleagues in Christchurch on that day, the weeks after the quake, and the many months of aftershocks. The endeavours of all those that continue to help the Christchurch community recover in big and small ways should also be acknowledged; recovery will be a long process and resilience will be built in part by life's positive messages—be they a quick chat or an in-depth conversation.

CASE STUDY 18.1

Lawrence

Lawrence, a 28-year-old triathlete, was knocked off his bicycle by a car on the way home from work. He sustained a fractured right femur, open fractured right lower leg, facial injuries that included an unstable mandible and chipped front teeth, and mild concussion. His road to recovery involved communicating with paramedics, the police, emergency department nurses, emergency physicians, house surgeons, a phlebotomist, a radiographer, a neurologist, the dental team, an orthopaedic specialist, operating room staff, ward clerks, orthopaedic nurses, physiotherapists, occupational therapists, outpatients' clinic staff, pharmacists, a pharmacy assistant, psychologist and a general practitioner.

His lower leg wound became infected and required daily dressings during the first three weeks. He found it very difficult to concentrate in the months after the accident and was depressed during the recovery period. His return to part-time work as a civil engineer took five months and started with office project work. Lawrence returned to full-time, active, on-site work in nine months. He is yet to return to cycling, but recently started training in the swimming pool. The driver of the car was charged with reckless driving causing injury, and was found guilty. One of the paramedics who cared for Lawrence gave evidence in court. Lawrence attended the court case and although the courtroom meant reliving the horrors of the crash, it did bring some closure for Lawrence.

The various people involved with Lawrence needed to communicate about specific information that related to their 'need to know' and the context in which they were working and interacting with him. The range of communications would have included conversation and chat, and many of them would have focused on delivering information while some of them would have also involved difficult messages about diagnosis and progress. Some of these conversations would have been casual and others more formal depending on the environment (that is, the site of the accident, the hospital, the clinic or a court of law). Adapting communication to these contexts requires a degree of skill and it is important to note that at no stage would gossip be appropriate.

{ SUMMARY }

When communicators are skilled they use a number of strategies or types of messages, depending on who they are talking to and the topic of conversation. Difficult messages may need to be reframed with information delivered in different ways to provide adequate understanding. The language of practitioners or the way the message is delivered may limit injured or ill people's understanding of their condition, and may also perplex their support network of family and friends. Words alone may be insufficient—diagrams or pictures may be needed to help demystify the medical jargon and ensure message clarity. Fear of the unknown can exacerbate pain and anxiety. Practitioners need to pick up the cues that a person does not fully understand the message and patiently repeat and reinforce messages on what is known about an individual's condition. Ongoing clear communication about difficult topics is imperative as knowledge empowers people to make informed decisions about their own health.

REFLECTION POINTS

18.1 Intention (motivation, message, meaning, emotion)

Particular types of situations alter how messages are conveyed. When there are concerns of safety, what influence is this likely to have on shaping the message?

18.2 Reception (received message, response, feedback)

In an emergency situation, what factors influence how well or accurately a message might be received?

18.3 Perception (style, manner, impression, analysis)

There are significant differences in communications between friends and in communications between clients/patients and health-care professionals. In what ways might you need to alter your personal communication style to fit your professional life?

QUESTIONS FOR REVIEW

1 Is ambiguity the result of the message itself or the way the receiver interprets the message?
2 Where were you when the Canterbury earthquake occurred? What difficult message strategies from key community figures do you recall from the Canterbury earthquake or a similar recent disaster?

3 Discuss the various conversations and details required by each health practitioner involved in the case of Lawrence (Case study 16.1). Where might light-hearted chat and in-depth conversation be appropriate?

4 Working in pairs, use the case study to take turns to deliver information using a systematic approach with one of the memory joggers (for example, MIST).

REFERENCES

Deuze, M. (2005). Popular journalism and professional ideology: tabloid reporters and editors speak out. *Media, Culture and Society, 27*(6), 861–82.

Holmes, J. (2000). Victoria University's language in the workplace project: An overview. *Language in the Workplace Occasional Papers 1*. Retrieved from www.victoria.ac.nz/lals/lwp/about-us/project.aspx.

Holmes, J. & Major, G. (2003). Talking to patients: The complexity of communication on the ward. *Vision—A Journal of Nursing, 11*(17), 4–9.

Lawrence, D. M. (2004). Preoperative safety briefing project. *The Permanente Journal, 8*(2), 21–7.

Talbot, R. & Bleetman, A. (2007). Retention of information by emergency department staff at ambulance handover: Do standardised approaches work? *Emergency Medicine Journal, 24*, 539–42.

WEBSITES

Communicate: www.communicationskills.co.nz

Health and Disability Commissioner: www.hdc.org.nz

Language in the Workplace Project: http://www.victoria.ac.nz/lals/lwp

{19}

Language and Vocabulary

Sue Raleigh and Susan Shaw

CHAPTER OVERVIEW

This chapter covers the following topics:

+ Intention
+ Meaning
+ Interpretation
+ Talking with and past each other
+ Colloquial communication
+ Formal language
+ The repercussions of poor communication
+ Responsibilities.

KEY TERMS

Message
Truth
Scientific communication
Opinion
Fact
Talking with
Language
Talking past
Vibe
Colloquial

All communication involves layers of **messages**. The most obvious messages are those that are clearly stated—either in writing or speech. This level of message is probably the least likely to be misunderstood as the actual words used are indisputable, even if their meaning may be contested.

Message The information contained within communication.

Intention

One of the most common assumptions in communication is believing that we understand what people intend to convey to us—or that they understand what we are conveying. However, the perspectives from which people view or experience situations may lead them to misinterpret messages. Intention is related to notions of genuineness and **truth**. Sometimes communication is misunderstood by, or upsetting to, the person receiving it. If the sender can justify that they sent the message in good faith and did not intend to offend the other person, then the communication can be considered to have been sent with good intentions.

Truth Information that is considered honest and accurate.

If a message causes offence or distress, and there is evidence that the sender intended to disregard the feelings or perspective of the recipient, then it may be deemed to have been sent with negative intent. Intention is also conveyed in tone and body language.

The four elements of praise, prohibition, attention and comfort have been identified as being understood by infants who may be too young to understand language in detail, but who can appreciate changes in tone of voice. Thus they take meaning from the delivery rather than the content of the communication (Papousek et al., 1990). This ability to understand 'communicative intent' has also been identified in children. Nuances of communication such as pitch appear to contribute to the development of young children (Kitamura & Burnham, 2003). The importance of intention has also been applied to the development of speech-directed robotics (Breazeal & Aryananda, 2002).

CASE STUDY 19.1

Misleading the public

There are high-profile examples within Aotearoa New Zealand and Australia of people misleading the public. All three of the examples outlined below include people falsifying information or 'embellishing' their curriculum vitae (CV) to secure high-profile and highly paid public positions. In each of these cases, the intention in terms of the written communication (the CV) may have been to mislead for their own advantage.

John Davy—chief executive of Māori Television, Aotearoa New Zealand
His CV allegedly included false claims about qualifications (Smith & Abel, 2008).

Linda Astor—psychiatrist, Aotearoa New Zealand
She allegedly represented herself as a specialist psychiatrist, but claims about her qualifications and experience could not be substantiated (Bonn, 1997).

Jayant Patel—surgeon, Queensland, Australia
He represented himself as a highly skilled surgeon and carried out many procedures (with high levels of complications, including death of patients). Limitations on his practice had been imposed in the USA, and these were not disclosed (Thomas, 2007).

The intention of communication should always be to convey accurate messages in an appropriate way.

Meaning

While we may convey similar messages on a regular basis, the context in which they are delivered and in which others receive them can easily change. There are several factors that may lead us into situations in which we do not say what we mean. Sometimes this is about how we code our messages, and other times it is about humour (including irony and sarcasm).

It is common for people to believe that some messages have more importance than others and it is these messages to which the most meaning is attributed. One of the prevailing beliefs in the Western world is that scientific information is likely to be truthful. However, information that is presented as scientifically valid may not be so. The popularity of the internet and electronic means of communication has led to changes in the way in which scientific information is presented and accessed. Information that may once have only been available to a small group of colleagues is now widely available and this has impacted on the quality and style of the information. The traditional scientific approach of communicating in rather austere, cautious and inaccessible terms is being challenged by postings that sensationalise research findings on the internet (Gonzalez-Pueyo & Redrado, 2003). **Scientific communication** can be as problematic as any other approach to sharing information.

Scientific communication The formal conventions for conveying scientific information.

CASE STUDY 19.2

'Truth' in scientific communication

Apparent connections between immunisation and autism

In 1998, an article was published linking the MMR vaccine and autism. Over a period of time, Andrew Wakefield, a clinician from the United Kingdom, became 'linked' to this theory and many parents of disabled children subscribed to his claims. Following an investigation, the *British Medical Journal* exposed the information as a 'fraud' (Godlee, Smith & Marcovitch, 2011).

The 'unfortunate experiment'

The understanding, provision and evaluation of health-care services in Aotearoa New Zealand changed dramatically following the investigation into the treatment of women with cervical cancer (and its precursors) at the National Women's Hospital in Auckland. Over the years that this 'experiment' took place, academics and practitioners published articles to draw attention to various concerns, but it was the popular media that brought the issue to the attention of the public and led to the official inquiry (Bunkle, 2010; Chang, 1990; McIndoe et al., 1984; Paul, 1988).

One of the big challenges in health and disability services is to make clear distinctions between **opinion** and **fact**. Practitioners generally give opinions that are based on their knowledge and experience. Because people and their well-being are so complex, it is often difficult to give absolute information or to categorically state what may be considered 'truth'. However, the understanding of concepts of truth and opinion vary in different contexts; this is particularly apparently when legal processes seek to define 'truth' based on the 'opinion' of practitioners (Ryan, 2003).

Opinion A belief based on knowledge and considered information.

Fact Information that is based on apparent truth.

Truth needs to be considered when patients have potential complications explained to them in terms of the percentage of risk (for example, 'There is a 50 per cent chance that this procedure may be successful'). For health practitioners and scientists, this language of risk and mathematical information (such as statistics) makes sense as they deal with this sort of information on a regular basis. However, for patients this language may be very foreign and make little sense to them at all. It has been suggested that this may be addressed by using different concepts to explain hypothetical scientific risks to patients; for example, how many patients would need to receive this care for one of them to benefit (or be harmed) (Bjerre & LeLorier, 2000).

Thinking of meaning in terms of 'what matters' for any particular individual is a good way to help ensure communication is relevant to people. In terms of explaining risk, it is appropriate to assume that 'what matters' for the patient is whether or not the procedure is going to be successful. To communicate in the most appropriate terms, we would need to consider what approach to explaining this is likely to make the most sense for the patient in that situation. An individual's sense of meaning is directly linked to their experience and understanding of well-being (Fjelland, Barron & Foxall, 2008).

Communicating with people who are terminally ill is an example of a field of health care that has carefully considered meaning from the perspective of the person receiving the message. The development of these approaches has been necessary because the dynamics in other communication settings with practitioners have been found to have a tendency towards being patronising or paternalistic (Rosner, 2004; Persson & Friberg, 2009). In terms of palliative and end-of-life care, meaning is considered in relation to how people perceive the life they have led and how they view death and dying.

Interpretation

Because there is so much specialised language and jargon used in the health and scientific fields, both practitioners and service users need to have reference points from which to consider messages. These may include lists of terms and their definitions or lists of terms that may or may not be used in order to reduce confusion and assist with understanding. When people use the same language but still appear to misunderstand each other, it is often because their tools for interpretation are different. This has been referred to as 'talking past each other' (Metge & Kinloch, 1995).

The most common form of verbal communication is the conversation. This approach to communication involves a mixture of informal language, coded messages and casual interaction. The availability of mobile phones emphasises conversation as a primary medium for communication. The significance of communication is demonstrated in research that found people involved in mobile phone conversations while driving were likely to make more driving errors than those not talking on a phone. However, those who partook in emotionally charged phone calls significantly increased the dangerous elements of their driving (Dula et al., 2011). Analyses of meetings between patients and practitioners indicate that while these interactions may have formal elements, conversational rules and interpretations also occur within them (Webb, 2009).

Respecting the use of conversational communication removes many of the barriers that may exist between professionals and service users. This may be considered risky by practitioners, as some of the mystique of their practice is lost when language is simple and widely understood. But such a change in communicative focus would reduce the risk of public health messages conveying racist or other unhelpful messages (van Ryn & Fu, 2003).

Talking with and past each other

Talking with another person involves listening as well as talking. It involves taking turns and listening with care to what is said. It may require putting aside ego—remaining silent yet attentive—in order to really hear the other person. This is likely to enable the other person to feel heard and to take turns and listen. Talking with may involve changing **language** or **vocabulary** so that the other person can understand. For example, small children aged 2 or 3 would be unlikely to understand the meaning of consequence, but would probably understand: 'If you do that, you will be put in time out.' Talking with is likely to involve acknowledging the reality for the other person, and sometimes this will include asking questions. The question may be about the content of the discussion and the impact this is having on the person involved.

Talking with Genuinely engaging in conversation and interaction with another person (rather than talking to or at that person).

Language Words and the way they are used by groups of people to communicate with each other.

Talking with another person takes energy, patience, thoughtfulness and skill. Bolton (1987) suggests talking with another involves giving them full attention, considering body posture, establishing and maintaining eye contact, and communicating in an environment free from distraction. It is possible to become skilful at communicating with people. Developing this skill requires perseverance, reflection and continual practice and refinement.

Occasionally people **talk past** each other because their time is limited and they want to end the conversation as quickly as possible. The other person is likely to pick up on this **vibe**, and participate in concluding the conversation. It is possible to interact with people who do not have this awareness or who choose to deliberately ignore the vibe. If they keep talking, the risk is that the conversation may then end abruptly. On other occasions people talk past each other when they do not understand a word or phrase and do not want to seek clarification.

Talking past The tendency for people to assume they agree with one another when their messages appear consistent but the intention or meaning differ.

Vibe An informal description for the sense of meaning conveyed between people when they communicate.

Talking past another person also might occur when one person expresses a concern or worry and the second person minimises the concern. For example:

> 'I'm worried about passing my driving test.'
>
> 'You'll be fine. A car licence—it's no big deal. Sitting my test to drive a crane will be a big deal.'

The person expressing the concern does not feel heard because the listener has diverted attention to themselves. Sometimes the listener will suggest that the talker look at the facts or to not worry (Bolton, 1987). When someone talks past another, it is common to feel diminished. Being 'talked past' can make people cautious about expressing themselves and this may affect the dynamic of a relationship and future conversation. When attention is lacking, eye contact minimal, body posture uninterested or closed and the environment full of distraction, talking past each other is common.

CASE STUDY 19.3

Talking past each other

Sometimes people talk past one another, as in these examples where a health practitioner asks questions using words the patient is not familiar with, and a student ignores a term they don't understand.

Treating a fracture

A health practitioner says to a patient: 'We need to reduce the fracture, elevate and put your fractured arm into a split POP.'
In this case, the practitioner has talked past the patient before establishing what they knew. It is important to find out what a person understands before talking to them. Then we can structure the conversation to ensure understanding. The health practitioner could ask, 'Can you tell me what you think is wrong with your arm?' The patient might say, 'I think I have a broken bone after falling down front my front steps.'

The health practitioner can then use the language used by the patient 'broken bone' and explain that a broken bone is called a fracture. Talking with people is more likely to facilitate trust and ensure future interactions are open.

Understanding terminology

A student interviewing a client does not know what 'hysterectomy' means. The student ignores the word and carries on with the interview. Later the student admits to not knowing what the term means. To establish trust and mutual respect during communication, we should acknowledge when we do not know something. The client who had the hysterectomy was diagnosed with cancer and the student did not find out this vital information from the interview. Clients can usually tell if the person they are talking with does not understand, and the client is often willing to explain things. Talking with people can be enhanced by the willingness to ask questions.

Colloquial communication

In Aotearoa New Zealand and Australia there are many **colloquial** phrases. These phrases riddle our spoken language and have evolved over time following input from many people who have migrated to this part of the world. It can be very challenging for visitors to Aotearoa New Zealand and Australia to understand what we may be talking about. For example one person may say to another, 'I'll just grab my cardi then let's go to smoko' and then follow with, 'I gave my bloke a good rark up last night'. The person listening may or may not understand that 'cardi' means cardigan, 'smoko' means go for a break from work, 'bloke' means man and that 'rark up' means to give someone a telling-off. Fortunately new migrants to Aotearoa New Zealand can go online and find resources such as New Zealand Slang by the New Zealand Information Network (De Hek, n.d.), which includes information on slang. In Australia, Koala Net (2010) offers explanation of Australia slang.

Colloquial Relating to acceptable casual language that is used in everyday settings by particular groups of people (it is not as informal as slang).

CASE STUDY 19.4

Australasian colloquialisms

Some slang is common to both Aotearoa New Zealand and Australia, such as these examples:

- ankle-biter: a small child
- bludger: a lazy person
- brass razoo: not having much money
- cockie: a farmer
- cut lunch: sandwiches
- dunny: an outside lavatory
- slash: a male term for 'urinate'.

The list of slang and colloquial expression is extensive so take a squiz online.

The use of colloquial expression is also prevalent in the health care and disability support sector. The word 'munted' has come into common usage and means wrecked or damaged. In some hospitals in Aotearoa New Zealand, staff may be instructed to 'call a code'—this means that a patient has 'gone off' and possibly stopped breathing or the patient's heart may have stopped beating. Calling a code will activate a team of emergency staff, including doctors and nurses, to arrive and assess and implement interventions to attempt to resolve the crisis. When a patient is 'not crisp' or 'fragile', their health status is uncertain and could change at any time. In the not so distant past, the term 'cabbage' was used in reference to patients who had received coronary artery bypass grafts (CABG). Being a 'vegetable' was a reference to limited brain function. One of the enduring aspects of such casual language is that it tends to be disrespectful.

Many surgical interventions, medical conditions and diagnostic tests have had the name of the procedure or condition abbreviated. Surgical interventions with abbreviated names include 'TURP', which is a trans-urethral resection of the prostate gland or a 'L) THJR', which is a left total hip joint replacement. Medical conditions such as hypertension get abbreviated to 'HP', 'CAD' refers to coronary artery disease and 'GORD' stands for gastric oesophageal reflux disease. Working in health involves learning the language of the field and that of medicine, surgery, pharmacology and diagnostic interventions. These concepts are important enough to impact on levels of risk. For example, 'NBM' or 'NPM' are frequently used abbreviations and mean 'nil by mouth' or 'nil per mouth'. These messages are commonly implemented prior to surgery, and failing to understand them may lead to harm. Teams of practitioners often develop their own coded messages that relate to their work; for example, antibiotic drugs are sometimes called 'antibugs' by nursing staff when they talk to each other.

Pharmacology has many abbreviations that have their origin in Latin; for example, 'a.c.', which is Latin for *ante cibum*, and means a medication is administered before meals. Other drugs are prescribed 'p.c.', which is after meals or *post cibum*. Administering a medication three times a day is abbreviated to 't.d.s.', which in Latin is *ter die sumendum*.

Diagnostic testing in health involves many procedures and technologies. For example, a person with a suspected brain injury or abnormal growth in the brain may have computed (or computerised) axial tomography undertaken, which is colloquially referred to as a 'CAT' scan. Many people have a blood test after visiting a doctor, and the names of blood tests are commonly abbreviated, such as the test called a full blood count/complete blood count (FBC/CBC) used to check levels of red blood cells (erythrocytes), white blood cells (leucocytes) and platelets. Familiarity with all this terminology and common abbreviations develops over time; no one is expected to know all of this automatically.

Unfortunately, sometimes abbreviations have more than one meaning. For example, FBC may mean either a full blood count or a fluid balance chart. If in doubt, always write the term in full, and if unsure of what something means, then ask.

Formal language

Formal language is often part of the culture or rituals of a profession and is also used in academic contexts. Many professions use formal language: law, medicine and information technology, to name a few. Monash University (2007) in Melbourne, Australia, has developed a website that compares formal and informal language. Formal language also occurs in cultural contexts. For example, in Aotearoa New Zealand being welcomed onto a marae involves specific formal Māori language (te reo).

The legal profession makes use of formal language and is very specific about the meaning of words. Some jobs have allocated formal titles to specific roles, and the people in those roles are addressed by the formal title; for example, a judge is addressed as 'Your Honour' and a medical consultant is addressed as 'Doctor', while a surgical consultant is addressed as 'Mr'. Until recent times, every adult patient admitted to hospital was called Mr or Mrs. Now many people are relaxed about being addressed by their first or given name. It is important to give people an opportunity to say how they would like to be addressed. Some older people find it insulting to be called 'Fred' or 'Margaret' and would prefer to be 'Mr Smith' or 'Mrs Brown'. When in doubt, the more formal approach of Mr, Ms, Mrs or Miss is recommended. This can then be followed by asking the person how they prefer to be addressed. Referring to people in terms such as 'Dear' or 'Sweetie' is not recommended as it suggests a lack of regard for them as an individual.

The repercussions of poor communication

Given the emphasis on good communication, and the effort that is involved in ensuring all people receive information in respectful ways, it is appropriate to consider the impact of poor communication. There is good evidence that poor communication is not only unfortunate but also may actually cause harm to people using health and disability services. In this context, poor communication describes communication that is more than just inaccurate; rather, it relates to communication failures between professionals and those they communicate with. A vast number of complaints about the delivery of health and disability services are directly linked to poor communication.

One of the enduring challenges is managing large amounts of information within and across complex organisations. Organisational cultures often include attitudes about service users and these are reflected in the communication of the organisation. In recent years in Aotearoa New Zealand, allegations have emerged that staff within the government agency responsible for collecting tax revenue actively bullied and harassed customers (Sawyer, 1999). This agency now has a charter outlined on its website that states standards for interacting with members of the public.

The ability to identify and address mistakes is essential in large organisations, and is preferable to asserting that problems have not occurred or they are someone else's fault. There is also a need to ensure that skills about communication are included in the education of practitioners (Orgel, McCarter & Jacobs, 2010).

Staff working in oncology services often convey difficult messages to patients, such as information about whether their cancer treatment is succeeding and what the information means in terms of their life expectancy. One study found that when oncologists are talking with patients who have incurable cancer, the language used when discussing negative outcomes was more likely to be general and indirect (Rodriguez et al., 2008). Thorne, Bultz and Baile (2005) analysed existing published information about the impact of ineffective communication between patients receiving cancer care and the doctors treating them. They found that that in addition to the psychological cost to patients there was a financial cost.

CASE STUDY 19.5

Missed opportunities

During a routine audit of a residential aged-care facility, an anomaly appeared in relation to the care of one resident. His care plan outlined a potential for him to become agitated and disruptive in the evenings, and this had been identified as being linked to tiredness and boredom. There was evidence that good communication between the resident and staff during these periods, the following of routines and the use of structured and familiar activities avoided him becoming unsettled.

This resident was prescribed sedative medication to be given as required to address his agitation. An analysis of his medication chart revealed that he was not given this medication for several days at a time and then he would receive it on a number of evenings in a row.

This information was compared with the staffing roster and it became clear that the medication was routinely administered when a particular staff member was working the afternoon duty in that unit.

A conversation with staff revealed that the majority of the staff appreciated the needs of this resident during evenings and followed the care plan to keep him occupied and settled. One staff member chose not to follow the suggested plan for supporting this resident. As a result he became unsettled on the evenings on which they worked and needed sedation.

This action amounts to 'chemical restraint' and is an example of inadequate care and also a failure to understand that meaningful communication and interaction could reduce the need for this resident to be medicated.

Responsibilities

There are significant risks involved in poor communication. It is essential that people appreciate their roles, the language that is relevant in any particular situation, and how to decipher messages and assist others to make sense of them. Taking responsibility for communications (both the content and delivery of the message) is important, and one of the hallmarks of professionalism.

CASE STUDY 19.6

Operating theatres

During 2003, researchers observed teams working in operating theatres. They recorded and analysed 421 communication events. A third of these events were considered to be communication failures. These failures were defined according to four categories:

- Failure of occasion—poor timing of communication (45.7 per cent)
- Failure of content—inaccurate in insufficient information conveyed (35.7 per cent)
- Failure of purpose—issues unresolved following communication (24 per cent)
- Failure in terms of audience—the wrong people receiving the message (20.9 per cent).

A third of these communication failures led to impacts including tension among the team, delays, waste of resources, inconvenience for patients and procedural errors.

Lingard et al. (2004)

In health care and disability support environments, patients and service users value authentic interaction and communication with providers. When interactions are considered as uncaring, the psychological needs of the patient or service user is put at risk (Wiman & Wikblad, 2004).

{ SUMMARY }

Even apparently clear written or verbal communication may include messages that require interpretation. The layers that require interpretation are often subtle and may only be understood by a particular audience.

A good deal of judgment is required to distinguish between formal and casual contexts, and therefore which language and style is appropriate. Words that have a clear meaning in one context may be completely inappropriate or misunderstood in another. Appreciating the intention and meaning of any communication helps us to interpret the information which is being conveyed. When first interacting with people it is wise to use more formal approaches to communication as this demonstrates respect. One of the key elements of good communication is to be certain that the information and manner in which it is conveyed are mutually understood. In many instances we also have professional responsibilities to ensure that we send unambiguous and respectful messages, and also provide support for people who are receiving them to ensure they understand.

REFLECTION POINTS

19.1 Intention (motivation, message, meaning, emotion)

In thinking about recent conversations you have been involved in, how were the verbal and non-verbal messages indications that you were communicating with 'good intent'?

What is colloquial communication and why is this type of communication used?

19.2 Reception (received message, response, feedback)

In thinking about a communication event where the message you intended was not well received, how might you have made your 'good intent' known more clearly?

What are advantages and disadvantages of using colloquial communication?

19.3 Perception (style, manner, impression, analysis)

What are the repercussions of poor communications in a health context?

How might your use of colloquial language or slang be interpreted by others?

QUESTIONS FOR REVIEW

1 What are the defining features of communicating with 'good intent'?
2 How might you communicate messages that are relevant and therefore more likely to be understood by a client?
3 In what ways does communicating as a professional differ from communicating as a friend?
4 What are the key elements of talking with someone and talking past someone?

REFERENCES

Bjerre, L. M. & LeLorier, J. (2000). Expressing the magnitude of adverse effects in case-controlled studies: 'The number of patients needed to be treated for one additional patient to be harmed'. *British Medical Journal*, *320*, 503–6.

Bolton, R. (1987). *People skills: How to assert yourself, listen to others, and resolve conflicts*. Sydney, NSW: Prentice Hall.

Bonn, D. (1997). Bogus psychiatrist dupes New Zealand. *The Lancet, 350*, 794.

Breazeal, C. & Aryananda, L. (2002). Recognition of affective communicative intent in robot-directed speech. *Autonomous Robots, 12*, 83–104.

Bunkle, P. (2010). Patient-centred ethics, the Cartwright Inquiry and feminism: Identifying the central fallacy in Linda Bryder, A History of the 'Unfortunate Experiment' at National Women's Hospital (2009, 2010). *Women's Studies Journal, 24*(2), 8–24.

Chang, A. R. (1990). Carcinoma in situ of the cervix and its malignant potential. A lesson from New Zealand. *Cytopathology, 1*, 321–8.

De Hek, (n.d.). *New Zealand immigration packs: Lifestyle: New Zealand slang*. Retrieved from www.nz-immigration.co.nz/lifestyle/slang-words.html.

Dula, C. S., Martin, B. A., Fox, R. T. & Leonard, R. L. (2011). Differing types of cellular phone conversations and dangerous driving. *Accident Analysis and Prevention, 43*(1), 187–93.

Fjelland, J. E., Barron, C. R. & Foxall, M. (2008). A review of instruments measuring two aspects of meaning: Search for meaning and meaning in illness. *Journal of Advanced Nursing, 62*(4), 394–406.

Godlee, F., Smith, J. & Marcovitch, H. (2011). Wakefield's article linking MMR vaccine and autism was fraudulent. *British Medical Journal, 342*, 64–6.

Gonzales-Pueyo, I. & Redrado, A. (2003). Scientific articles in internet homepages: Assumptions upon lay audiences. *Journal of Technical Writing and Communication, 33*(2), 165–84.

Kitamura, C. & Burnham, D. (2003). Pitch and communicative intent in mother's speech: Adjustments for age and sex in the first year. *Infancy, 4*(1), 85–110.

Koala Net. (2010 April). *Australian slang*. Retrieved from www.koalanet.com.au/australian-slang.html.

Lingard, L., Espin, S., Whyte, S., Baker, G. R., Reznick, R., Bohnen, J., Orser, B., Doran, D. & Grober, E. (2004). Communication failures in the operating room: An observational classification of recurrent types and effects. *Quality and Safety in Health Care, 13*, 330–4.

McIndoe, W. A., McLean, R., Jones, R. W. & Mullins, P. (1984). The invasive potential of carcinoma in situ of the cervix. *Obstetrics and Gynecology, 64*(4), 451–8.

Metge, J. & Kinloch, P. (1995). *Talking past each other: Problems of cross-cultural communication*. Wellington, NZ: Victoria University Press.

Monash University. (2007). *Language and learning online: Formal language*. Retrieved from www.monash.edu.au/lls/llonline/writing/general/academic/3.1.xml.

Orgel, E., McCarter, R. & Jacobs, S. (2010). A failing educational model: A self-assessment by physicians at all levels of training of ability and comfort to deliver bad news. *Journal of Palliative Medicine, 13*(6), 677–83.

Papousek, M., Bornstein, M. H., Nuzzo, C., Papousek, H. & Symmes, D. (1990). Infant responses to prototypical melodic contours in parental speech. *Infant Behavior and Development, 13*, 539–45.

Paul, C. (1988). The New Zealand cervical cancer study: Could it happen again? *British Medical Journal, 297*, 533–9.

Persson, M. & Friberg, F. (2009). The dramatic encounter: experiences of taking part in a health conversation. *Journal of Clinical Nursing, 18*, 520–8.

Rodriguez, K. L., Gambino, F. J., Butow, P. N., Hagerty, R. G. & Arnold, R. M. (2008). It's going to shorten your life: Framing of oncologist-patient communication about prognosis. *Psycho-Oncology, 17*, 219–25.

Rosner, F. (2004). Informing the patient about a fatal disease: From paternalism to autonomy—The Jewish view. *Cancer Investigation, 22*(6), 949–53.

Ryan, M. (2003). The adversarial court system and the expert medical witness: 'The truth the whole truth and nothing but the truth?' *Emergency Medicine, 15*, 283–88.

Sawyer, A. J. (1999). A comparison of New Zealand taxpayers' rights with selected civil law and common law countries—Have New Zealand taxpayers been 'short-changed'? *Vanderbilt Journal of Transnational Law, 32*(5), 1345–1400.

Smith, J. & Abel, S. (2008). Ka whawhai tonu matou: Indigenous television in Aotearoa/New Zealand. *New Zealand Journal of Media Studies, 11*(1), 1–14.

Thomas, H. (2007). *Sick to death: A manipulative surgeon and a health system in crisis—A disaster waiting to happen*. Sydney, NSW: Allen and Unwin.

Thorne, S. E., Bultz, B. D. & Baile, W. F. (2005). Is there a cost to poor communication in cancer care? A critical review of the literature. *Psycho-Oncology, 14*, 875–84.

van Ryn, M. & Fu, S. S. (2003). Paved with good intentions: Do public health and human service providers contribute to racial/ethnic disparities in health? *American Journal of Public Health, 93*(2), 248–55.

Webb, H. (2009). 'I've put weight on cos I've bin inactive, cos I've 'ad me knee done': Moral work in the obesity clinic. *Sociology of Health and Illness, 31*(6), 854–71.

Wiman, E. & Wikblad, K. (2004). Caring and uncaring encounters in nursing in an emergency department. *Journal of Clinical Nursing, 13*, 422–9.

WEBSITES

A Dictionary of Slang: www.peevish.co.uk/slang/links.htm
Chemistry & New Zealand: http://chemistry.co.nz
Language & Learning Online: www.monash.edu.au/lls/llonline/writing/general/academic/3.1.xml
New Zealand Immigration Packs: www.nz-immigration.co.nz
The Online Slang Dictionary: http://onlineslangdictionary.com

{20}

Style and Manner

Tony MacCulloch

CHAPTER OVERVIEW

This chapter covers the following topics:

+ Professional communication
+ Casual communication
+ Intimacy issues
+ Integrity
+ Dysfunctional styles to avoid.

KEY TERMS

Presence
Transactional analysis
Interaction

Communication can be said to be the life-blood of interpersonal relationships. If it is lacking, relationships are likely to struggle, founder and eventually seize up. When **present** and carefully cultivated, it can enable relationships to flourish and all to benefit. Within the day-to-day process of living, working and interacting, it can be said that individuals each have a responsibility for the quality of their communication. In this sense, it is the responsibility of practitioners to ensure that they convey the message they want to get across to others in a clear, effective, unambiguous and respectful manner. Good-quality communication is more likely to occur when people take the trouble to think about what they wish to say and how they need to say it, and to anticipate how it might be received by the other person. It means carefully selecting the most appropriate language, choosing how to phrase the points to be conveyed and considering the other person's perspective. While for many people, life experience together with learning throughout childhood enables this process to become almost automatic, this is not the case for everyone. The different roles people find themselves taking on throughout a typical day can require skilful change or modification of communication style at particular moments. Of necessity it requires that people become more aware of communication skills they use well, of skills they use awkwardly, and of skills they really need to develop.

Presence The state of accompanying others in a meaningful way.

CASE STUDY 20.1

Communication style flexibility

Charge Nurse Mary Smith arrives to begin her Monday morning shift at the surgical unit. In the staff room she greets a long-time colleague in her usual light and friendly manner: 'Hi Jenny, how was the weekend and your daughter's wedding? I know you were a bit worried about some of the guests coming to the reception. It must have been a proud day for you.' Jenny's response echoes the warmth and friendship between them: 'I couldn't have wished for a better day, and I didn't need to worry about his friends. They were very polite and well behaved.' Mary concludes the exchange: 'I did tell you last week you worry too much.'

Later in the morning, Mary observes Jane, a junior staff member, repeating a serious error in the preoperative patient identity checking process and needs to firmly correct the omission: 'Jane, I notice that when you gave your patient his preoperative medication, you didn't check his wrist identity name and number. As it happens we have two male patients with the same surname on the list today, so the risk for error is even higher. You must always follow our formal checking process and understand how important this is. Do not let that happen again.'

Just prior to concluding her shift of duty, Mary sees an experienced team member crying in the staff room. She sits down beside her, and quietly asks: 'What's the matter? It's not like you to let things get to you like this.' Her colleague replies: 'For some reason, today when one of my patients was given a terminal diagnosis, it felt like we do so little to help. It's not fair that life is so cruel for some people. I feel so inadequate.' Mary responds: 'Sometimes it is very painful to be so close to your patient's experience, particularly when the prognosis is grim. I guess tears are one way of expressing how sad it is and how much you care.'

This case study illustrates how important it is to be able to change communication style in response to very different situations. In this instance, Mary's communication shifted from a casual, friendly, informal style to a serious, formal and disciplinary style, and then later to a compassionate, empathic and deeply caring style. Each was appropriate to the needs of the situation and yet at the same time demonstrated how Mary was professional in her communication.

Professional communication

When linked with communication, the term 'professional' implies something quite specific about the quality and nature of that communication. At its best it can refer to a quality of communication that is utterly appropriate and fitting for the context in which it occurs. It draws on motivation, language and intent to inspire trust, safety and appropriate authority. There is a clear intent to initially connect with the recipient, perhaps by making reference to something that both parties can relate to.

CASE STUDY 20.2

An example of communication

There are many reasons for practitioners and patients to communicate. Commonly these interactions include a beginning (or opening), some indication of the purpose of the message and an invitation to discuss.

Opening the interaction:

Hello Peter, it's good to see you again after what has clearly been a difficult time since I saw you last week.

What follows is likely to refer to the central purpose of the communication:

> Today we need to review how things are progressing for you since you had surgery and decide how best to manage the next stage of your recovery process. Tell me how it's been for you with the management of your pain and coping with activities such as getting dressed and having a shower?

There may then be some discussion about options and decisions that need to be made followed by clarification about different approaches:

> I'm thinking about whether it might be better for you if, rather than initially going straight home and managing by yourself, you could stay with your family for a few weeks first. That would mean if you have any complications there would be someone on hand to support you. How would that work for you?

At their worst, interactions between practitioners and patients or clients can illustrate communication that is saturated by the power and authority of the profession from which it originates. It may become detached and alienated from the real world of those outside the profession, positioning the client as passive with a duty to comply unquestioningly with the health practitioner's instructions.

Greater access to information available via the internet and other media has nourished the rising voice of consumer groups. This shift in power has been attributed to a rejection of oppressive 'power over' that can characterise some professional groups. Emerging challenges to the knowledge and work of practitioners illustrate how professional communication has the capacity to either perpetuate social injustice and serve political agendas or contribute to empowering consumers and encouraging stronger mutually beneficial alliances between those involved.

Professional communication carries important positive connotations of adherence to ethical standards that protect the recipient, which may serve to reassure patients. Ethical standards outline the need to honour the role of boundaries, which are of particular importance in health care and disability support. In this context, health practitioners have a significant power advantage over clients or patients who, by virtue of their state of well-being at the point of needing to engage professionals, can be highly vulnerable.

Casual communication

Casual or informal communication can be described as the lubricant of social intercourse. The essential point relates to the value of 'small talk' in establishing and maintaining a relatively superficial level of relationship with another person. It is the kind of conversation that frequently focuses on the weather, sport, news of the day or other topics that carry minimal risk and can be considered common ground. While they are safe topics and reveal little about what really matters to both parties involved, there is an art to using such casual conversation in a way that is genuine, sincere and conveys real interest in the world of the other. Part of this skill is about sensing other people's awkwardness or discomfort with silence and then having the assurance to 'break the ice' in a natural way using safe 'small talk'. As this process proceeds, both parties can become more comfortable and feel safer revealing more significant aspects of themselves, and in so doing make it possible to move towards greater levels of intimacy.

Intimacy issues

Like so many words in the English language, 'intimacy' can convey different meanings and is thus open to misinterpretation or misunderstanding. In a marital context, for example, it refers to physical, emotional and sexual closeness between partners. By its very nature, nursing practice frequently requires physical and emotional closeness between nurse and patient. Assistance with the patient's personal bodily functions, such as toileting and washing the genital area, are examples of how the role of the nurse embodies intimacy. 'Communication intimacy' in this context describes a quality of safety carried with the role of nurse that enables the discussion of very personal and intimate matters within a professional relationship that transcends usual social constraints. Erikson (1968) connected the term with a stage in emotional development: 'intimacy versus isolation'. In this context, he alluded to how the individual needs to achieve or master the ability to experience real depth and closeness in relationships with others. Orlofsky, Marcia and Lesser (1973) confirmed that those who had successfully resolved this stage were more able to experience intimacy. Berne (1972), the originator of **transactional analysis**, identified intimacy as one of six ways that people may choose to structure their use of time. He characterised it as an ability to use our 'natural child' ego state in a spontaneous way to give unconditional positive strokes (Steiner, 2003) and in so doing experience a mutually rewarding level of closeness with another human being. In transactional analysis terms, the alternative is to engage in other time-structuring modes that maintain distance and superficiality in relationships with others.

Transactional analysis An approach to psychotherapy that emphasises interactions and relationships between people.

Intimacy in communication between practitioners and their patients, then, requires the practitioner to have the ability to engage comfortably and closely with the private, personal and frequently hidden world of the patient—as the moment or situation requires it. The patient dying alone needs a nurse who is willing to listen and talk about what really matters to them in that moment. The mother grieving over the loss of her baby needs someone to hear her anguish. The paraplegic rugby player needs someone who will be there as he struggles to find new meaning for his life. Intimacy means being able to be close to others' pain and suffering without becoming overwhelmed, while remaining open enough to accurately empathise with their experience. Intimacy within the bounds of a therapeutic nurse–patient relationship must be profoundly respectful and acutely sensitive to the subtle and frequently unstated needs of the patient. It requires the practitioner to be absolutely trustworthy in the eyes of the patient, and securely confident in their own ability to respond appropriately.

Integrity

Health-care contexts by their very nature involve practitioners caring for patients who are in some way vulnerable, whether it be physically, emotionally, mentally, socially or spiritually. Among the many ethical and professional competencies required of such practitioners is integrity, sometimes also referred to as honesty or trustworthiness. Qualities such as these are the critical foundations of trust. Good-quality professional practice can only happen if all involved are guided by values, of honesty and truth. These values, when consistently upheld by practitioners, demonstrate integrity.

It becomes clear that for a practitioner to win the trust and respect of those in their care, their communication style, manner and behaviour must at all times reflect integrity. It is interesting to note that when surveys are conducted to assess who people most trust in the community, practitioners rate very highly: 'Most trusted are ambulance officers (89.8%), fire fighters (82.1%), nurses (79.9%) and doctors (71.2%)' (HorizonPoll, 2011).

This professional regard reflects well on the adherence to ethical standards practitioners set for themselves, and does much to inspire trust and respect among those who are served in the community by these groups. On a personal level, it requires that individual practitioners make a conscious choice and decision to ensure their personal and professional behaviour, together with their communication, is at all times congruent with appropriate ethical and moral standards.

Dysfunctional styles to avoid

Interaction Mutual influence or reciprocal action between people.

Relatively few people have the opportunity to attend formal education to learn the complex skills required to communicate effectively, and yet many people do amazingly well in navigating their way through the maze and complexity of human **interaction**.

CASE STUDY 20.3

Learning to communicate

Depending on the nature of our personal upbringing and life experiences, it can be something of a gamble just what communication skills we do learn. Confused and mixed messages can lead to failed personal relationships that are hurtful and sometimes damaging to all parties. Conti-O'Hare (2002) discusses such experiences within what she terms 'the wounded healer' concept, which acknowledges the possibility that many of those who enter healing professions have at some time in their life become emotionally 'wounded'. This proposition echoes the same notion described by Heron (2001). When replayed in health-care contexts, similar dysfunctional communication can undermine relationships with colleagues, contaminate our responses to the patients we care for, and distort the messages we give to those around us. The risks of such unclear communication causing confusion and irritation are easy to imagine. More seriously, there is the added risk that in some situations lives can be put at risk if critical clinical information about a patient is not accurately and promptly passed on to other team members.

Individuals learn communication skills from their parents and those they live with, as well as from teachers and the media, with varied degrees of sophistication. When looking to effectively upskill in communication (and perhaps also attend to previously avoided 'emotional damagedness') there are three key steps.

Step one requires reflection, feedback and self-awareness of how we communicate. It is critical for practitioners to regularly critically reflect on their practice and to take note of feedback from colleagues in order to deepen their awareness of how previously learnt patterns of communication can, albeit unintentionally, put colleagues or patients at risk. For some, reflection on communication or engagement with others is almost automatic—they do it often and thus know their communication strengths and weaknesses well. For others, such reflection is somewhat foreign and these people might find it difficult to specifically name their strengths and weaknesses.

Step two requires a decision to unlearn old dysfunctional patterns and motivation to learn a new, expanded range of more effective communication skills. In some instances, this may require some counselling with a view to working through what Heron (2001, p. 14) refers to as 'the wounded child'. The principle at work here is that it is common to experience a variety of traumatising events in an earlier stage of one's life. It is equally common to not have the opportunity to effectively address or resolve such things. The result is that, unbeknown to us, communication, relationships and the work that we do can become contaminated and distorted (Heron, 2001).

Step three requires that we refine our ability to be flexible and tailor our communication style to best fit the multiple roles we play. This means becoming more conscious of those roles and reflecting on those that we use easily and those we find difficult. It may also mean seeking opportunities to expand our repertoire of role skills.

CASE STUDY 20.4

Peter

Peter, a recently qualified registered nurse, was covering the night shift in the coronary care unit. Throughout the evening, the condition of all his patients had been stable and he had successfully dealt with a few minor disruptions. He was feeling somewhat relieved about this because he had grown up believing that it was essential to manage things yourself and not bother other people even if you needed help. As a child his father had frequently beaten Peter for bothering him when he was busy.

Just after midnight, Mr Johnson, a man in his late fifties, started showing distinct signs of ventricular tachycardia, a serious cardiac arrhythmia that can occur following a heart attack. Peter had been advised earlier by the senior nurse on the unit to immediately call the medical registrar if this patient should develop any arrhythmia. However, Peter was so apprehensive about troubling the registrar that he decided to administer an appropriate 'use as needed' PRN medication. An hour later Mr Johnson's condition deteriorated into ventricular fibrillation, quickly followed by full cardiac arrest. The 'code blue' team rushed to the scene to commence cardiac resuscitation. After a series of attempts, cardiac rhythm was re-established.

When advised of the sequence of events, the registrar was emphatic that he should have been summoned immediately when Mr Johnson's condition changed, stating 'that lack of communication and failure to follow specific instructions could have caused this patient's death'. Peter learned a powerful lesson about the importance of not letting his own emotional needs get in the way of appropriately calling upon colleagues when needed. He later sought some personal counselling and successfully worked through the issues of his 'wounded child' (Heron, 2001).

Self-awareness of this kind becomes an amazing strength because it opens the door to change, development, enhanced emotional competence (Heron, 2001) and the possibility of improving the quality of communication not only at work but also in all areas of life.

{ SUMMARY }

Communication style and manner is not something most people think about, partly because it has an automatic unself-conscious quality about it. In health care, however, the manner and style of our communication with colleagues, patients and their family/whānau profoundly influences the effectiveness of information exchange, the development and maintenance of therapeutic relationships, and the degree to which patients will trust and respect us. By examining aspects of professional communication—such as responsibility, intimacy, integrity and dysfunctional styles—it becomes possible to significantly deepen self-awareness and to review natural communication style assets. This process also enables people to identify particular aspects of professional communication that may be problematic and take steps to address any deficiencies in their skill set.

REFLECTION POINTS

20.1 Intention (motivation, message, meaning, emotion)

Think about your personal communication style. Is it casual, informal, quiet, reserved, calm, confident, extrovert or dominating? How might this have been shaped by your culture, family upbringing or your personality?

When considering the communication styles needed as a health practitioner, what changes might you need to consider? How could you approach such a task?

20.2 Reception (received message, response, feedback)

Consider previous occasions when you have needed to see a health practitioner. Did this health practitioner demonstrate professionalism in their style of communication with you (both personally or in writing)?

20.3 Perception (style, manner, impression, analysis)

Compile two lists: one that identifies what you consider to be your communication strengths and one that identifies the communication skills you believe a health practitioner should have. What aspects of your communication style might need to change? Reflecting on Heron's (2001) proposition about 'unresolved emotional distress', are there issues that are unresolved?

QUESTIONS FOR REVIEW

1 Why is the art of casual conversation useful for a professional?

2 Whose responsibility is it to ensure that communication between the professional and the client is of a good quality?

REFERENCES

Berne, E. (1972). *What do you say after you say hello?: The psychology of human destiny*. New York, NY: Grove Press.

Conti-O'Hare, M. (2002). *The nurse as wounded healer: From trauma to transcendence*. Sudbury, MA: Jones and Bartlett.

Erikson, E. H. (1968). *Identity, youth and crisis*. New York, NY: W. W. Norton.

Heron, J. (2001). *Helping the client* (5th edn). London, UK: Sage.

HorizonPoll. (2011). *Who Kiwis most trust and distrust*. Retrieved 27 February 2011 from www.horizonpoll.co.nz/page/97/who-kiwis-most-trust-and-distrust.

Orlofsky, J., Marcia, J. & Lesser, I. (1973). Ego identity status and the intimacy versus isolation crisis of young adulthood. *Journal of Personality and Social Psychology, 27*, 211–19.

Steiner, C. (2003). *Emotional literacy: Intelligence with a heart*. Fawnskin, CA: Personhood Press.

WEBSITES

Emotional Intelligence: http://danielgoleman.info/topics/emotional-intelligence
Good Communication Skills: www.goodcommunicationskills.net
Introducing Transactional Analysis: www.nztaa.org.nz/page/6-introducing-transactional-analysis

{21}

Receiving the Message

Kirk Reed

CHAPTER OVERVIEW

This chapter covers the following topics:

+ Interpretation
+ Evaluating the message
+ Options for responding
+ Feedback
+ Complaints.

KEY TERMS

Empathy
Active listening
Critical listening
Information triage

Receiving a message requires well-developed listening skills that include paying careful attention to what is being said as an active, empathetic or critical listener. Interpreting and evaluating messages that are received, along with ways of responding, are key elements in effective communication and of particular importance in the health and disability sector. Feedback is essential to evaluating communication, and this logically includes complaints and how to make and address them as they inevitably arise.

Interpretation

Empathy The ability to appreciate the thoughts, feelings and perspectives of others.

Active listening The process of listening with the intention to understand and to treat the communication with respect.

Receiving the message involves good listening skills, especially listening with **empathy** to another person. This is an active rather than a passive process. To listen passively is to avoid displaying any behaviour that lets the speaker know they are being listened to. Passive listeners sit with a bland stare or frozen facial expression and do not show any interest in what the person is saying. Engaging in **active listening**, by contrast, involves responding verbally, non-verbally and emotionally to the speaker's message. Responding in this way serves several purposes and determines how the message is received and interpreted by the listener. First, it can be a measure of how accurately the message is understood. Second, responses indicate whether the listened agrees or disagrees with the message. Finally, responses tell the speaker how they are affecting the listener or receiver of the message.

Listening to empathise is only one possible listening goal, as it will not always be necessary to seek out and interpret messages in response to a person's emotions. Listening and responding empathically requires focusing on the person speaking and is also about attempting to understand the message from his or her perspective. Carl Rogers, a psychologist, summarised the value of empathy by highlighting that 'a high degree of empathy in a relationship is possibly the most potent factor in bringing about change and learning' (Rogers, 1980, p. 139).

Developing active listening skills enables appropriate decisions to be made that influence the service being provided. However, there are many barriers that exist when it comes to listening effectively, which in turn can distort how the information is interpreted. An awareness of these barriers—whether they are internal or external—will assist in avoiding potential hazards that might negatively affect the listening process. External factors are those in the environment and might include such things as noise, distraction, unrelated activity in the space where the interaction is occurring, a ringing telephone or mobile phone, or someone knocking at the door. It is important that time is taken to remove or reduce these barriers as much as possible. An active listener also attends to the internal factors: the things about a person that may influence the receipt of a message. These types of factors might include being in touch with or attending to the speaker's emotions, putting ideas and assumptions to one side to avoid making judgments, and avoiding identifying a solution or course of action before having listened to the message.

The language of the listener may also hinder the effectiveness of the communication and the interpretation of the message. If the language of the speaker is poor—for example, when there is a health condition that affects speech or when there is a strong accent that others might find difficult to follow—this can hinder effective communication. Mutual understanding requires both communicators to have some level of competence in a common language. Mutuality of understanding is especially important across cultures, as some skills associated with active listening may not be appropriate in some cultures; for example, eye contact or touch. In some cultures, age and gender will impact on what the speaker says and how they respond to the listener. For others, the language barrier may mean that an interpreter is required. An interpreter adds a level of complexity in transmitting, receiving and interpreting a message: in the process of interpretation there is a risk that the meaning of the message may be lost or non-verbal communication misunderstood. In addition, having a translator adds further levels of complexity regarding privacy and trust.

Evaluating the message

While being an active empathetic listener is one listening goal, it is also important to listen critically and to evaluate the message being received. **Critical listening** involves listening to evaluate the quality, appropriateness, value and importance of the information that is heard. The goal of a critical listener is to use information to make choices and inform decision-making. This might include listening for personal details, key facts and events; indentifying signs, symptoms and conflicting details; and evaluating if a person's choices have worked for them in the past.

Critical listening
The process of listening with the intention to evaluate and form an opinion.

A critical listener does not necessarily offer negative comments. Rather, they seek to identify both good information and information that is flawed or unhelpful, constantly making decisions about which information is useful and relevant. This process has been termed **information triage**. Before evaluating information that has been received, it is vital to consider the logic and reasoning used in the message.

Information triage
The process of analysing and refining information that is received in order to discern what is of value.

A number of authors (Davis, 2006; Devito, 2007; Egan, 2007; Harms, 2007, Purtilo & Haddad, 2002) have considered a range of factors that should be either avoided or implemented to ensure that critical listening skills are put to their best use. It is useful to avoid:

+ stereotyping the other person, regardless of their appearance or communication skills
+ losing concentration because of thoughts on other matters
+ interrupting the other person with your own thoughts or ideas
+ engaging in passive listening and showing a lack of interest in what the speaker is saying
+ making judgments based on your own personal values or beliefs.

In preparation for active, empathetic or critical listening, the following strategies are useful:

+ 'Tune in' to what the speaker is saying.
+ Pay attention to the facts and the accuracy of information.
+ Adjust the physical environment to reduce distractions.
+ Carefully observe all non-verbal messages.
+ Consider how useful the information is. Is it accurate, factual and relevant?
+ Search for the meaning in verbal and non-verbal messages.
+ Consider cultural variations in listening.
+ Schedule an interpreter if required.

Effective listening is beneficial to build relationships between practitioners and patients or service users. Effective listening allows for evaluation of the messages that are received and decisions about the usefulness and relevance of the information. It is also important to be aware of the barriers that can hinder effective listening and work to reduce these.

Options for responding

Regardless of the communication goal, there are several strategies that can be used to respond to others. The timing of the response, usefulness of the information, amount of detail and descriptiveness of the response are all important to consider when responding to others. Effective responses for clear communication are those that are perceived as being empathetic, caring, warm and thoughtful.

The responses identified below can be effective depending on the context in which they are used.

1 Understanding—the understanding response is most likely to create a climate where honest, frank communication can occur. It is a feelings-oriented response that conveys sensitivity and understanding. Strong feelings can become a barrier to communication; this response can diminish those feelings. Understanding is empathetic—it implies listening beyond the words and reflecting on the feelings and emotions. Focusing on

others feelings enables recognition of the other person as an individual and worthy of attention and concern. This type of response can reduce hostile feelings and can be used when someone is over-emotional, crying or fearful. Examples of understanding responses:

- ~ It sounds to me like you're feeling pretty down about this.
- ~ I can tell that this is really upsetting you.
- ~ You seem pleased with that decision.
- ~ You seem excited by that option.

2 Clarification—the clarification response indicates intent to comprehend what the other person is saying or to identify the most significant feelings or key points in the message that is emerging. It indicates a genuine desire to check that perceptions are correct. This can be done in several ways: echoing the last few words, summarising the points that seemed most relevant, and paraphrasing. A response of this nature can be followed by a period of silence, which gives the other person a chance to get their thoughts together or to correct your perception, and encourages the other person to explain more fully. The clarification response also serves to focus the discussion. Examples of clarification responses:

- ~ You seem to be saying …
- ~ If I hear you correctly, you are saying that you could develop a better way of doing that.
- ~ So what you want to do is …

3 Self-disclosure—the self-disclosure response shows your attempts to give others insight into who you are. It is sharing something about yourself that relates directly to the conversation; for example, your personal beliefs, attitudes and values or an event from your own life that is relevant to the conversation. Self-disclosure is useful in connecting with another person, but overuse can be unhelpful as it focuses the attention on the wrong person. It also risks altering the relationship between the communicators, which can be very confusing. Examples of self-disclosure responses:

- ~ Like you, I never felt like anyone accepted me for the way I was.
- ~ I lost my father about three years ago.
- ~ When I was younger, the kids at school always made fun of me because of my weight.

4 Questioning—the questioning response seeks to elicit information. Open questions tend to focus on the other person's general thoughts and feelings, and tend to promote communication. Closed questions, on the other hand, focus on specific facts and generally get a 'yes' or 'no' answer. Open questions are recommended for exploring a broad topic, while closed questions can be interspersed to get specific facts or can be used to cut off long explanations. Caution is need with questions beginning with

'why' as they pressure the other person for an explanation and may result in the person becoming defensive. Examples of questioning responses:
- Do you like your new house? (closed)
- What do you like about your new house? (open)
- Are you confused about something? (closed)
- What is confusing you? (open)

5 Information giving—the information-giving response involves relating facts in an objective manner without judgment or evaluation. It allows the other person to accept or reject the facts and to take responsibility for using the information. This kind of response is useful in giving both positive and negative feedback. Examples of information giving responses:
- The support group can be used to meet others with similar problems.
- We only have a budget of $500 for the project.

6 Reassurance—the reassurance response aims to reduce anxiety, diffuse intense feelings and express confidence, and is often used by people who come upon a situation that is beyond their depth of experience. Reassurance may be used as an expression of sympathy and is sometimes used when people do not know what to say or do. If this kind of response is to be used, think carefully about the words that may be used. For example, rather than saying 'You will manage', instead say 'I have confidence in you'. Examples of reassurance responses:
- Hang in there—that feeling is normal.
- Things have not always felt this bad. Even though you are feeling low at this point, things do change. With depression it's about holding on to hope—it wasn't always like this, so a future can be different also.
- You managed it last time, so you know you can do it, even though it's hard.

7 Analytical—the analytical response seeks to analyse, explain or interpret the other person's behaviour and feelings. It goes beyond what the person has said in an attempt to explain or connect ideas and events. This type of response can lead to resentment and is more appropriate for use when there is an ongoing counselling relationship, where the person needs to become aware of certain behaviour or reaction patterns. Examples of analytical responses:
- Perhaps you see her as an authority figure, and that could be why you cannot relate to her.
- You often come late. Perhaps it is because you don't really feel comfortable here.
- You are lonely because you are afraid to risk getting involved with people.

8 Advice giving—the advice-giving response is usually unproductive as it implies that you are in a position of power and know the reasons for the other person's problems, and what he or she should to do about them. Telling people what to do takes away

their responsibility for decision-making and problem-solving, can create a sense of dependency and often leads to resistance and resentment. Rewording advice into an information-giving response or a question is much more productive. Examples of advice-giving responses:

- ~ Instead of arguing try and see the other person's viewpoint.
- ~ You shouldn't say things like that.

Developing effective skills in responding to another person will ensure that clear, honest and frank communication takes place. Knowing how and when to use different responses develops over time and with practice—some will work well and others will not. Options for responding will depend on the person, the context and the purpose of the interaction. Having a repertoire of responses available to use, and tailoring these to specific contexts and people, enables lines of communication to be maximised.

CASE STUDY 21.1

Responsible communication

You have a very busy day ahead, with more than the usual number of people to see. Tanya, a 40-year-old woman, has turned up for her follow-up appointment with you. She is usually optimistic and relaxed, and is nearly ready to be discharged from your service. Today she looks tired and begins to tell you about all the things that are wrong in her life: the pressures at work, separating from her husband three weeks ago, not being sure about what the future holds and how depressed she has been feeling.

You are extremely busy and not that interested in hearing much more because you have your own problems, and you don't want a reminder of those things at work. You are finding it difficult to concentrate because of the building work happening down the corridor, which has been going on for two days, and you don't want to fall behind because you have a dentist's appointment straight after work. What professional priorities do you have in this situation and how could you manage the issues that are competing for your attention?

Feedback

Feedback is when a two-way process of honest interaction takes place, in contrast to a monologue, or a one-way flow of information. The process of feedback enables a dialogue, ensuring that the listener becomes a part of the communication process. As a result, the listener is more likely to be engaged in reasoning, responding and reflecting on the message being received. Feedback can help improve the accuracy of the communication and help keep the conversation personally relevant.

Feedback is retrospective and its purpose is to raise awareness about strengths, weaknesses and omissions in recent behaviour or communication between two or more people (Heron, 2001). It is likely that feedback will focus on verbal or non-verbal communication and generally distinguishes between what the person was aware of and those actions that were unintended or that they were not aware of. In terms of verbal communication, the feedback might focus on the content or meaning of the message, the intention of what was said, the choice of words, the tone of voice, the volume, pitch or speed of the voice, or pauses and silences. Feedback might also focus on why a message was interpreted in a particular way, any value judgments that came into play, or particular professional or personal knowledge that influenced the interpretation of the message.

In terms of non-verbal communication, feedback might include eye contact, touch, facial expressions, gestures (with arms, hands, legs, the head or the neck), a particular action, breathing style or physical positioning in relation to the other person (standing, sitting, near, far, beside, opposite, etc.). Feedback on behaviour or communication might be subjective, objective or descriptive. Subjective feedback is based on an impression (right or wrong) or an emotional reaction. This kind of feedback is not supported with evidence and may provide useful information for the recipient to consider. Objective feedback, on the other hand, is an objective judgment that is supported by reasons or evidence; it is generally based on something observed or tangible. Finally, descriptive feedback gives a description. It might be a description of posture, speech patterns or a particular action. This kind of feedback allows the recipient to become aware of their actions and provides a point for discussion.

As feedback is retrospective, it has no immediate effect on current behaviour and can only be applied to modify future behaviour or communication. However, there is a more fundamental sort of feedback that is more dynamic. This is the feedback a person gives to themself about their own behaviour while it is occurring, and can be used to influence and modify ongoing behaviour. This kind of feedback is called self-monitoring and is a creative, flexible, adaptive and forward-looking means of making change that is action-oriented.

Complaints

There are many reasons why someone might complain about a person or a service provided. These can include a personality clash, miscommunication, error, injury, damage to equipment or (in the worst-case scenario) a fatality. A complaint is often in response to a mismatch between a person's expectations and their experience. Therefore, it is important to be honest and transparent when dealing with a complaint. Complaints are not necessarily a bad thing—if a person is complaining, the chances are there is a problem. Finding out what the problem is and fixing it can lead to improved customer or client satisfaction, improved service, upskilling or professional development, and systems to ensure that the errors do not recur.

Complaints should not be ignored and need to be managed effectively and efficiently. If working for an organisation, there is likely to be a complaints policy and procedure; this is something to become familiar with and adhere to before taking action. When dealing with people who are making a complaint, they are likely to be unhappy, angry or upset and it is easy for problems to escalate. Listen patiently, respectfully and calmly to what a person has to say and do not respond on an emotional level. LEAD is a useful acronym to remember when dealing with a complaint:

+ L = Listen
+ E = Empathise
+ A = Act
+ D = Document

Aside from policies and procedures, in the New Zealand context there are two pieces of legislation that are relevant to patients or clients making a complaint: the Health Practitioners Competence Assurance Act 1992 and the Health and Disability Commissioner Act 1994.

The Health Practitioners Competence Assurance Act establishes the need for registration as a health practitioner. Each discipline has its own authority that oversees a particular profession; for example, the Nursing Council, the Occupational Therapy Board of New Zealand, the Physiotherapy Board and the Psychologists Board. In terms of dealing with a complaint about a member of a particular profession, the registration board has the authority to appoint a professional conduct committee. The role of this committee is to investigate complaints and make recommendations or determinations in response to the complaint.

The Health and Disability Commissioner Act created the office of the Health and Disability Commissioner, which has a role of promoting and protecting the rights of health disability consumers. The Health and Disability Commissioner Act made provision for the establishment of the Code of Health and Disability Service Consumers' Rights. The code contains ten rights for consumers; right number 10 is the Right to Complain, where 'every consumer has the right to complain about a provider in any form appropriate to the consumer' (Health and Disability Commissioner, 2004).

CASE STUDY 21.2

Responding to a complaint

Today, John has come in to see you. He is 71 years old and recently had a fall at home and has his leg in a cast. He looks annoyed. John is pretty sure that he has the correct time to come and see you, but he is not sure. Before you can start the interview, John tells you that he wants to make a complaint. As he talks, his voice sounds angry and upset and he is shaking. He lets you know that he has had four telephone calls in the last three days from the receptionist changing the day and time of his appointment, with no reason given for the changes. He is annoyed because at the moment he cannot drive, so has to call on his daughter to drive him to the appointment. She works full time and finds it difficult to get away from work, so she is also annoyed about all the changes.

{ SUMMARY }

Receiving the message requires good listening skills as an active empathetic or critical listener, ensuring that the listener is evaluating, interpreting and responding to the message in a way that promotes clear, honest and frank communication. Giving and receiving feedback is a useful tool to change future behaviour or communication styles. Different ways of giving feedback, including how to respond to a complaint, are important skills. A complaint may be perceived as being a negative message; however, complaints have the potential to change and improve service delivery and contribute to professional development. It is essential to be aware of policies and procedures related to complaints, and to respond to a complaint in a calm and respectful manner, ensuring that action is taken and a clear process of documenting the complaint is implemented.

REFLECTION POINTS

21.1 Intention (motivation, message, meaning, emotion)

In Case study 21.1, what are the barriers to listening to Tanya's problems?

21.2 Reception (received message, response, feedback)

If you are unable to empathise with Tanya, or are unable to set aside the time to talk with her, in what other ways might you manage this scenario professionally?

21.3 Perception (style, manner, impression, analysis)

In Case study 21.2, how would you deal with John's complaint?

QUESTIONS FOR REVIEW

1 What options for responding have you used in the past? Why did they work?
2 Consider your usual style of listening. Are you naturally an active or passive listener?
3 What effect might your use of active listening have on the emotional response of a person talking with you?
4 How do you know someone is listening to you? What verbal and non-verbal behaviours indicate they are listening?

REFERENCES

Davis, C. M. (2006). *Patient practitioner interaction: An experiential manual for developing the art of health care* (4th edn). Thorofare, NJ: Slack.

Devito, J. A. (2007). *The interpersonal communication book* (11th edn). Boston, MA: Pearson.

Egan, G. (2007). *The skilled helper* (8th edn). Belmont, CA: Thomson.

Harms, D. (2007). *Working with people: Communication skills for reflective practice*. Melbourne, Vic: Oxford University Press.

Health and Disability Commissioner. (2004). *Code of health and disability services consumers' rights*. Wellington, NZ: Author.

Heron, J. (2001). *Helping the client: A creative practical guide* (5th edn). London, UK: Sage.

Purtilo, R. B. & Haddad, A. (2002). *Health professional and patient interaction* (6th edn). Philadelphia, PA: Saunders.

Rogers, C. A. (1980). *A way of being*. New York, NY: Houghton Mifflin.

WEBSITES

Effective Communication Skills for Health Professionals: www.ehow.com/way_5544230_effective-communication-skills-health-professionals.html

Health and Disability Commissioner: www.hdc.org.nz

New Zealand Legislation: www.legislation.govt.nz

{22}

Written Communication

Kate Diesfeld

CHAPTER OVERVIEW

This chapter covers the following topics:

+ The legal terrain
+ The fundamentals of record keeping
+ Elements of a consent form
+ Formal submissions
+ The writing process.

KEY TERMS

Documentation
Records

Record keeping is a fundamental function of professional life, and substandard reporting can have significant repercussions for providers. This chapter examines a recent legal case to illustrate the potential legal and professional impact of inadequate record keeping, and reviews recent legal cases to offer important and concrete lessons for the prevention of similar errors.

The legal terrain

By way of background, both registered and non-registered providers of health and disability services in Aotearoa New Zealand are bound to protect specific rights of the people they serve. Non-registered providers take note! In Aotearoa New Zealand, people who *hold themselves out* as providing health or disability services (including students and volunteers), are bound by the ten rights contained within the *Code of Health and Disability Services Consumers' Rights* (Health and Disability Commissioner, n.d.).

CASE STUDY 22.1

Failure to report an error

The following case is emblematic of many cases that resulted in legal proceedings because of poor record keeping. A complaint was filed with the Health and Disability Commissioner regarding a non-registered health-care assistant who was responsible for the care of an elderly man with dementia and challenging behaviours (Case 06HDC10115).

The rest home dismissed the assistant for breaching its policy on administration of medication, failing to document and report a medication error, and failure to inform the resident's family. Instead of administering a particular medication at 5 pm, the assistant gave it at midday. Then the assistant decided that, as she had already made the error, she would 'trial' this practice because the resident was very agitated in the evenings.

The assistant told the evening staff about the incident and asked them to give the resident his midday medication at 5 pm as an experiment. Employees reported the matter to the manager and, after an investigation, the assistant was dismissed. The assistant claimed the conduct was an accidental error.

In the Commissioner's opinion, the assistant failed to provide the resident with the appropriate standard of care and therefore breached Right 4(1). Also, in failing to alert the family, the assistant breached Right 6(1). The case progressed to the Human Rights Review Tribunal (New Zealand Legal Information Institute, 2010). The Tribunal found that the assistant did not deliberately alter the resident's medication. However, having made an error, her decision to experiment and not report the error was a breach of Right 4(2) for failure to comply with relevant standards and 4(5) for failure to cooperate with other providers to ensure quality and continuity of service.

Documentation Written information that often follows a prescribed format.

What is the lesson regarding **documentation**? This case sends a strong message to the broad audience of registered and non-registered providers that appropriate care includes 'competent reporting' and applies to all who hold themselves out as providing a health or disability service. The rights apply to the constellation of paid and volunteer non-registered providers, including providers of complementary medicine (Paterson, 2000), paramedics, massage therapists and counsellors.

Registered health practitioners are governed by the Health Practitioners Competence Assurance Act 2003. Many registered health practitioners were found guilty by the Health Practitioners Disciplinary Tribunal (HPDT) for misconduct related to 'inadequate, inaccurate or misleading recordkeeping'. For example, poor documentation featured in the misconduct of a chiropractor (Chiro09/131D) (HPDT, 2009a), a doctor (Med08/102) (HPDT, 2008a), midwives (Mid08/82D and Mid10/146P) (HPDT, 2008b), a nurse (Nur09/138D)(HPDT, 2009b) and a physiotherapist (Phys09/130D) (HPDT, 2009c). In addition to potential name disclosure, the penalty may include costs, a fine, conditions placed on practice, suspension and the ultimate penalty of de-registration (HPDT, 2011).

The fundaments of record keeping

Records Documented information about what has occurred.

Record keeping in the health-care context aids the provision of safe and appropriate care. We should also be mindful that **records** may be used in a variety of legal proceedings and may be viewed by consumers and their representatives (Burgess, 2008). Records may be relevant for a spectrum of legal proceedings by the review bodies discussed above and investigations by employers, police, the Privacy Commissioner and the Ombudsman (Burgess, 2008). Thorough documentation is particularly important when multiple services and providers are involved.

Burgess (2008) observes that it may be appropriate to relay information verbally in some instances, but *important* information should always be in written form. The written record is more reliable because verbal communication relies on memory that may fade or become distorted over time. Burgess (2008, p. 175) published guidance for nurses and midwives, which is equally relevant for all providers.

Written records should be:

+ factual, accurate, concise, legible and indelible
+ signed (or initialled as appropriate) and dated
+ written as soon as possible after care or events occur
+ a documentation of:
  ~ objectively described relevant facts such as observations, decisions and events
  ~ substantiated professional opinion
  ~ future plans or directions for care and treatment
+ completed by the person who delivered the care or witnessed events
+ completed before the person responsible leaves work
+ conform to legal and employer requirements
+ made and kept confidential, thus respecting the client's right to privacy.

It is advisable to use ink and it may be wise to spell out the month when dating a document because, for example, 10/2/11 could be interpreted outside Aotearoa New Zealand as October 2, 2011 rather than 10 February 2011. Providers also need to be careful when using abbreviations because they may not be universally understood (Dalziel & Johnson, 2010).

Regarding content, report writers should avoid ambiguous, subjective and judgmental statements. Objective reporting is essential. If a provider 'did not see, hear, feel, smell or taste something' but intends to report its occurrence, the provider should state the source of the information (Dalziel & Johnson, 2010, p. 207). For example, if the provider did not observe an alleged fall, the provider should report: 'Ms Jones stated that she fell out of bed.' Vague reports on the consumer's status, such as 'usual day', are of limited value in court and other legal proceedings (and may indicate the provider's carelessness) (Dalziel & Johnson, 2010, p. 207).

Generally, when asked to give evidence in court or in a sworn statement, individuals are required to give only an account of what was experienced by their senses: 'Reporting what one was told and asserting the truth of what was said is hearsay evidence and is not usually admissible' (Dalziel & Johnson, 2010, p. 210). Therefore, providers should avoid documenting hearsay or, alternatively, record that the information was reported or experienced by a specified *other* person.

Mistakes should be identified and the corrections clearly recorded, with inclusion of the erroneous words. Errors should be crossed through with a single line and initialled because erasure could raise questions regarding the alterations. In relation to the alteration, 'an error which, although corrected, is still readable will remove any suspicion of wrongdoing' (Burgess, 2008, p. 175). If the correction is made on a separate sheet, it should be attached to the original, signed and dated (Dalziel & Johnson, 2010).

Providers should 'avoid rewriting or transcribing any documentation made by another health professional' (Burgess, 2008, p. 175). To establish accuracy in recording telephone orders, the order should be written down immediately and repeated back to the person issuing the order. Then the order should be signed and dated by the person, and countersigned and dated by the prescribing person as soon as possible.

A variety of resources on professional report writing are freely available on the internet, including advice for specific professions such as psychology (McGee, 2010), along with instructions for documentation of specific procedures, such as consent forms.

Elements of a consent form

The concept of informed consent needs to be fully understood by all who work in the health care and disability support sector. Because people are complex and their decisions may change, consent should be seen as a process rather than a single event. However, it is also good practice to have a way of documenting consent and this generally involves the use of a consent form. It should include:

+ name and full identification of consumer
+ name and procedure agreed to
+ name of place for carrying out the procedure
+ consent to specified associated treatments; these could presumably have been discussed as part of the procedure
+ consent to or statement acknowledging possible need for emergency treatment
+ a statement of what information had been given; for example, what the procedure involves, why it is required and why it is recommended in preference to alternatives.

Further items can be added per those in the *Code of Health and Disability Services Consumers' Rights* (Health and Disability Commissioner, 2009):

+ a list of specific risks and advantages, which have been discussed
+ agreement to another person carrying out the procedure, or any other necessary procedure, if circumstances require this (Johnson & Keenan, 2010, p. 106).

It is essential to document a consumer's refusal. Among the range of guidance available on record keeping is the topic of factors to document when a consumer *refuses* services. It is advisable to document the efforts taken on the consumer's behalf with responses to the following types of questions (Johnson & O'Brien, 2010, p. 177):

+ Where is the consumer going?
+ Does the consumer know how to take care of himself or herself?
+ Does the consumer know what symptoms indicate the need for further medical attention?

+ Does the consumer know how to seek further attention?
+ Does the consumer know what complications can occur?
+ How does a provider demonstrate that she or he engaged in this process with the consumer?

CASE STUDY 22.2

Document, document, document!

Guidance from the Health Information Privacy Code

Another somewhat unexpected source of guidance in Aotearoa New Zealand is the *Health Information Privacy Code* (HIPC) (Privacy Commissioner, 2008). The HIPC's twelve detailed rules articulate the principles that reflect sound clinical practice and New Zealand law.

The HIPC applies to a range of activities conducted by a 'health agency'. This term is widely defined to include, for example:

- providers of health and disability services
- professional bodies that are responsible for training, registering and disciplining practitioners
- agencies that provide advocacy services for health and disability consumers.

Of particular relevance to students and their clinical supervisors, 'health agency' includes 'a school, faculty or department of a tertiary educational institution that provides the training or a component of the training necessary for the registration of a health practitioners' pursuant to Clause 4(2)(d).

'Health records' include a variety of documents, including 'assessment, investigation and results; diagnosis; care plans; health promotion activities; treatment and medications; patient progress; referrals and support services; evaluation and follow-up' (Dalziel & Johnson, 2010, p. 205).

A few examples will illustrate the guidance offered by the HIPC. Rule 4 requires that health information must be collected without unreasonable intrusion on the person's private affairs and must be collected lawfully and fairly. Violations may include 'digitally recording (audio or video) a consumer without consent, collecting information in an overbearing or threatening manner, or asking a consumer to provide personal details in a public area, such as at a front counter or hospital bed in a ward' (Dalziel & Johnson, 2010, p. 204).

Rule 8 aims to protect individuals by requiring agencies to take reasonable steps to ensure information is accurate, up-to-date, complete, relevant and not misleading. Reasonable steps for ensuring accuracy will vary depending upon the proposed use. For example, rigorous checks may be appropriate if decisions regarding health-care entitlements (for example, through the Accident Compensation Corporation) or treatment alternatives depend upon that information. Reasonable steps might also include having the affected individual check the accuracy of health information at the time it is collected from another agency, or as soon as is practicable. The Privacy Commissioner acknowledges that health agencies may face difficulties in ensuring accuracy and completeness of information provided by another health agency. Consideration should be given to recording the *source* of the information on the file.

For providers and students, the HIPC's additional, detailed commentary will answer most questions regarding management and protection of health information (Privacy Commissioner, n.d.). For example, a 'legitimate use of information where the individual is not identified might be where a student sees a patient (with consent) and later writes up the notes as a case history without identifying the patient' (Privacy Commissioner, n.d., p. 51). Regarding mental health consumers' information, more specific guidance was recently produced in consultation with the Mental Health Commission (Privacy Commissioner, 2010).

In summary, legal guidance is available from the HIPC for health agencies that handle health information. More specific advice regarding matters such as consent forms and documentation of consumers' refusal of services are also accessible.

Formal submissions

New Zealanders have the opportunity to engage in the political process, and written submissions are a potentially powerful method to participate in public debates. Many governmental departments invite written submissions to survey the public's views on governmental proposals (Ting, 2002). The submission process allows community members to have equitable opportunities to voice their opinions. This opportunity applies to individuals involved in disability and health reform. For example, New Zealand scholars and paramedics made submissions regarding the debate surrounding registration of paramedics (Costa-Scorse, 2008). While international guidance is available (Ting, 2002), more occupation-specific advice within Aotearoa New Zealand is also accessible (New Zealand Association of Occupational Therapists, 2006).

Generally, there are two types of submissions. The first is an invitation by a governmental body to canvass public opinion on a specific topic. The second is when the governmental body's decision has already been made but submissions are invited to substantiate the decision. The aim of both types is to influence the governmental body. The submission explains why the specific governmental proposal should be supported or rejected, while illuminating the underlying reasoning.

The New Zealand Association of Occupational Therapists (2006) suggests the following approach for submissions to select committees:

+ Write clearly, order your message and make it easy to read.
+ State clearly what it is about.
+ State clearly who it is from.
+ Clarify any intention to appear before a select committee.
+ If writing on behalf of an organisation (with their authority), state their aims and give background information (who they serve, when it began, how many they serve/represent, their interest in the topic).
+ State who has been consulted with.
+ Address five basic factors: relevancy, clarity, conciseness, accuracy and conclusion.

The argument should be succinct, fair and accurate (which is wise advice for all forms of professional writing). A moderate and persuasive style is recommended that is presented in good English and without any abusive or foul language. Fair criticism is acceptable and where appropriate this should be followed with suggestions for constructive alternatives.

A well-researched argument is a more persuasive argument. We can only respond to opposing arguments if we fully appreciate their views, which requires research (good submissions anticipate opposing arguments). To bolster the argument, incorporate regional, national and international perspectives. It is advisable to quote experts (where appropriate) because it gives experts their due and adds authority to the submission. The New Zealand Government website includes information and links to assist with developing and presenting submissions.

The writing process

Report-writing advice for members of health and disability professions would not be complete without acknowledging the real challenges we all face at the beginning of the writing process. Many people who write as part of their education and professional lives face remarkably similar challenges, although these may not be readily recognised or admitted (Becker, 1998, 2007). Yet a spectrum of wonderful resources is available to guide and inspire those who are developing and refining their writing skills.

Academic and professional writing is an acquired skill. Like the skills required for a triathlon (or even a 10-km run), writing requires practice and resilience. Many expert writers admit the discipline and patience that is involved in the writing process

(Becker, 2007; Neale, 1992). One source of inspiration is the eloquent revelation by Pamela Richards that she experienced a tremendous sense of risk and insecurity as a postgraduate student when committing her thoughts and research to the written word (Richards, 2007). Her story and advice is invaluable.

Guidance is available on how to focus (Sellers, 2007) and how to overcome writing blocks (Mack & Skjei, 1979). For reassurance that the challenges we face are universal and surmountable, we have the words from Chaucer to Shakespeare, from Orwell to Austen (Neale, 1992). And for those who experience 'punctuation deficits', we have the recommendations of Watson (2003) and Truss (2006). Practical exercises help refine writing skills (Glaser, 1999) and style guides abound (Strunk & White, 2007; Williams, 2006).

{ SUMMARY }

Documentation matters for members of health and disability occupations and the people they serve. Best practice requires competent documentation. Our moral and legal obligations to the people that we serve include professional report writing. Understanding how to record, what to record and when to record will improve professional practice. It will also reduce the likelihood of a complaint related to documentation. Happily, a range of resources (both legal and non-legal) is available.

REFLECTION POINTS

22.1 Intention (motivation, message, meaning, emotion)

Why is accurate documentation of client care important?

22.2 Reception (received message, response, feedback)

How might you check the accuracy of material you are documenting about a client?

22.3 Perception (style, manner, impression, analysis)

Health practitioners sometimes make mistakes with documentation. How should these be managed?

QUESTIONS FOR REVIEW

1 Under what circumstances may a practitioner be concerned about information that they include in patient records?
2 How would you differentiate between objective and subjective assessment data?
3 What elements are considered essential to document when gaining informed consent?

REFERENCES

Becker, H. S. (1998). *Tricks of the trade: How to think about your research while you're doing it*. Chicago, IL: University of Chicago Press.

Becker, H. S. (2007). *Writing for social scientists: How to start and finish your thesis, book, or article*. Chicago, IL: University of Chicago Press.

Burgess, M. (ed.) (2008). *A guide to the law for nurses and midwives* (4th edn). Auckland, NZ: Pearson Education.

Costa-Scorse, B. (2008). Submission on the provision of ambulance services in New Zealand. *Journal of Emergency Primary Health Care, 6*(3). Article 990321. Retrieved from www.jephc.com/full_article.cfm?content_id=492.

Dalziel, K. & Johnson, S. (2010). Health information. In R. Keenan & L. Clery (eds), *Health care and the law* (4th NZ edn) (pp. 199–240). Wellington, NZ: Thomson Reuters.

Glaser, J. (1999). *Understanding style: Practical ways to improve your writing*. Oxford, UK: Oxford University Press.

Health and Disability Commissioner. (2009). *Code of Health and Disability Services Consumers' Rights Regulations 1996*. Retrieved from www.hdc.org.nz/the-act—code/the-code-of-rights.

Health and Disability Commissioner. (n.d.). *Code of Health and Disability Services consumers' rights*. Retrieved from http://www.hdc.org.nz/the-act—code/the-code-of-rights/the-code-(full).

Health Practitioners Disciplinary Tribunal. (2008a). *Tribunal Decisions (Doctors): Med08/102*. Retrieved from www.hpdt.org.nz.

Health Practitioners Disciplinary Tribunal. (2008b). *Tribunal Decisions (Midwives): Mid08/82D*. Retrieved from www.hpdt.org.nz.

Health Practitioners Disciplinary Tribunal. (2009a). *Tribunal Decisions (Chiropractors): Chiro09/131D*. Retrieved from www.hpdt.org.nz.

Health Practitioners Disciplinary Tribunal. (2009b). *Tribunal Decisions (Nurses): Nur09/138D*. Retrieved from www.hpdt.org.nz.

Health Practitioners Disciplinary Tribunal. (2009c). *Tribunal Decisions (Physiotherapists): Phys09/130D*. Retrieved from www.hpdt.org.nz.

Health Practitioners Disciplinary Tribunal. (2011). *Tribunal statistics: All professions*. Retrieved from www.hpdt.org.nz/Default.aspx?tabid=86.

Johnson, S. & Keenan, R. (2010). Consent. In R. Keenan & L. Clery (eds). *Health care and the law* (4th NZ edn) (pp. 85–117). Wellington, NZ: Thomson Reuters.

Johnson, S. & O'Brien, A. (2010). *Liability for personal injury*. In R. Keenan & L. Clery (eds), *Health care and the law* (4th NZ edn) (pp. 149–97). Wellington, NZ: Thomson Reuters.

Mack, K. & Skjei, E. (1979). *Overcoming writing blocks*. Los Angeles, CA: JP Tarcher, Inc.

McGee, S. (2010). *Key research and study skills in psychology*. London, UK: Sage.

Neale, R. (1992). *Writers on writing: An anthology*. Auckland, NZ: Oxford University Press.

New Zealand Association of Occupational Therapists. (2006). *How to write a submission*. Retrieved from www.nzaot.com/publications/submissions/how.to.php.

New Zealand Legal Information Institute. (2010). *New Zealand Acts*. Retrieved from www.nzlii.org/nz/legis/consol_act.

New Zealand Legislation: Acts. (2003). *Health Practitioners Competence Assurance Act 2003*. Retrieved from www.legislation.govt.nz/act/public/2003/0048/latest/DLM203312.html.

New Zealand Legislation: Regulations. (n.d.). [Database] Wellington, NZ: Parliamentary Council Office. Retrieved from www.legislation.govt.nz/regulation/browse.aspx.

Paterson, R. (2000). *Medicine for today: Professional responsibility and complementary medicine*. Presented to Otago University, Dunedin, New Zealand. Retrieved from www.hdc.org.nz/education/presentations/medicine-for-today—professional-responsibility-and-complementary-medicine.

Privacy Commissioner. (2007). *Health Information Privacy Code 1994*. Auckland, NZ: Office of the Privacy Commissioner. Retrieved from http://privacy.org.nz/assets/Files/Codes-of-Practice-materials/Health-Information-Privacy-Code-1994-including-Amendment.pdf.

Privacy Commissioner. (2008). *Health information privacy code 1994 including amendment*. Auckland, NZ: Office of the Privacy Commissioner. Retrieved from http://privacy.org.nz/assets/Files/Codes-of-Practice-materials/Health-Information-Privacy-Code-1994-including-Amendment.pdf.

Privacy Commissioner. (2010). *Guidance material for health providers and mental health consumers*. Auckland, NZ: Office of the Privacy Commissioner. Retrieved from http://privacy.org.nz/guidance-material-for-health-practitioners-on-mental-health-information/?highlight=.

Privacy Commissioner. (n.d.). *Health information privacy code with commentary*. Auckland, NZ: Office of the Privacy Commissioner. Retrieved from http://privacy.org.nz/health-information-privacy-code-1994-incorporating-amendments-and-including-revised-commentary.

Richards, P. (2007). Risk. In H. S. Becker (ed.), *Writing for social scientists: How to start and finish your thesis, book, or article* (pp. 108–20). Chicago, IL: University of Chicago Press.

Sellers, H. (2007). *Chapter after chapter: Discover the dedication and focus you need to write the book of your dreams*. Cincinnati, OH: Writer's Digest Books.

Strunk, W. & White, E. B. (2007). *The elements of style* (4th edn). New York, NY: Penguin.

Ting, H. (2002). *Writing a submission*. Retrieved from www.lawlink.nsw.gov.au/lawlink/legislation_policy/ll_lpd.nsf/vwFiles/Writing%20a%20Submission%20-%20Helen%20Ting.pdf/$file/Writing%20a%20Submission%20-%20Helen%20Ting.pdf.

Truss, L. (2006). *Eats, shoots and leaves: The zero tolerance approach to punctuation*. New York, NY: Gotham Books.

Watson, D. (2003). *Death sentence: The decay of public language*. Sydney, NSW: Knopf.

Williams, J. (2006). *Style: Towards clarity and grace*. Chicago, IL: University of Chicago Press.

WEBSITES

Guidelines for Medical Record and Clinical Documentation: www.searo.who.int/LinkFiles/2007_Guidelines_for_Clinical_Doc.pdf

Health and Disability Commissioner's Case Notes: www.hdc.org.nz/decisions—case-notes

Health Practitioners Disciplinary Tribunal: www.hpdt.org.nz

Making a Submission to a Parliamentary Select Committee, New Zealand Parliament: www.parliament.nz/en-NZ/AboutParl/HowPWorks/Procedures/4/9/e/00CL00CMakingSubmission1-Making-a-submission-to-a-Parliamentary-select.htm

Patient Safety Checklists, World Health Organization: www.who.int/patientsafety/implementation/checklists/en

{23}

The Electronic Message

Ailsa Haxell

CHAPTER OVERVIEW

This chapter covers the following topics:

+ Technology as more than a tool
+ Mobile phones
+ Text messaging
+ Internet
+ Social networking sites
+ Discussion boards
+ Blogs
+ Twitter
+ Virtual reality environments.

KEY TERMS

Technology
Conversation
Social networking

What we consider new and emergent today will seem commonplace in just a few short years. As we become used to technologies, they tend to slip into the background as if they had always been there. **Technology** in this chapter is defined as practice—as 'the way we do things'—rather than the artefacts of electronics, computers, mobile phones or pixels on a screen. In taking this approach to technology, emphasis is placed on practice, on the ways of working and talking when this is mediated by communication and computer technologies. In applying this understanding of technology, the focus is to foreground practice, utilising stories that trace the ways communicating changes, and avoiding the trap of seeing technology as 'just a tool'.

Technology
Tools that enable communication and access to information.

To see new communication devices or computer technologies as 'just a tool' denies their mediating effects. The implication is that we can pick up or put down such objects with no change to our way of being. As will be seen, this is a flawed account.

Technology as more than a tool

The evolution of humankind is commonly linked with when our earliest ancestors could first use opposable thumbs to manipulate a stick, and each age of humankind has been named for the artefacts that epitomised the technologies of the age: stone, bronze, iron, industrial and digital. This is the first evolution of humankind that places a means of communicating as central to what identifies us as people.

Just as every other age transformed humankind, so too will this one. Unlike our predecessors we can be heard, in real time, the world over: voice has been amplified, as has hearing. What has changed in the last fifty years is this can be achieved anywhere, anytime with ease. We expect to find wireless access to the internet in airports, cafes and malls, and recognise that wireless access will soon be as much a background of expectation as access to television, radio and mobile phones. This availability changes us; and changes our patterns of relating. Whether this is a good or bad thing remains disputed; however, such disputes are not new, as Marvin (1988, p. 1) points out:

> New technologies is a historically relative term. We are not the first generation to wonder at the rapid and extraordinary shifts in the dimension of the world and the human relationships it contains as a result of new forms of communication, or be surprised by the changes those shifts occasion in the regular pattern of our lives.

Marvin (1988) had studied the histories of electricity and of telephones. In investigating *When Old Technologies Were New*, she asserts new technologies are suspect precisely to the extent that they lessen control (p. 76). Using different mediums in different patterns of relating inevitably changes the social order. In her analysis of the moral panic associated with the development of telephones, she noted the literature focused on how particular groups of people should behave, and that these expectations were being transgressed. The new technologies resulted in new kinds of encounters, meaning relationships needed to be reconfigured; or, as Marvin (1988, p. 5) states, 'some people were suddenly too close while others were much too far away'. What was being negotiated was less about how to use a device and more about one's social positioning: was it right or proper, and who had authority on such matters? Who would speak on behalf of others, who would be listened to, and who might not?

As Marvin showed, fears regarding the effects of telephones predated fear regarding internet use, mobile phone use and texting. Frequently, the discussion positions new technologies as good or bad, while the complexity gets neglected. Such normative evaluation of communication and computer technologies is a bit like asking 'Is talking to strangers a good or bad thing?', 'Is talking quietly or loudly a good or bad thing?' The answer must be: *it depends*.

Technology shapes the message and the messenger

There are alterations in the ways we connect, and in the ways in which technologies are involved in this connecting. Such alterations influence not only how we do things but also how we think about things. In a YouTube clip, *The Machine is Us/ing Us*, Wesch (2007) presents a thoughtful piece on how differently we function in digital spaces. It is also a provocation to think differently about things: not only might we reconsider 'tools' but also how digital spaces have influence on relating and thereby influence on identity.

Sherry Turkle (2006), a psychoanalytical psychologist, argues human development may suffer. With reference to the teenage years, where identity and independence are forming, she argues that ready access to parents and friends by mobile phone enables dependency. In contrast is the view of Broadbent (2009), who argues from a social justice perspective that mobile phones provide for a 'democratising of intimacy', especially for those who are time or resource poor. For those who are socially disadvantaged—whether because of poverty, shift working, holding multiple jobs or travelling long distances for work that takes one away from family and loved ones—a mobile phone can reduce the isolation effects and ameliorate alienation.

Despite the seeming contradictions between mobile phone use being positioned as both good and bad, both Turkle and Broadbent might be correct. People are not homogenous, measures of good and bad are not necessarily mutually exclusive, and renegotiating the ways in which we communicate provides opportunities for seeing both the complexities involved and how we might deliberately use the technologies we have at our disposal to make a positive difference.

That we do alter in response to the tools we use, and that we also reconfigure the tools that we use, led self-proclaimed cyborg Donna Haraway to state: 'Technology is not neutral. We're inside of what we make, and it's inside of us. We're living in a world of connections—and it matters which ones get made and unmade' (Kunzru, 1997, p. 33).

Haraway's self-proclaimed cyborg status provokes consideration for the ways we as people are enhanced (or not) by the technologies we use. The provocative statement is also an important political statement. In establishing new ways of communicating, we need to look at who is advantaged or disadvantaged, and the pros and cons involved in using these 'new' technologies. This chapter now explores some of the specific media currently being used.

Mobile phones

Use of mobile phones has increased dramatically. Mobile phone ethnographer Jan Chipchase identifies that a mobile phone is now among the top three objects people do not leave home without: keys, money and mobile phone (Palmer, 2008). In Aotearoa New Zealand, mobile phones now outnumber people, with 104 per cent saturation reported by Nelson and Shepheard (2008). The 2009 Census showed 85 per cent of New Zealanders had a mobile phone and that the largest percentage increase between the 2006 Census and 2009 Census was for the group aged between 65 and 74 years. Mobile phones can no longer be considered a phenomenon of young people. Nonetheless, the age groups most likely to have a mobile phone are 20–24-year-olds (93 per cent) and 15–19-year-olds (89 per cent) (Statistics New Zealand, 2009). The saturation level of more than 100 per cent indicates that a significant number of people have more than one mobile phone.

It is not that phones are new but that newness results from their being used differently now that they are mobile. The anywhere, anytime feature enables what Gergen (2002) calls absent presence. He suggests that this risks depth to relationships; that a lowering of cues risks the authenticity of a message being conveyed.

Text messaging

The patterns of mobile phone use in Aotearoa New Zealand are unique. Young people have taken to text messaging (also called short message service or SMS) at a much higher rate than comparable countries such as Australia or the USA. Reasons for this include the comparative costs of mobile phone plans, with prepay plans being considerably more prevalent in Aotearoa New Zealand than in the USA. New Zealand mobile phone calls are among the most expensive in the OECD (Nelson & Shepheard, 2008). It is cost-savvy young people in particular who are more likely to text than to call.

The text capacity of a mobile phone was developed as a 'backchat', through which companies could tell customers when a call had been missed or when credit was due to expire. In other words, the space was designed for extraordinarily brief messages (Wray, 2002). And because the mobile phone was not designed as a writing medium, the keyboard is typically based on the numerical keys, where each key does the work for up to four letters. Mobile text messages are also usually constrained to the small screen, with a width of 28 characters and a depth of 10 lines, with the first line allocated to the recipient's name and the total message not exceeding 160 characters, including spaces. There's work, then, in crafting a message succinct enough to be carried by SMS messaging. An SMS message longer than 160 characters is sent as two messages, effectively doubling costs for the sender. Brevity in messages, even when not required, has become a convention associated with the medium. The common practice is to be brief, shorten, k? A staccato of short sentences and short words has become the norm.

Most of the time, conveying a succinct message takes into account a reduction in key strokes as well as ensuring the message fits the character limit per message. The work taken to craft a message suggests playfulness with the medium rather than illiteracy. For example, there is less physical effort in writing 'yup' than writing 'yes'. 'Yup' only takes six key strokes on a numeric keyboard performing an alphabet, and 'yes' takes nine.

It takes longer to text than it does to talk, and getting the message across quickly and with minimum fuss seems to contribute to shortening of words and dropping vowels out of words, even where the space for a message would have allowed full spelling. However, unique to the very small screen of conversations is the apparent paradox of saying more with less. To say more with less, in a texting medium, cuts into the conventions of most health-service related conversations and particularly counselling relationships. The texting medium reduces the cues one has to work with. Not only is the person invisible, and so no body language cues are available, but they are also inaudible, and so no paralinguistic cues are available either. Who is present in a texting **conversation** is an unknown: young, old, male, female, even the number of people present can only be inferred from what is shared. Removing paralinguistic cues means age, gender, urgency or distress is similarly masked. Paradoxically, the apparent anonymity afforded by fewer social cues being present is counterbalanced by there being undeniable visible digital traces of a text-based conversation. Messages sent and received stay on a person's mobile phone sim card until they are deleted, while the mobile phone company service provider can also store the message. Anonymity is therefore more assumed than actual. The effect that others cannot hear a conversation gives a semblance of privacy that is actually not warranted. Risks to privacy are therefore reasonably high.

Conversation An informal exchange of ideas.

With the absence of visual and auditory cues, textually based interactions present emotional content in more deliberate and sometimes exaggerated ways. The use of emoticons such as ☺ or :-) or the Asian emoticon of similar meaning (^^) are used to reduce the ambiguity that might occur with the absence of other social cues. The use of capital letters is used to suggest extra volume or force behind a message. In the absence of body language to provide further cues for a message, emotions tend to be deliberately added into the conversation, and are also frequently exaggerated to provide a sense of what is or is not important; ROFL or 'rolling on the floor laughing' is an example of this. Ambiguity of abbreviated messages is also problematic when well-known acronyms such as 'lol' may mean both lots of love and laughing out loud.

CASE STUDY 23.1

Txt-counselling

New Zealand's Youthline is a world leader in 'txt-counselling', having provided counselling by text messaging since December 2004. The mobile phone texting medium significantly alters how counselling can occur. The lack of space typically results in text messages that move straight into the main content of a message, rather than checking out availability to talk or setting up trust in the relationship. Youthline notes that young people who initiate a text-based counselling interaction tend to go straight to the heart of what concerns them. Establishing rapport and trust do not appear as a separate phase in such interactions. This is not because the 'relationship' does not exist—it clearly does—but because building of rapport is integral to each interchange rather than being a discrete step at the start of the counselling conversation. The minimum and sufficient conditions for establishing a working therapeutic relationship are tested and altered within a medium that privileges brevity. The counselling responses, in turn, are reshaped. It is an art to demonstrate the equivalent skills to active listening, empathy, affirming strengths and inviting further interactions all in a 160 character response:

> Hi there, its g8 that u
> hav txt us. Sounds
> like there r some
> thngs u mite wnt 2
> tlk about, u culd call
> us 0800211211 tlk
> thru options.

What appeared to make phone counselling attractive to young people—its anonymity and ease of access—is potentiated through text counselling. Recipients can exercise more control over their composure, there is less pressure for an immediate response, the trace of messages seems to have a positive effect in not going over the same material repeatedly, and affirmative statements can be kept on the phone as a useful reminder of strengths or strategies.

For those providing counselling, the disembodiment requires working with fewer cues. However, it is important to remember that this is a conversation, and just as with any conversation there is no need to attempt everything in one response. The use of text messaging alters the performance of counselling but not the intent. The intent of helping people find their own solutions to problems remains. While mobile phones (and texting in particular) have received significant negative media coverage, there are health-related examples that also demonstrate effective, empowering applications (Haxell, 2010).

In health promotion, the sending of affirmative messages seems to have a positive effect in part because it is imminently portable, is already accepted, has little outlay of costs, has low maintenance costs and is widespread. Health promotion applications of text messaging have included interventions to assist people in their resolve to stop smoking (Bramley et al., 2005) and to provide knowledge on sexual health services (Levine et al., 2008).

Sending text message reminders of appointments has also been shown to significantly increase attendance and to reduce non-attendance rates. The use of text reminders is more cost effective and less labour intensive than traditional appointment reminders such as letters or phone calls. For example, the sending of text reminders in a UK ophthalmology clinic resulted in a 38 per cent reduction in non-attendance (Koshy, Car & Majeed, 2008), while at a paediatric outpatient clinic in Australia, the non-attendance rate dropped from 29.4 per cent to 19.5 per cent (Geraghty et al., 2007).

With the advent of further changes in the technologies available by mobile phone—such as phones increasingly being used to access the internet, and the use of qwerty keyboards rather than a numeric-based alphabet—the phenomenon of text messaging may date quickly. Nonetheless, the knowledge of how to do more with less can still be utilised. If text messaging evolves with greater use of internet access (with a shift from 160-character messages to unlimited-character emails) and if associated costs come down further, then issues of absent presence and of being invisible and inaudible will probably continue to make the medium attractive particularly for young people. However, having more space in which to talk will make the medium easier to negotiate. The future looks strong for the continued development of mobile technologies. With the advent of mobile phones that can take health-related apps, there is increased likelihood of having health strategies and information close at hand.

Internet

The internet has had wide-ranging ramifications for the delivery of health-care information. Health information is now readily available to anyone with access to the internet. In addition, information can be placed on the internet by anyone with the capacity to build a website, make use of a social networking site or contribute to a discussion group.

Though health information via the internet is readily available (Powell et al., 2005), there is also evidence that people often do not know how to evaluate the credibility, bias or relevance of health websites (Gauld & Williams, 2009; Murray et al., 2003).

The study by Gauld and Williams (2009) across Australia and Aotearoa New Zealand found 17 per cent of those they surveyed had sought health information online in the preceding year (p. 154). They also found that 90 per cent of those who had accessed health information online believed the information they accessed was reliable, although only one-third checked the credentials of information providers (p. 155). Of those who had accessed the internet for health information, 15 per cent described the discussion with their doctor about what they had located on the internet as uncomfortable (p. 152) and 4 per cent thought that doing so had worsened their relationship with their doctor (p. 155). Clearly there is a need for practitioners to be able to listen, explain, interpret and discuss, in a supportive and constructive way, the relevance of the information clients are bringing with them.

Social networking sites

Social networking The process of people interacting, often through the medium of technology.

Social networking provides a means to connect with people. On the internet this may occur in virtual spaces such as discussion boards, blogging, micro-blogging sites such as twitter and virtual reality sites such as Second Life. This is not a finite list. Social networking sites, just as with any other type of community, have a natural cycle of coming and going, of growth and attrition, and of movement between communities.

The composition and shape of a social network helps to determine a network's usefulness to its members. Smaller, tighter networks can be less useful to members than networks with a lot of loose connections or weak ties. More open networks, with many weak ties and social connections, are more likely to introduce new ideas and opportunities than closed networks. In other words, a group of friends who only do things with each other already share the same knowledge and opportunities, whereas a group of people with connections to other social worlds is likely to have access to a wider range of information.

Discussion boards

An internet discussion board, or message board, is an online discussion site where people can hold conversations in the form of posted messages. They differ from other types of online chat, such as instant messaging, because the messages are at least temporarily archived. Some discussion boards are open to anyone who is able to access the discussion board through the internet, others require specific group membership. Some allow total anonymity, while others require membership to be verified. Some discussion boards allow posted messages to be immediately visible, while others require moderation. For health-related discussion boards set up by a health service provider, it is likely that such moderation is undertaken by a health practitioner, but this is not always the case. In some discussion boards it is the anonymity provided that allows expression of feelings and questions that, because of embarrassment or shame, might otherwise not be asked.

A discussion board can provide a sense of community by sustaining contact with people who are going through similar experiences. The advantage in health care is that there are groups of people who might otherwise be unable to meet due to access concerns. Access might be limited by illness or disability, or because of the need to care for someone with a disability. It also may be linked to there being relatively low numbers of people with a particular health concern who are geographically widespread, or because of anxiety or fears of marginalisation. A supportive online environment has the added advantage of being able to pose a question and receive advice or support without having to make an appointment, arrange transportation and take time off work. The asynchronised nature of discussion boards allows for leaving a message when the question arises, and coming back to it later when others may have responded. International time zones can therefore be bypassed.

Blogs

Blogs are one form of social networking where people can upload their own material to the internet. A blog is short for 'web log' and is the name for an online diary or journal, or the activity of writing thoughts in that journal. In a health-care context, these are often a personal account of what is going on for someone: sometimes the experiences of caring for someone with significant health-care needs and sometimes a personal story of living with a disability or illness. Blogs also allow people to 'meet online' with others who might share similar experiences and so establish a community of support. Following Pennebaker and Beall's (1986) ground-breaking work on emotional support having a protective influence on survival, Pennebaker continued research into the therapeutic benefits of externalising feelings. Writing about traumatic experiences results in individuals talking more to their friends, laughing more, and being more positive in their conversations (Pennebaker, 2000). In writing of the health benefits of narrative he states:

> In an ideal world, upsetting experiences are transformed into stories that are shared with others. This process helps us to understand the events and, at the same time, alerts our friends to our emotional and psychological state. Such storytelling ultimately helps us maintain a stable social and emotional life. In our less-than-ideal existence, however, we often keep important personal experiences to ourselves. Holding these secrets can be biologically taxing, can block the natural cognitive work of coming to terms with the secrets, and can distance the secret-keeper from friends and family. Translating personally upsetting experiences into language in a story format, even when the story is written rather than spoken, may accomplish for us what oral storytelling must have accomplished for our ancestors—improvements in physical and mental health as well as the development of closer social bonds.
>
> *Pennebaker (2000, p. 18)*

This is similar to the benefits identified by Tan (2008) who suggests blogging is a means for self-reflection, provides symptomatic relief in the expression of emotions, and provides a venue where a person is safely able to develop 'voice' through which she or he can speak about what they are going through without feeling judged.

Twitter

Twitter (http://twitter.com) is a form of microblogging. Each posted comment is limited to 140 characters. The posts tend to be a response to the permanent question of 'What's happening?' as this is the header of a twittering page. Such tweets (posted comments) can be read by anyone who has elected to 'follow' you, meaning that your tweets will show up in a stream of tweets that others read. They can also be forwarded with one push of a keypad to that person's followers and so on. Tweets have a much more immediate presence than blogs, and are often used to link to other material on the internet as a pointer for others. The ability to send tweets via SMS also makes this form of microblogging useful for providing short messages to a wide audience.

People who want to follow a particular subject, rather than a person, can group together subjects of their choice by doing a search using the hashtag (#) function. Similarly, the hashtag function can be used to establish a live synchronised conversation with multiple users contributing concurrently. This provides for a very odd way of talking, as each participant in each utterance has a maximum of 140 characters to 'speak' with, and the posting of tweets usually occurs concurrently rather than consecutively as there is no indication of who might be writing a message at any one time.

Twitter has been considered a trivial medium, with one study (Pearanalytics, 2006) labelling 40 per cent of posts as pointless babble, 38 per cent conversational, 9 per cent having 'pass along' value, 6 per cent being self-promoting, 4 per cent comprising advertising, and 4 per cent news. People who tweet have contested this labelling. A less biased and preferred term for pointless babble is 'social grooming': the activities that maintain social links (Boyd, Golder & Lotan, 2010).

Despite previously being regarded as a marginal form of communication, Twitter gained respectability as a rapid way of disseminating information following the Christchurch, New Zealand, earthquake of February 2011. Messages could be sent directly by text messaging from a mobile phone and be disseminated widely at great speed and little cost. With the Central Business District no longer functioning, and with the absence of electricity, phone lines, computers and even offices and buildings, Twitter became a mechanism for efficiently disseminating important civil defence and police messages.

Virtual reality environments

Developing out of massive multiplayer online platforms, virtual spaces such as Linden Laboratories' Second Life (http://secondlife.com) have developed as a venue for synchronised, or real time, interactions between people represented as avatars.

CASE STUDY 23.2

Virtual reality and health care

Applications for virtual reality in health-care environments include the following:

- Simulated hospital and clinic environments allow for a particular procedure to be known in advance.
- Conferences can occur anywhere that individual guest speakers and an audience can convene. For example, if a conference occurs in Second Life, there is no need to travel in 'real time' or in 'real space', incurring 'real costs'.
- Simulations of potential real-life events can be 'played out' in Second Life; for example, an epidemic following the outbreak of an infectious disease.

FIGURE 23.1 *The author's Second Life avatar*

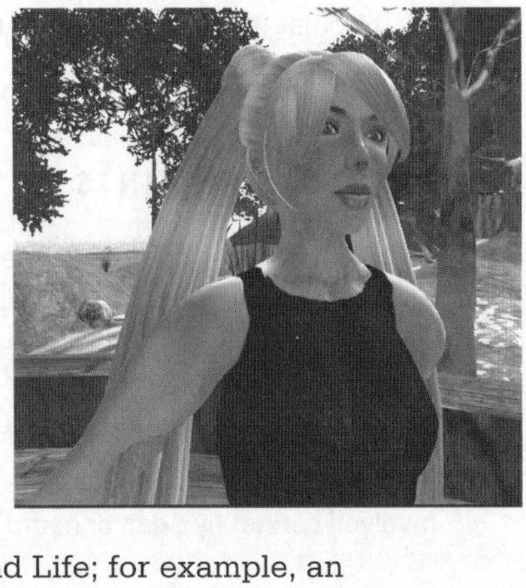

AILSA HAXELL

- 'Real' appointments occurring in 'real time' can involve textually based interactions with health practitioners, such as nutritionists, counsellors and psychotherapists (for further examples, see Linden Laboratories, 2011).
- The advantages include anonymity. Using an avatar, which represents oneself as one would like to be seen rather than how one is, may lower stigmatisation. In addition, experimentation with identity can occur without harm or judgment.

Choices in using different technologies need to take into account how the medium works—what are its good or bad attributes? For example, in the absence of visual cues how is the identity of a person verified before any private information is disclosed? Consideration also needs to be given to the nature of the material being conveyed—is it something the person needs to be prepared for? Can they can be supported? The medium chosen needs to suit the message.

{ SUMMARY }

In focusing on technology as a medium for practice, the emphasis has been on how the technology has influence. However, technology is not just a tool—it also affects how we interact, and it would be a mistake to consider it merely as the bearer of a message. Communications alter with different media, and these alterations, for better or for worse, affect professional practice. There are many modalities to consider in terms of communicative technology. It is reasonable to assume that the prevalence of these technologies requires that practitioners are not only familiar with texting, blogs and social networking but that they also consider using them to interact with patients, service users and colleagues.

REFLECTION POINTS

23.1 Intention (motivation, message, meaning, emotion)

What advantages might there be for a client using a communication medium in which they cannot be seen or heard?

23.2 Reception (received message, response, feedback)

What are some of the difficulties involved in using media where the people involved cannot be seen or heard?

23.3 Perception (style, manner, impression, analysis)

What challenges then occur for health practitioners when working in situations where the identity of the person they work with may be unknown?

QUESTIONS FOR REVIEW

1 In media representations of mobile phone use, how are young people usually portrayed?
2 Applying the concept of absent presence in social networking, what are the advantages and disadvantages involved?

REFERENCES

Boyd, D., Golder, S. & Lotan, G. (2010). *TweetTweetRetweet: Conversational aspects of retweeting on Twitter*. Paper presented at the 43rd Hawaii International Conference on System Science. Retrieved from http://doi.ieeecomputersociety.org/10.1109/HICSS.2010.412.

Bramley, D., Riddell, T., Whittaker, R., Corbett, T., Lin, R.-B. & Wi, M. (2005). Smoking cessation using mobile phone text messaging is as effective in Maori as non-Maori. *New Zealand Medical Journal, 118*(1216). Retrieved from www.nzma.org.nz/journal/118-1216/1494.

Broadbent, S. (2009). How the internet enables intimacy [Video webcast]: TEDGlobal. Retrieved from www.ted.com/talks/stefana_broadbent_how_the_internet_enables_intimacy.html.

Gauld, R. & Williams, S. (2009). Use of the internet for health information: A study of Australians and New Zealanders. *Informatics for Health and Social Care, 34*(3), 149–58.

Geraghty, M., Glynn, F., Amin, M. & Kinsella, J. J. (2007). Patient mobile telephone 'text' reminder: A novel way to reduce non attendance at the ENT out-patient clinic. *Journal of Laryngology and Otology, 122*(3), 296–8.

Gergen, K. J. (2002). The challenge of absent presence. In J. E. Katz & M. A. Aakhus (eds), *Perpetual contact, mobile communication, private talk, public performance* (pp. 227–41). Cambridge, MA: Cambridge University Press.

Haxell, A. (2010). Empowerment in tight spaces: Youth counselling in a text-messaging medium. Paper presented at the E-Youth Multidisciplinary Conference Balancing between opportunity and risk.

Koshy, E., Car, J. & Majeed, A. (2008). Effectiveness of mobile-phone short message service (SMS) reminders for ophthalmology outpatient appointments: Observational study. *BMC Ophthalmology, 8*, 9.

Kunzru, H. (1997). You are cyborg. *Wired*. Retrieved 14 September 2010 from www.wired.com/wired/archive//5.02/ffharaway.html.

Levine, D., McCright, J., Dobkin, L., Woodruff, A. J. & Klausner, J. D. (2008). SEXINFO: A sexual health text messaging service for San Francisco youth. *American Journal of Public Health, 98*(3), 393–5.

Linden Laboratories. (2011). *Second Life healthcare*. Retrieved 28 February 2011 from http://wiki.secondlife.com/wiki/Healthcare#Articles.

Marvin, C. (1988). *When old technologies were new. Thinking about electric communication in the late nineteenth century*. New York, NY: Oxford University Press.

Murray, E., Lo, B., Pollack, L., Donelan, K., Catania, J., White, M. et al. (2003). The impact of health information on the internet on the physician-patient relationship: Patient perceptions. *Archives of Internal Medicine, 163*(14), 1727–34.

Nelson, R. & Shepheard, T. (2008). *Market analysis. New Zealand Telecommunications Market 2008–2012 Forecast and Analysis*. Retrieved 7 February 2011 from www.tig.org.nz/library/e6a3855d-6e5b-4a6b-8c67-9c0be9ae1e27.cmr.

Palmer, J. (2008). Interview: The cellphone anthropologist. *New Scientist, 2660*.

Pearanalytics. (2006). *Twitter study—August 2009*. Retrieved 31 March 2011 from www.pearanalytics.com/blog/wp-content/uploads/2010/05/Twitter-Study-August-2009.pdf.

Pennebaker, J. W. (2000). Telling stories: The health benefits of narrative. *Literature and Medicine*, *19*(1), 3–18.

Pennebaker, J. W. & Beall, S. K. (1986). Confronting a traumatic event: Toward an understanding of inhibition and disease. *Journal of Abnormal Psychology*, *95*, 274–81.

Powell, J. A., Lowe, P., Griffiths, F. E. & Thorogood, M. (2005). A critical analysis of the literature on the internet and consumer health information. *Journal of Telemedicine and Telecare, 11*(1), 41–3.

Statistics New Zealand (2009). *Household use of information and communication technology*. Retrieved 6 February 2011 from www.stats.govt.nz/browse_for_stats/industry_sectors/information_technology_and_communications/hhold-use-of-ict.aspx.

Tan, L. (2008). Psychotherapy 2.0: Myspace® Blogging as self-therapy. *American Journal of Psychotherapy, 62*(2), 143–63.

Turkle, S. (2006). Always on/Always on you: The tethered self. In J. Katz (ed.), *Handbook of mobile communications and social change* (pp. 121–38). Cambridge, MA: Massachusetts Institute of Technology Press.

Wesch, M. (2007). Web 2.0 … The machine is us/ing us. Retrieved 16 January 2011 from www.youtube.com/watch?v=6gmP4nk0EOE.

Wray, R. (2002). First with the message: Interview Corr Stutterheim, executive chairman CMG. *Guardian*. Retrieved 28 February 2010 from www.guardian.co.uk/business/2002/mar/16/5

WEBSITES

Second Life: http://secondlife.com

Twitter: http://twitter.com

Unsolicited Electronic Messages Act 2007: www.legislation.govt.nz/act/public/2007/0007/latest/DLM405134.html

{24}

Creative Messages

Deb Spence and Liz Smythe

CHAPTER OVERVIEW

This chapter covers the following topics:

+ Poetry
+ Story
+ Image
+ Sound
+ Understanding as ontology.

KEY TERMS

Poetry
Story
Music
Ontology

This is an opportunity to explore and reflect on the practice of health practitioners in a different way. Let these words and images speak and broaden understandings of what is already known, and that which is still to be known. The invitation is to experience poetry, story, images and other aesthetic encounters that awaken knowing and extend understanding.

Poetry

Poetry The construction of language in an artistic manner.

> Poems are not … simply emotions … they are experiences. For the sake of a single poem, you must see cities, many people and things … and know the gestures which small flowers make when they open in the morning. You must be able to think back to streets in unknown neighbourhoods, to unexpected encounters, and to partings you have long seen coming: to days of childhood whose mystery is still unexplained …; to childhood illnesses … to mornings by the sea, to the sea itself, to seas, to nights of travel … and it is still not enough.
>
> *Freedman (1996, p. 5)*

To be human is to live in a never-ending stream of experience, most of which is never captured in words. How does one talk about vulnerability without feeling like a fool? How does one hold the insight of a moment? How does one impart fledgling wisdom to others? Glenn Colquhoun is a New Zealand general practitioner who writes poetry, sharing his experiences of health practice (see Case study 24.1).

CASE STUDY 24.1

A note of warning to patients when all else fails

Sometimes the needle is too blunt.
The stethoscope is too quiet.
The scalpel will not cut.
The scissors chew like old men's gums.
Sometimes the book has not been written.
The pill cannot be swallowed.
The crutches are too short.
The x-rays hide like dirty windows.

Sometimes the thermometer will not rise.
The plaster will not stick.
The stitches cannot hold.
The heart conducts a normal ECG.

Then I have to ask you what to do.

Which is what you might
have wanted all along.

Colquhoun (2002, p. 94)

Health-practice writing would normally come in the form of policy, a research report or a scholarly paper. Colquhoun brings us his warning using poetry. He reminds us that the skills and strategies, technology and teachings of health-care practice do not always work. Even when people do the right thing, even if they follow best practice guidelines, even though it should work—it may not. When all else fails, he asks for guidance. There is a sense of relief in this sharing.

Colquhoun brings us back to the heart of the practice encounter to the moment when professional expertise reaches it limits. The poem stirs memories of similar encounters in the reader. Maybe it was a time when a health practitioner did not listen, did not ask or did not realise that a patient had an understanding of their condition that was more than 'standard care' could ever discern. Poetry calls us back to the essence of being human. It opens up our vulnerability. It helps us to laugh at ourselves. It lingers in our minds, gently nudging us when we, too, one day experience equipment that fails. Poetry is succinct, yet it has much to teach us.

In Case study 24.2, poetry lets us stop and think about what 'she' said, how it was for her, and what was said, or might one day be said, in reply.

CASE STUDY 24.2

She asked me if she took one pill for her heart and one pill for her hips and one pill for her chest and one pill for her blood how come they would all know which part of her body they should go to.

I explained to her that active metabolites in each pharmaceutical would adopt a spatial configuration leading to an exact interface with receptor molecules on the cellular surfaces of the target structures involved.

She told me not to bullshit her.

I told her that each pill had a different shape and that each part of her body had a different shape and the pills could only work when both of these shapes could fit together.

She said I had no right to talk about the shape of her body.

I said that each pill was a key and that her body was ten thousand locks.

She said she wasn't going to swallow that.

I told her they worked by magic.

She asked me why I hadn't said that in the first place.

Colquhoun (2002, p. 14)

These words take us to the heart of a conversation that reveals the complex nature of interpersonal communication. Patients often ask for explanations relating to their treatments and we try to assist their understanding in numerous ways. This woman is wondering how her pills work. The first response is scientific. Practitioners have knowledge of underlying physiology and often use these terms to explain mechanisms of action. But the words are foreign and have no meaning for most patients. The second attempt also misses the mark because the woman feels invaded. She is sensitive about references to her body. And the third suggestion is clearly too fantastical.

The acceptance of the final explanation, although inappropriate from the perspective of being a practitioner, teaches us that we usually need to provide a range of explanations before being successful. Furthermore, even though we understand the scientific reasons for interventions, there is a sense that these, too, work as if by magic. Stories like this help us to see the thinking behind human interaction. They show importance of dialogue: its to and fro nature and the different interpretations that can be drawn from it. Effective communication is less about the health practitioner providing information to patients and more about finding understanding together.

Practice encounters often go by unnoticed for their significance. While both parties leave with memories and mood, the fine details are not recorded and often undervalued. Colquhoun provides an example in a dialogue that unfolds in Case study 24.3.

CASE STUDY 24.3

Aunty Flu

'Kia ora.'
'Tena koe pakeha.'

There is no conversation in the next line.
There is a kiss.

'How are you?'
'I am well.'
'Where have you been?'
'I have been working.'
'Which way did you come?

'I came the long way.'
'I was looking but did not see you.'

'What have you been doing?'
'I have been to the doctor. He is a pakeha doctor.
He said that I smoke too much.
I said "Well doctor it is like this,
If I walk out of here I'm still going to smoke—you're not
Paying for my smokes." He said "Are you taking your pills?"
I said I hadn't taken them for a week and I'm not dead yet.

He said "O—Mrs Rewiti."

Well I did, I said that, it is not his fault.
He is a good doctor. I took him a kete.

You look too skinny. Do you want a cup of tea?'
'I would.'
'The kettle is over there.'

Colquhoun (2003, p. 61)

In this encounter, each person has their own culture, understandings and ways. Colquhoun puts the spotlight on a simple conversation that on the one hand says 'nothing much', and on the other 'speaks volumes'. Aunty Flu has been to see a 'good' Pakeha doctor but makes her own decisions about whether or not to take his advice and his pills. Now Colquhoun enters. The encounter starts with a greeting and a kiss. But before that was the waiting and the watching. There is respectful caring on both sides. This is revealed in the openness, the trust, the honesty; each person accepting the other as they are. Aunty Flu makes it clear that she will keep smoking if she wants to, and with some pride declares that she is doing well without the pills. Then she turns her attention to this 'skinny' Pakeha doctor, ordering him a cup of tea. The care is reciprocal and building trust takes time.

Practice always happens in a context, encountering variations in culture, age, gender, interests, social status and myriad other differences. It almost always involves one person seeking to connect with the other, at the same time expecting the other to join the dialogical interplay. While health practitioners might come with a plan, opening themselves to the other means responding to the unfolding of what happens. It is to become humble and in so doing to be gifted with the trust of other.

Poetry, such as this, allows us to experience a conversation as though we were there. In 'being there', with time to watch and an opportunity to ponder, we find our own questions:

+ How would 'I' be going into the home of a kai awhina [elderly Māori woman] whom I sensed was not going to take my professional advice?

+ How would I feel greeting and chatting with someone whose way of living might be very different from my own? How would I respond to feedback about my physique?
+ Would I put the kettle on with enthusiasm?

There are no right answers—only the responses that come from everything that has shaped people to be as they are. This poem is a reminder of shared humanity.

Story

Story The explained perspective of an individual.

Stories are usually longer than poems. Their words are connected into paragraphs, but can equally capture an experience and provide vivid insight. Used imaginatively, they help us to understand the experiences of others, as in Case study 24.4.

CASE STUDY 24.4

The power of story

She started with a story.
A story that called us in.
And there was this quietness that permeated the room, the night.
Almost a reverence that I recall in church as a young child, a call,
not an expectation … to speak softly, reverently, respectfully …
Because something was important, was to be honoured. Something
was worthy of respect.

Moules (2006, p. 7)

In Case study 24.5, Janet Frame writes powerfully about a woman having a bath. Listen to fragments of it and imagine that she is a precious elderly relative.

CASE STUDY 24.5

The bath

When she was sure that the water was hot enough … she ventured from the kitchen through the cold passageway to the colder bathroom. She paused in the doorway to get used to the chill of the air then she walked slowly, feeling with each step the pain in her back, across to the bath, and though she knew that she was gradually losing the power in her hands she managed to wrench on the stiff cold and hot taps … Sitting upright, not daring to lean back or lie down, she soaped herself, washing away the dirt of the past fortnight ... Then when her washing was completed she found herself looking for excuses not to try yet to climb out ... How slippery the surface had become! ... She leaned forward, feeling the pain in her back and shoulder. She grasped the rim of the bath but her fingers slithered from it almost at once. She would not panic, she told herself; she would try gradually, carefully, to get out. Again she leaned forward; again her grip loosened as if iron hands had deliberately uncurled her stiffened blue fingers from their trembling hold. Her heart began to beat faster, her breath came more quickly, her mouth was dry. She moistened her lips. If I shout for help, she thought, no one will hear me. No one in the world will hear me. No one will know I'm in the bath and can't get out ...

Then she told herself sternly that she must have no nonsense, that she had really not tried to get out of the bath. She had forgotten the strong, solid chair and the grip she could get on it ... She tried to do this; she just failed to make the final effort. Pale now, gasping from breath, she sank back into the bath. She began to call out but as she had predicted there was no answer. No one heard her, no one in the houses or the street or Dunedin or the world knew that she was imprisoned. Loneliness welled in her ... for over half an hour she stayed alternatively struggling and resting until at last she did succeed in climbing out and making her escape into the kitchen. She thought, I'll never take another bath again. This is the end or the beginning of it. In future a district nurse will have to come to attend me. Submitting to that will be the first humiliation. There will be others, and others.

Frame (1983, pp. 180–3)

Stay with the feelings evoked by the story. Imagine how it might feel to be the nurse, or the therapist, who gets the referral that draws them into this woman's life. Would they see a lonely old woman who was slow and cranky, who would not move fast enough for the time that had been allocated for her? Or would there be space to pause and recognise the vulnerability, the courage, the hard-fought resilience that has finally cracked? Perhaps the practitioner would begin to understand that their well-meaning, competently executed care may be experienced as humiliating. How can people show they understand? It might help to remember this story and ask people to share their story. But asking is not enough; it is the listening that matters.

In Case study 24.6, Patricia Grace, another New Zealand author, gives us a first-person reflection on what it was like to go nursing in an earlier era of training and hospital life. One person's story so often takes us back to 'my' story. Listen to the impact.

CASE STUDY 24.6

Nursing as a vocation

So nursing was my vocation. I loved, most of all, to work in the wards, attending to the needs of the patients, although it was difficult for me sometimes. I was lucky that I had Kui Hinemate beside me, or inside me, or wherever it is that she speaks to me from. First of all there was her disapproval to deal with, but I'm a daughter who always had her own way. I had to make her know that this was something I really wanted to do. After that she helped me.

When there were things that felt wrong for me—touching the dead who were not my own dead to touch, shifting the bed of the dead into a ward for the living, handling the linen of the dead and depositing it with all the other linen without any clearing, preparing the room where someone had died for karakia to say and to do my own cleansing. They were the customs I had observed so well as I journeyed about with old ones when I was a child, everything that Kui Hinemate and the grandmothers had taught me would keep me safe during my life. But I did them surreptitiously. Being thought a princess was enough, I didn't want any more rumours circulating about me.

So it was a double life, as my life always has been in the city, but it became less difficult as I understood it more. It's an absorbing and interesting life as long as you are certain, and as long as you keep hold of who you know you are.

There were other areas of difficulty for me. Māori patients would see me, perhaps just as I passed by, and would call to me or send for me and want me to attend to them. They would want only me to touch their heads or attend to personal matters. I longed to do what they wanted, and sometimes did, but the hospital was a place of territories that were strictly and jealously guarded.

Grace (1992, pp. 204–5)

Stories are not simply to be read. They are conversational partners that draw us to reflect. They help us to ask the hard questions of ourselves, to see parallels, to understand what otherwise might only have been a gut feeling. We become a little wiser, and so are better prepared to face the challenges that undoubtedly lie ahead.

Image

Just as words create pictures in our mind, so, too, in our daily experience we are surrounded by images, be they real, photographic or created. Sometimes in the midst of a tough experience, knowing comes from escaping the busyness and going out into the world of nature. When we open ourselves to look, see and dwell with meaning, understanding can come, as illustrated in Case study 24.7).

CASE STUDY 24.7

FIGURE 24.1 *The tree*

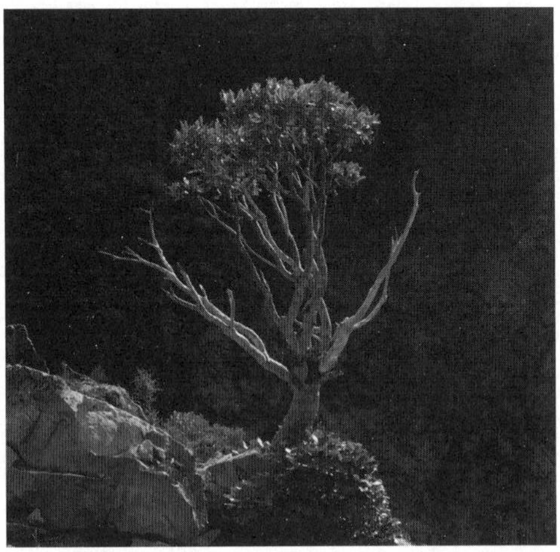

Photo: Norton (2010)

Engaging with an image

One seeing: my attention goes immediately to the new and luxuriant growth flanked by the branches that have died. The cliff edge resilience of the tree, the slanting light on the rocks and the dark/sombre background convey a sense of beauty, hope and quiet strength. I think about the need for fortitude. I see the outstretched arms that hold the wisdom of endurance. I see the flourishing growth in the midst of struggle. I take hope. I feel courage stir in my bones.

And another: how can that tree grow in such a place? How can it hold on against the storms that have shaped it so dramatically? How can it defy the forces that rage against it time after time? I think of the roots, the unseen part of this weathered old tree. How far down do they go? What do they cling to? What gives them such strength? I take that question into my own life. And then I remember the person I met the other day who had faced so much pain and despair, yet still was calm and gracious. I did so little for her, but she made me feel like I had given her a precious gift. Her 'roots' were akin to the roots of this tree.

FIGURE 24.2 *The moment*

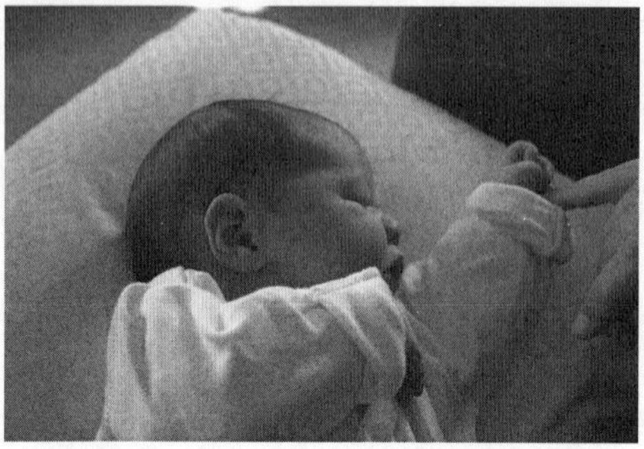

Now look at Figure 24.2. What does the touch show? The mother's finger gently engages with her newborn baby. Is it a touch of deep relief, the crying settled, the baby finally asleep? Or is it a touch that hopes to gently stir the long-slept baby into wakefulness? How does it feel to be a new mother, called to this baby day by day—morning, afternoon, evening and night? What happened to days off? Remember when once one's days were ordered, with some semblance of control? Is this touch a connectedness that has changed this woman's life beyond anything she imagined? How do health professionals understand the huge transition a woman makes to motherhood? How do they discern the bigger picture of understanding that lies behind this image?

Engaging in conversations about the visual arts can help understanding, assist to develop empathy and facilitate reflective thinking: 'Because artwork expresses thoughts and evokes emotions, it also has a great influence on our spiritual and moral growth' (Yrjo Hirn, in Blomqvist, Pitkala & Routasalo, 2007, p. 92).

Sound

Sound is another powerful means of capturing our attention, mood and sense of being. Sound speaks. It can soothe, calm and lull us to sleep. It can invigorate, challenge and awaken our attention. Meyer talks of musical suspense, when we are kept waiting in a moment of unknowingness:

> It makes us feel something of the insignificance and powerless of man ... The low foreboding rumble of distant thunder on an oppressive summer afternoon, its growing intensity as it approaches, the crescendo of the gradually rising wind, the ominous darkening of the sky, all give rise to an emotional experience in which expectation is fraught with powerful uncertainty.
>
> *Meyer (1956, p. 28)*

Music The organised composition and presentation of sound.

Music is used therapeutically in health: relaxing and easing distress, unlocking memories and opening channels of communication. It can change mood from despair to hope, bring peace in the midst of anxiety, and relieve pain (Munro & Mount, 1978). Music can also be a political tool, often being associated with civil rights movements. Songs convey the issues of the time, creating a 'travelling text' (Nyairo & Ogude, 2005), which may be steeped in political agendas.

CASE STUDY 24.8

Goodnight nurse

Goodnight nurse, you've done all that you can
Thank-you for the kindness when the rest of them ran
Who says there are no angels?
I can see them—And I can hear them
And I sure feel them in this room
Thank you for the silence when I needed you to be
Thank you for listening without judging me
Thank you for speaking out when my voice eluded me
Thank you for just being here and sitting with me
Goodnight nurse

Neufeld (2010)

In Case study 24.8, music gave nurse Michael Neufeld the freedom to share his experience in a way that words alone could not. It captured an essence or way of being far beyond mere description, allowing the sharing of emotions such as joy, sadness, love, anger and gratitude. The verse above was written after caring for a man who shared his life story on the eve of his death.

The man, by his own admission, was someone whom many would not want to know. He was angry and alone, and 'being' alongside him was very challenging. Yet he chose to share his life, the experience changing the nurse both personally and professionally. The intensity of the relationship and granting of simple human acts is communicated through the music.

Understanding as ontology

This chapter has taken a journey of interpretation. Words, pictures and experience of sound can be taken into a personal reservoir of knowing, and make unique interpretations of meaning. The aim has been to offer an **ontological** perspective (as opposed to an epistemological, theoretical one), as discussed by Harman (2007) in Case study 24.9.

Ontology Concerned with the nature of being or existence.

CASE STUDY 24.9

Insights

While the science of practice is essential, there is equally a place for ontological insights. Harman (2007) puts it this way:

> In order to gain knowledge of things, any science has to objectify them, and to objectify things means to 'de-live' them. In other words, knowledge always cuts things down to size or turns them into caricatures through some sort of oversimplification ... To treat [things] scientifically means to 'cut them off at the knees', converting them from mysterious and multifaceted things into concepts whose basic features can be clearly listed in a glossary. While this distortion is inevitable, it is a distortion nonetheless.
>
> *Harman (2007, p. 23)*

One cannot function within the complexity of the world of health care without general, theoretical understandings that pertain to 'everyone' who fits within a category. But Harman's point is that such generalisations always distort individual experience. A referral that requests 'assistance with bathing', for example, hides the huge loss and vulnerability that led to this situation. Harman reminds us that 'what things really are is events' (p. 24). 'An' event is always unique, always in a context and always shaped by what happened before and possibilities that lie in the future. Practice happens in a world of human events, not in a sanitised, orderly and necessarily predictable way according to theoretical models. We can learn much about the experiences of clients and our fellow practitioners through their poetry, their stories, their music and their art.

In research literature, such understanding falls within the brief of phenomenology, hermeneutics, narrative analysis and other qualitative approaches. The wisdom of practice is born of such insights.

{ SUMMARY }

The arts in all their many and varied forms seem to relieve us of the need to pretend to be perfect. We are only human, and to be human is to not always get it right. Learning from mistakes grows rich wisdom. Poets, authors, painters and other creative artists often bring insights from the struggles of life. They allow us to absorb some of their wisdom without necessarily enduring the experience. We encourage wide reading because it exposes people to the world of the arts and to know that anything that touches on what it means to be human will help individuals develop as thoughtful and mindful practitioners. Personal engagement with writing, painting and composing provides profound opportunities to reflect on and develop practice. Drawing from the lived experience of health practitioners and clients complements the learning gained through the 'emotionally devoid textbook' (Begley, 1996, p. 188).

REFLECTION POINTS

24.1 Intention (motivation, message, meaning, emotion)

How do you express yourself? What does this tell others about you? What do other people know of you? What are the sounds that soothe or inspire you? Is there some favourite music? Is it the sound of waves on a west coast beach, or the tuis amid the bush? What are the sounds that disturb and irritate you?

24.2 Reception (received message, response, feedback)

What do you know of others around you by how they express themselves? How do you honour the diversity of others and their self-expression?

24.3 Perception (style, manner, impression, analysis)

How might you consider and/or use sound as a therapeutic strategy or expression of experience?

QUESTIONS FOR REVIEW

Do the perfect thing; make some mistakes. One of the biggest mistakes you can make is to try not to make any mistakes. However hard you work at everything right, sometimes you'll say the wrong word or make the wrong move. You're only human. And it's precisely your humanity that makes you approachable and believable. So relax and be natural. Your goofs will also signal an important truth: there is a limit to your dependability. No one should ever put their entire trust in you.

Millar (in Schmit, 2002, p. 77)

1 What has contributed to you saying the wrong thing?
2 How can images and creative messages assist with communication and why are they valuable?
3 What are the challenges for you in relation to creative messages?

REFERENCES

Begley, A. M. (1996). Literature and poetry: Pleasure and practice. *International Journal of Nursing practice, 2*, 182–8.

Blomqvist, L., Pitkala, K. & Routasalo, P. (2007). Images of loneliness: Using art as an educational method in professional training. *Journal of Continuing Education in Nursing, 38*(2), 89–93.

Colquhoun, G. (2002). *Playing god*. Wellington, NZ: Steele Roberts.

Colquhoun, G. (2003) *The art of walking upright*. Wellington, NZ: Steele Roberts.

Frame, J. (1983). The Bath. In *You are now entering the human heart* (pp. 180–183). Wellington, NZ: Victoria University Press.

Freedman, R (1996). *Life of a poet: Rainer Maria Rilke*. New York, NY: Farrer, Strauss & Giroux.

Grace, P. (1992). *Cousins*. Auckland, NZ: Penguin.

Harman, G. (2007). *Heidegger explained: From phenomenon to thing*. Chicago, IL: Open Court.

Meyer, L. (1956). *Emotion and meaning in music*. Chicago, IL: University of Chicago Press.

Moules, N. (2006). A whispered story. In C. Dinkins & J. Sorrell (eds), *Listening to the whispers. Re-thinking ethics in healthcare* (p. 7). Madison, WI: The University of Wisconsin Press.

Munro, S. & Mount, B. (1978). Music therapy in palliative care. *CMA Journal, 119*, 1029–34.

Neufeld, M. (2010). *Goodnight nurse*. Retrieved from www.youtube.com/watch?v=dl8dGZDBXCU.

Norton, A. (2010). Finding cadence. *Blurb*. Retrieved from www.blurb.com/bookstore/detail/1702454.

Nyairo, J. & Ogude, J. (2005). Popular music, popular politics: Unbwogable and the idioms of freedom in Kenyan popular music. *African Affairs, 104* (415), 225–49.

Schmit, C. (2002). *Too deep for words*. Louisville, KY: Westminster John Knox Press.

WEBSITES

Artist in Residence, Southern Health, Victoria: www.southernhealth.org.au/page/About_Us/Arts_in_health/Artist_in_residence

British Columbia Medical Museum: www.bcmamedicalmuseum.org/collections

London Museums of Health and Medicine: www.medicalmuseums.org

MAP Foundation: www.mapfoundation.org/index.html

{PART 3}

Professional Communication

Chapter 25 Professional Communication ... 299
Chapter 26 Therapeutic Engagement ... 309
Chapter 27 Care at a Distance ... 322

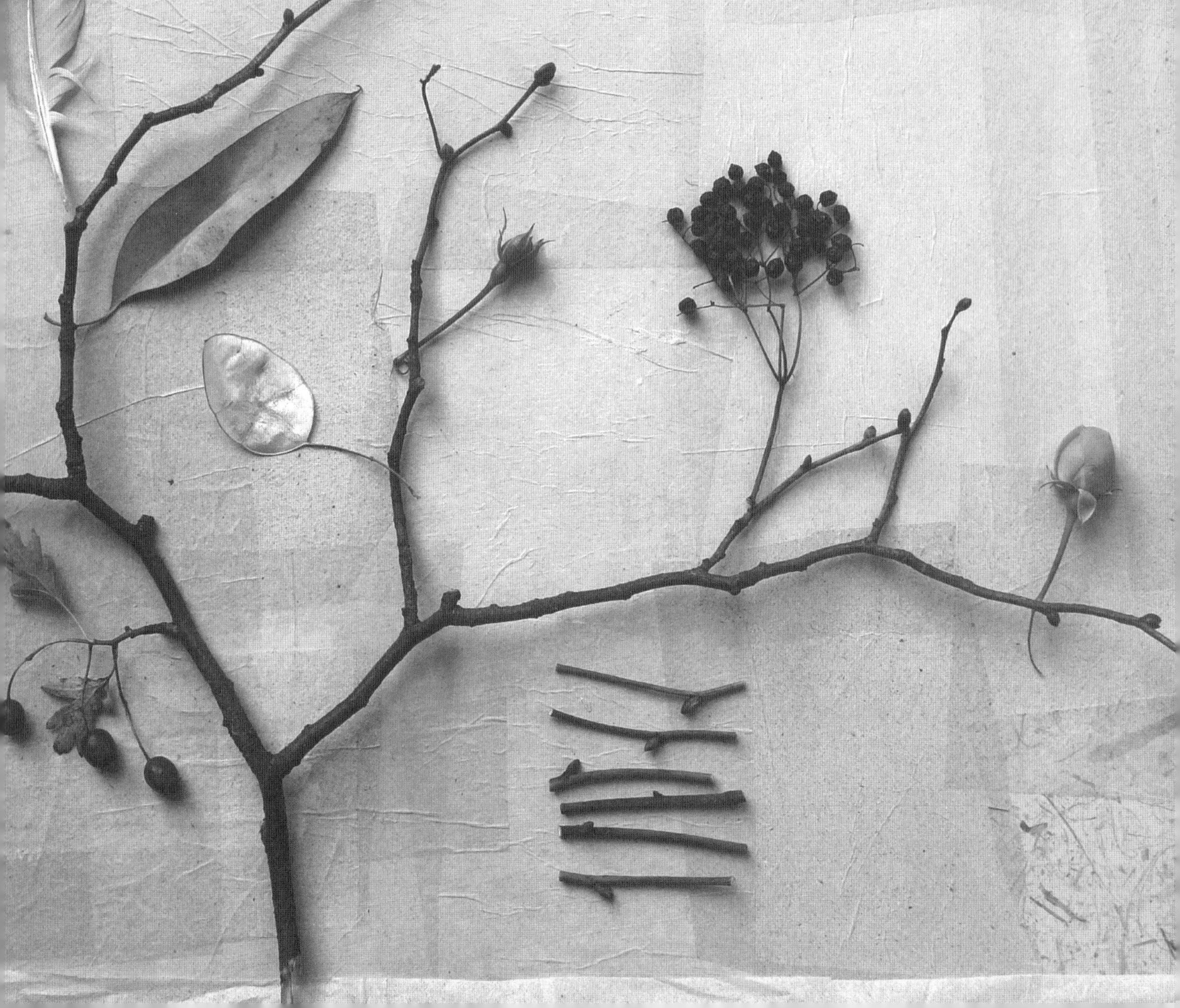

{25}

Professional Communication

Susan Shaw

CHAPTER OVERVIEW

This chapter covers the following topics:

+ Communication codes
+ Costs of inadequate communication
+ Professional responsibilities
+ Interprofessional communication
+ Communicating in organisations.

KEY TERMS

Abbreviations
Person-centred
Slang
Serious and sentinel events
Interprofessional
Professional accountability

Communication is one of the fundamental activities of human existence and is more complex and dynamic than people generally think. This is because so much of communication is based on accepted culturally and socially laden concepts, many of which are subtle. At any point in their lives, people are involved with groups that are related to age, physical location, occupation, family, beliefs and interests. All of these have their own culture—expectations about how people should behave to respect and remain in the group—and these are evident in obvious and silent rules about how they should communicate.

CASE STUDY 25.1

Knowledge and power

It is appropriate to consider the power that educated people have in society and to be mindful of the responsibilities this entails. It is convenient but not accurate to assume that people who have power and knowledge will necessarily behave in ways that are honourable.

> Dear Teacher
>
> I am a survivor of a concentration camp. My eyes saw what no man should witness:
>
> Gas chambers built by learned engineers; children poisoned by educated physicians; infants killed by trained nurses; women and babies shot by college and high-school graduates; so I am suspicious of education.
>
> My request is: help your students to become human. Your efforts must never produce learned monsters, skilled psychopaths, educated Eichmanns. Reading, writing and arithmetic are important only if they serve to make our children more human.
>
> *Ginott (1972, p. viii)*

Communication codes

Communication is often described with reference to written and verbal ways of passing on messages. Appreciating the language that is used in any communication helps people to assemble the messages that are conveyed. The words (spoken and written) that professionals and groups use have specific meanings, and the differences in terminology and the need to have differential language exists for a range of reasons. These language peculiarities between people and professional groups include terms that may be relatively easy to decode (such as talking about 'upper limbs' or 'lower limbs' instead of 'arms' and 'legs'). However, there are considerable risks attached to any communication that requires decoding, as confusion over the meaning or the message compounds when the possibilities for interpretation increase. Language used in one context may not be meaningful, or may even be offensive, in another situation. The use of **abbreviations** is an example of a risky communication situation as there can be different interpretations for the same code. The interpretation of the code depends on the understanding and perspective of the professionals involved, and inaccurate interpretations can lead to serious consequences for the patient or service user.

Abbreviations Brief or shortened form of words or phrases.

TABLE 25.1 *Interpretations of abbreviations*

Code	*Interpretations from Wear et al. (2006); Parvaiz et al. (2006)*				
HV	*Hallux valgus*	High velocity	Home visit	Health visitor	High vaginal swab
MT	Metatarsal	Mental test score	Management team	Medical technician	Multidisciplinary team
TT	Tendon transfer	Tetanus toxoid	Treatment	Tourniquet time	Thrombin time
LP	Lumbar puncture	Luer plug			
BPD	Borderline personality disorder	Bronchopulmonary pneumonia			

The particular communication codes that groups of people use form part of their identity and culture. The members of the group understand the code, so being able to interpret the information makes individuals legitimate members of the group. Often the codes have emerged from the desire to have a shorthand type of documentation. However, these coded messages serve other purposes such as circumscribing the membership of the group and limiting the involvement of others who are not members and do not understand the information. Many professional groups (including law and medicine) create a level of mystery round their knowledge and practice by using complex communication that requires some guidance or interpretation in order for others (including patients) to understand.

At this current point in world history, it is considered desirable that patients and those around them are informed and understand what is going on in any situation. A good test of communication in the health care and disability support sector is to ask whether or not it is **person-centred**. If the person at the centre of the situation (the patient or client) can understand the communication and experience it as respectful, then it is probably appropriate.

Another form of coded message is the **slang** vocabulary of messages that build up meaning within professional groups over time. Slang is casual in the

Person-centred An emphasis within relationships that focuses on the person receiving or seeking support, rather than the people, systems or organisations providing it.

Slang Informal and popular use of language.

extreme and generally conveys judgmental messages about people or situations. Some slang presents strongly coded messages. Slang is often only understood in relatively small groups of practitioners.

TABLE 25.2 *Examples of slang messages*

Ash cash—money paid for completing cremation forms
Bash cash—money paid for completing forms in emergency clinics
Departure lounge—geriatric ward
FLK—funny-looking kid
Freud squad—psychiatric team
GPO—good for parts only
LONNH—lights on, nobody home
PFO—pissed, fell over
PPP—piss-poor protoplasm
PRATFO—patient reassured and told to 'go away'
SGKB—single girl keeping baby

Costs of inadequate communication

It is rather simplistic to insist that good communication is important because it plays a role in ensuring that people are treated respectfully. While a primary motivation should be to provide good care, it is common for people and organisations to use potential negative consequences to appreciate the need for them to behave in a certain way. Reports about things going wrong in the course of delivering health and disability services include analyses of **serious and sentinel events**. In Aotearoa New Zealand these reports provide insights into communication issues.

Serious and sentinel events Incidents that lead to unexpected outcomes such as injury (serious) or death (sentinel).

TABLE 25.3 *Examples of sentinel and serious events in Aotearoa New Zealand 2009–10*

Type of adverse event	*Description of event*	*Communication issues (cause or recommendations)*
Serious	Delayed recognition of deteriorating condition—patient recovered following prolonged care and rehabilitation	• Handover and referral to senior medical staff delayed • Clinical communication processes reviewed with the team
Serious	Unauthorised removal of baby from hospital	• Adoption policy not followed • Communication failures
Serious	Delay in escalation of treatment for patient with respiratory deterioration	• Emergency escalation process not followed • Poor communication between staff members

Type of adverse event	*Description of event*	*Communication issues (cause or recommendations)*
Serious	Retained surgical swab not identified for five days after operation	• Interruptions and distractions during the count processes • Poor communication between the team members regarding the swabs placed inside the patient
Serious	Delayed and misdiagnosis of fractured hip for several days, resulting in additional days in hospital	• Need to strengthen multidisciplinary team communication
Serious	Patient self-harm requiring surgical intervention	• Patient's mental state required use of the Mental Health Act and locked unit status • Communication failure between admitting team and hospital staff regarding risk status of patient
Serious	Delayed treatment for lung cancer that was not reviewed or reported at the time of X-ray	• Copy of chest X-ray report not sent to general practitioner • General practitioner did not follow up on chest X-ray report as requested to do
Serious	Delayed diagnostic procedures for three patients (all subsequently diagnosed with cancer)	• Discrepancy found on Ministry of Health website with two sets of national guidelines for triage times • All three patients have been directly contacted and an apology offered for the delay in being seen
Serious	Medication error	• There is no place to document blood results in urokinase protocol, therefore heparin chart was used to document blood results and heparin changes • Mismatch between urokinase blood thinning protocol (heparin) and standard hospital heparin chart; patient given standard dose that was too low for condition
Serious/ sentinel	Patient with infection was not identified, required resuscitation and later died (inadequate and delayed diagnosis)	• Swabs taken two days prior to delivery not checked • Need to Identify and communicate risk factors • Review systems to check laboratory results
Sentinel	Patient admitted with infection, which deteriorated over 16 hours with muscle damage and organ failure. Condition critical and patient died despite treatment	• Need to review on-call clinical communication processes
Sentinel	Baby died following delay in identifying foetal distress during labour	• Baby monitoring machine alarm was switched off by automatic default, unbeknown to the staff • No staff member allocated to patient care during lengthy handover • Implement a standardised communication process during handover

(Continued)

TABLE 25.3 *Examples of sentinel and serious events in Aotearoa New Zealand 2009–10 (cont.)*

Type of adverse event	Description of event	Communication issues (cause or recommendations)
Sentinel	Baby suffered cerebral palsy potentially as a result of the labour and birth	• Improved communication between staff in rural areas and tertiary units while awaiting retrieval
Sentinel	Patient inhaled stomach contents when anaesthetic given, subsequently died	• A lack of communication led to naso-gastric tube not being inserted prior to the patient being anaesthetised
Sentinel	Delayed response to deterioration potentially contributing to death	• Need to review intensive care unit guidelines for admission • Strengthen communication between critical care services
Sentinel	Suicide of a community mental health patient within seven days of contact	• Identified the opportunity for improved primary/secondary/NGO mental health services communication and collaboration
Sentinel	A patient presented to ED with severe pain and apparent vomiting; she was HIV positive with diagnosed shingles. She was discharged and returned to ED later that day when she was admitted. She died soon after admission	• Emergency department staff should be reminded of the process to call interpreters and use of communication cards
Sentinel	Death of a patient with reduced immunity following a delay in antibiotic administration	• Inadequate processes for the recording of telephone referrals and internal communication of this information
Sentinel	Pregnant woman involved in motor vehicle accident; her unborn child suffered distress and was born dead	• Problems identified with communication systems for contacting key health practitioners • Additional communication systems to contact staff in an emergency
Sentinel	Patient death due to a rare complication following a biopsy procedure	• Communication regarding treatment options could have been more comprehensive
Sentinel	Unexpected death of a patient undergoing plasma exchange from overwhelming infection	• No effective process for communicating urgent after-hours laboratory results for outpatients
Sentinel	One dose of radiation therapy administered to patient due to incorrect diagnosis	• A major cause of this incident was the incorrect interpretation of imaging results • Encourage the responsible clinical staff to jointly review and discuss the images with a radiologist (if the formal report of the investigation is not available) before proceeding to active treatment • Encourage staff to gain back-up/second opinions from colleagues in difficult clinical situations to apply accurate clinical judgment

An adverse event: health care event causing patient harm that is not related to the natural course of the patient's illness or underlying condition.
Serious event: requires significant additional treatment but is not life threatening and has not resulted in major loss of function.
Sentinel event: life threatening, or has led to an unanticipated death or major loss of function.

adapted from Health Quality & Safety Commission (2010)

Professional responsibilities

Professional groups and organisations often have policies and codes about practice that make reference to communication. Problems with communication feature strongly in complaints from patients and families, and many poor outcomes and experiences can be addressed through sound and honest communication.

Key elements of good quality professional communication include the following:

+ honesty and integrity (this includes recognising and responding to mistakes)
+ explanation (it is a good idea to give people a 'commentary' about what is happening)
+ feedback (seeking and listening to compliments and complaints)
+ reflection.

Honesty appears to be universally valued; however, there are examples in all fields in which less than honest communication is tolerated or condoned. For example, the tendency to emphasise research findings that have positive outcomes over those with negative or contrary results (Hirsch, 2004) raises questions about honesty. In terms of individual practitioners, there are examples of deliberate misrepresentation of qualifications or skills, failing to demonstrate reflection or failing to acknowledge feedback. In extreme situations this has led to injury and death.

CASE STUDY 25.2

Professional misrepresentation

A surgeon in Australia

Jayant Patel was employed as a surgeon in a rural setting. Over a period of time, problems emerged in relation to his skills and interactions with colleagues and patients. The negative outcomes included serious harm for some patients and the deaths of others. Lack of communication and systems to respond to concerns played a role in the escalation of these problems and delays in having them addressed.

Thomas (2007)

A psychiatrist in Aotearoa New Zealand

Linda Astor was employed within Aotearoa New Zealand as a psychiatrist. Over a period of time, concerns about her practice emerged. Investigations revealed that there was very little truth in how this practitioner had represented herself.

Bonn (1997)

Members of the public today have more access to information about health and disability care and support than they have done in the past. This democratisation of information means that health practitioners and other professionals are no longer the arbiters of power and information, and they are likely to be questioned and challenged. It is important to know that information needs to be accompanied by good-quality communication in order for it to be meaningful and relevant.

Interprofessional communication

While communication between patients or service users and those interacting with them is of prime importance, challenges in relation to communication between practitioners and groups cannot be underestimated. Some obvious challenges exist in relation to coded messages. Good quality **interprofessional** communication is essential to the well-being of those receiving services.

Interprofessional Interaction between two or more professionals.

CASE STUDY 25.3

Talking past each other

There are many examples of poor communications between practitioners. A particularly entertaining video clip (*Orthopaedics vs. anaesthesia*, n.d.) gives some insight into how professionals can assume they are communicating meaningfully with one another for the good of the patient, when in fact they are just reciting messages they are familiar with.

TABLE 25.4 *Orthopaedics vs. anaesthesia—parallel messages*

Orthopaedic messages	*Anaesthetic messages*
There is a fracture—I need to fix it.	Who is the patient? What are the issues?
I can fix it quickly—I am good at this.	The patient is at serious risk.
I am being obstructed from doing my job.	It is too dangerous to give an anaesthetic.

Communicating in organisations

When people interact there are complex interpersonal and other contextual issues that influence their experiences, interpretations and communication. When these interactions take place within organisations, other layers of complexity are added. It is essential that documentation honestly represents the communication that has taken place and that people have access to information about them. The policies or conventions for communicating and recording interactions need to be followed as they demonstrate **professional accountability**.

Professional accountability The expectations that professionals should be able to defend or account for their actions.

{ SUMMARY }

It is essential to ensure that sent messages are understood. Health and science environments have very particular conventions and expectations in relation to communication. Problems with communication in these contexts have the potential to detrimentally impact on others. There are a number of key points to consider in relation to professional communication. Understanding codes, professional responsibilities, and professional and interprofessional communication helps with making sense of messages and provides insight into respectful communication with colleagues and those accessing health and disability services.

REFLECTION POINTS

25.1 Intention (motivation, message, meaning, emotion)

In what ways do health practitioner communications differ from communications between friends?

25.2 Reception (received message, response, feedback)

How might you minimise the risk of communications between clients and health practitioners being misinterpreted?

25.3 Perception (style, manner, impression, analysis)

How might a person-centred approach alter how clients are valued and treated?

QUESTIONS FOR REVIEW

1 What are key aspects of good communications in health care?
2 What are some of the risks involved in using slang or abbreviations?
3 What are some of the risks in coding and decoding messages?

REFERENCES

Bonn, D. (1997). Bogus psychiatrist dupes New Zealand. *The Lancet, 350*, 794.

Ginott, H. G. (1972). *Teacher and child*. New York, NY: MacMillan.

Health Quality & Safety Commission. (2010). *Making our hospitals safer: Serious and sentinel events 2009/2010*. Wellington, NZ: Author.

Hirsch, L. (2004). Randomized clinical trials: What gets published and when? *Canadian Medical Association Journal, 170*(4), 481–3.

Orthopaedics vs. anaesthesia. (n.d.) Xtranormal. Retrieved from www.xtranormal.com/watch/6752641.

Parvaiz, M., Singh, G. K., Hafee, R. & Sharma, H. (2006). Do multidisciplinary team members correctly interpret the abbreviations used in the medical records? *Scottish Medical Journal, 51*(4), 49.

Thomas, H. (2007). *Sick to death: A manipulative surgeon and a health system in crisis—A disaster waiting to happen*. Sydney, NSW: Allen and Unwin.

Wear, D., Aultman, J. M., Varley, J. D. & Zarconi, J. (2006). Making fun of patients: Medical students' perceptions and use of derogatory and cynical humor in clinical settings. *Academic Medicine, 81*(5), 454–62.

WEBSITES

Annotated Bibliography on Patient-Provider Communication: www.patientprovidercommunication.org/index.cfm/bibliography.htm

Serious and Sentinel Events 2009/2010, Health Quality & Safety Commission New Zealand: www.hqsc.govt.nz/page/22534/serious-and-sentinel-events-2009-2010-full/?tab=2349&contentType=486

{26}

Therapeutic Engagement

Elizabeth Finn

CHAPTER OVERVIEW

This chapter covers the following topics:

+ Consumers' involvement in their care
+ Communication
+ Communication in a health-care setting
+ Effective communication
+ Barriers to effective communication
+ The therapeutic relationship when things go wrong.

KEY TERMS

Consumers
Rapport
Empathy

When a health service practitioner interacts with a consumer for the purpose of providing health care—whether in a general practice or dental surgery, a pharmacy, any kind of clinic or consulting room, or a residential facility or hospital ward—the practitioner and consumer together embark upon a dialogue. This is a two-way communication process that is intended to result in a health benefit for the consumer. The process that occurs during such an interaction, where both the practitioner and the consumer are actively involved, may be considered therapeutic engagement. Therapeutic engagement requires a partnership between practitioner and consumer in an effective communication process to reach an optimal health outcome.

Although the concept that health service practitioners and consumers should be involved in a partnership during an episode of health-care delivery may seem fundamental today, this has not always been the case. It is useful to consider earlier models of health-care delivery in order to recognise the importance of effective communication in facilitating the provision of good-quality, safe and appropriate health care.

Consumers' involvement in their care

Prior to 1987, in Aotearoa New Zealand health services were delivered in the context of a patriarchal model of health care. Clinicians who had, by virtue of their extensive training and experience, a body of knowledge beyond that of their patients tended to make decisions about the care and treatment of their patients based solely on their own professional judgment and preferences, without consideration of the views of their patient. The patriarchal model was widely accepted and patients trusted their doctors to make decisions for them in their best interests. Sometimes patients knew very little about their condition, treatment or prognosis.

This model of health care was challenged in 1987 when serious concerns about the treatment provided to some patients at Auckland's National Women's Hospital were exposed. An inquiry resulted in the publication of a report (the Cartwright Report) that would have far-reaching effects on the way health care was delivered in Aotearoa New Zealand. The report (Cartwright, 1988) stated that the rights of patients to a good standard of care—including full information and the ability to make choices about their care—were of such importance that they should be enshrined in legislation. In line with these recommendations, the Health and Disability Commissioner Act was passed into legislation in 1994. The Act required a new model of care, and set out providers' responsibilities in the *Code of Health and Disability Services Consumers' Rights* (Health and Disability Commissioner, 2009a). It promoted a model where providers need to work in partnership with **consumers**, engaging with them in a

Consumers people who use goods and services.

consultative manner and responding as appropriate to their individual circumstances; in other words, a consumer-centred model of care.

The increasing responsibility of consumers for their own care has also been influenced by social, political and economic changes. These have altered the way health care is delivered (Nettleton, Harding & Taylor, 1994). These factors include the increasing costs of health care, and political polices designed to shift costs from third-party payers (government-funded agencies and insurers) to health consumers themselves (Sclar, Robison & Skaer, 1996). Other factors are the increasing incidence of lifestyle diseases—such as cardiovascular disease, cancer, HIV/AIDS, cirrhosis of the liver, obesity, depression and hypertension—which encourages individuals to make health and lifestyle changes (Maguire, 2001); and a growing trend for consumers to move away from the traditional medical treatments and choose therapies such as herbal medicines, acupuncture, osteopathy or other complementary or alternative treatments (Canter, 2001). The availability of reports about health, disease and treatment options on internet sites and in the popular press provides information that individuals can use in making decisions about their own care.

In general medical practice, the recognition that patients wished to be more involved in their own care was addressed by Laine and Davidoff (1996), who introduced the concept of patient-centred medicine. Since then, the consumer-centred philosophy has become widespread, and there is increasing evidence that the involvement of consumers in their own care contributes to better health outcomes (Kravitz & Melnikow, 2001). Further, the nature of the interactions of a consumer with his or her provider is known not only to be an important part of health-care delivery (Landis, 1996), but also to influence treatment outcomes (Parasuraman, Zeithaml & Berry, 1988). Therefore, effective communication and therapeutic engagement are key principles in the provision of appropriate, good-quality health care.

Communication

Communication is a complex interactional process. It may be described as a *two-way* process of sharing information. The process is characterised by turn-taking, where each message bears a relationship to the message preceding it. Each participant acts and reacts to the other, backwards and forwards, so the dialogue generally maintains an aspect of symmetry (McGregor, 1994).

In a conversation or dialogue between participants, meaning is conveyed not only by talking and listening, but also by non-verbal aspects of communication such as eye contact (or lack of it), tone and inflection of the voice, as well as posture (open or confrontational) and movements including nodding, smiling, shrugging and other gestures, often referred to as body language. Studies have suggested that only about 7 per cent of the meaning of what is communicated by an individual comes from the words spoken. The remaining 93 per cent comes from the context, including body language (Bolstad et al., 1992).

The contribution of body language to successful communication is very powerful. For example, maintenance of eye contact, nods, smiles and an interested facial expression signify active listening and encourage a speaker to continue; a speaker who notices that the listener's attention is elsewhere quickly feels he or she is not being listened to and will lose interest in maintaining the conversation, or even become angry. Confusion may result where a person's verbally transmitted message does not match the body language that accompanies it. Consider the child who steals a biscuit: her mother notices her contradictory body language (she 'looks guilty') even though the child is saying: 'Someone else took the biscuit.'

As well as the contribution of body language, and the separate acts of speaking and listening, communication involves the reciprocal understanding of meaning between the participants. For communication to satisfy the goals of the participants, each must agree that they understand, or share the interpretation of, the messages that are passed between them. Participants need to actively monitor for this understanding, and a speaker may need to modify what they say in response to verbal or non-verbal feedback from their listener.

Communication in a health-care setting

Conversations that occur in institutional settings have been found to differ from ordinary conversational interactions (Heritage, 1997). Within these settings, participants' interactions are focused on achieving specific and pre-defined goals that are a function of the institutional setting in which they are interacting. In health care, the goal is to facilitate optimal health outcomes for the consumer through the provision of safe, quality health care.

For this to be achieved, both the practitioner and the consumer need to be actively involved in both a partnership (therapeutic engagement) and an effective communication process. The *Code of Health and Disability Services Consumers' Rights* sets out the right of health services consumers to effective communication (Right 5), and states that this requires a 'form, language, and manner that enables the consumer to understand the information provided' and 'an environment that enables both consumer and provider to communicate openly, honestly and effectively'. Right 6(1) of the Code also requires that consumers are given all the information that a reasonable consumer, in that consumer's circumstances, would expect to receive (Health and Disability Commissioner, 2009a).

Rapport The basis for mutually respectful interactions between people.

Empathy The ability to appreciate the thoughts, feelings and perspectives of others.

Interactions in a health-care setting generally follow a structure that may facilitate the development of good communication. First, the participants meet and greet each other, making eye contact, perhaps shaking hands, and establishing **rapport**. The concept of rapport incorporates ideas of harmony as people understand one another. It indicates the presence of respect and trust, and opens up the opportunity for consumers to share their concerns with the practitioner, and for the practitioner to develop empathy for the consumer. **Empathy** is the ability to understand and sensitively appreciate the predicament (thoughts and feelings) of another person, without these necessarily being directly communicated. Empathy also involves the communication of that understanding back to the consumer in a supportive way. When a consumer feels at ease, accepted and heard in such an environment, and feels that his or her concerns are acknowledged, he or she is more likely to respond openly and actively, in a two-way communication process, allowing therapeutic engagement.

Effective communication

Effective communication is characterised by the development of an open, trusting and respectful relationship between the practitioner and consumer. Consumers who feel rapport with a provider—who feel listened to and understood; who feel comfortable about asking questions, voicing concerns and fears; who feel they can express emotion; and who perceive empathy in their practitioner—are more likely to provide full information and to enable the provider to respond more effectively.

Practitioners are more likely to develop a working partnership and work with consumers to reach mutually agreed treatment outcomes if they:

+ show real interest in consumers
+ develop good relationships
+ show warmth and acceptance
+ question skilfully to draw relevant information from consumers
+ read body language
+ listen attentively to what consumers say (and be alert to what they do not say)
+ check back with consumers to clarify what they have heard
+ happily receive questions
+ respond to discussion
+ avoid medical terms and jargon.

Communication is concerned with the practitioners' relationships with consumers, as well as the information that needs to be gathered, given and discussed.

CASE STUDY 26.1

Being too familiar

Janet is recounting her morning visit with a locum doctor. 'He called me Janet! Never met the man before! I'm Mrs Sheppard to him! What's happened to respect these days?' She takes another sip of coffee. Then continues slowly, affronted: 'And then as if that wasn't bad enough, he called me "dear", and he spoke really slowly and loudly, as if I was deaf and couldn't understand. I am only 70 after all.' She sipped her coffee again, while Annie looked at her with empathy, appreciating that Janet felt patronised by the locum. Janet said, 'I don't have much faith in a doctor who makes me feel small. It's just as well that he didn't suggest any new treatment because I wouldn't have followed it. I'm glad Dr Scott will be back next week. I always feel very confident with him.'

The importance of effective communication cannot be overestimated. Good communication matters because it is strongly correlated with better outcomes for consumers—both directly and indirectly. First, without effective communication supporting the necessary exchange of information between consumer and practitioner, misdiagnosis and inappropriate treatment selection are more likely. Second, consumers' experience of 'being heard' is one of the greatest determinants of consumer satisfaction, and influences consumers' views of the competence of their practitioner. Research has shown that the way practitioners communicate with consumers, and how responsive they are, can influence the way they accept and act on advice, and the way they perceive the quality of the health service encounter (Finn, 2003). Satisfaction with the service is positively related to how consumers follow up with treatment plans and, consequently, on the effectiveness of the treatment provided (Ley, 1982; Parasuraman, Zeithaml & Berry, 1988).

Furthermore, engagement in effective communication needs to be an essential aspect of the delivery of health care because it is set down as a responsibility for all practitioners under the *Code of Health and Disability Services Consumers' Rights*.

CASE STUDY 26.2

Doctor and consumer

Following a screening test (prostate-specific antigen or PSA test) that raised suspicion of prostate cancer, a 70-year-old man received a form from his doctor reminding him to have a further test. The man did not understand what the test was for and did not attend for the test. No further attempt was made by the general practice to remind him to have the repeat test. A year later, the man consulted his doctor again and at this time the test showed a higher level of PSA. The man was immediately referred to a specialist and then to a hospital urology service. Eighteen months after his first presentation, the man underwent a biopsy that revealed prostate cancer that had spread into most of his bones. A complaint was made to the Health and Disability Commissioner. The Commissioner's view was that the clinic should have informed the man what PSA tests are for, and what the results of his test were, so he could understand and appreciate why he needed a follow-up test.

This case illustrates the need for practitioners to develop a therapeutic relationship with consumers to ensure partnership in the health-care process, so consumers understand the status of their health and what their responsibilities are (Health and Disability Commissioner, 2008).

Barriers to effective communication

There are many barriers to effective communication in our health-care institutions, whether they are clinics, consulting rooms or hospitals. Barriers can arise from the physical environment, and the personal attributes and behaviours of the people concerned.

First, health-care communication involves practitioners (such as doctors, dentists and pharmacists) who are perceived to possess the power of knowledge and professional skill, and lay people (consumers), who are perceived not to posses knowledge or skills. Not only may practitioners seem daunting because of their professional status, but (in contrast to the 'equal participation' of speakers in ordinary conversation) practitioners are also more likely to take the initiative and dominate the conversation (Heritage, 1997). Opportunities for consumers to make a contribution may then be limited; they may be deprived of the chance to let the practitioner know their concerns and fears, what they understand about their situation, or what they are seeking from the consultation. Unless practitioners are clear about a consumer's understandings and needs, they cannot 'get into the consumer's shoes', consider the situation from the consumer's perspective, and decide the appropriate information, advice or treatment to offer. Power differentials (both real and perceived) can be minimised by engaging in an open, respectful, consumer-centred communication process.

Second, there may be differences in the personal background, knowledge, experience and understanding of the practitioner and consumer; for example, differences in their values, preferences, ethnicity, cultural background, sexual orientation or spiritual beliefs and practices. Participants need to be aware of differences, and avoid making assumptions or judgments based on their own life experience. They need to work together during the interaction, using questioning and discussion to ensure mutual understanding of differences and to arrive at mutually acceptable goals (Morrow, 1997). For example, some consumers of Polynesian decent may nod when given information by a practitioner, but this nod may indicate respect for the practitioner, rather than the European interpretation that the information has been accepted and will be acted upon. A European practitioner who relied on the familiar interpretation of the nod would be likely to miss the opportunity to ensure the consumer understood and would follow the recommended treatment, meaning the anticipated outcome may not be achieved.

Where a consumer speaks a language different from that of their practitioner, the practitioner has a responsibility to ensure communication is provided in a manner that enables the consumer to understand what is said. This may involve the need for an interpreter to ensure the appropriateness, safety and quality of the care provided.

Third, the specialised words used in health care (jargon) may not be understood by consumers. Sometimes consumers may feel embarrassed about asking for an explanation, in case they appear ignorant, but practitioners have a responsibility under the *Code of Health and Disability Services Consumers' Rights* (Right 5(2)) to provide information in a form that consumers can understand. They have an obligation to ensure consumers are familiar with all the terms used, and that they completely understand what is being discussed.

Fourth, physical factors may impede the effectiveness of communication. Any of the following examples could reduce the effectiveness of the communication between practitioner and consumer, and consequently jeopardise the quality of the health-care goals each participant is working towards:

+ a large office desk between the practitioner and a consumer, obstructing an open aspect to communication
+ a computer at which a practitioner takes notes throughout the consultation, hampering important eye contact between practitioner and consumer
+ interruptions of phone calls during a consultation that threaten concentration and demonstrate a lack of respect for the consumer.

Further, the pressure of time on either the practitioner or the consumer has been shown to reduce the effectiveness of communication. Practitioners may arrive at a diagnosis on the basis of symptoms disclosed by a consumer early in the consultation—without exploring further or considering all possible diagnoses—or they may close a consultation without giving a consumer time for questions or providing adequate advice about what to do if the situation does not improve. Equally, consumers may believe that 'the doctor is too busy to listen', and provide only partial details about their complaint, with the result that the doctor may reach a diagnosis on the basis of inadequate information, and instigate incorrect treatment. Similarly, a consumer may be unwilling to spend the necessary time required for an appropriate consultation.

Finally, the disposition of either the consumer or the practitioner can have a negative impact on the communication process. Consumers may be very unwell or debilitated, frightened or distressed, or angry and harassed by issues that are not associated with their health care in any way. Any such issues may impact on the way the consumers behave and communicate. Practitioners' communication also may be affected by surrounding issues, such as the effect of staffing shortages, a difficult consultation earlier in the day or an unrelated personal matter.

The therapeutic relationship when things go wrong

The therapeutic relationship provides the basis for the open and honest discussions that are needed between practitioners and consumers when things go wrong, especially when consumers experience harm as a result of medical error. A large number of adverse events (unintended or unexpected outcomes of care that could have, or did, lead to harm for a consumer) occur in the delivery of health care. A study of adverse events in Aotearoa New Zealand public hospitals found an incidence rate of adverse events in almost 13 per cent of sampled admissions. These findings were consistent with those of studies undertaken in Australia and Britain (Davis et al., 2001).

When consumers experience unexpected outcomes of health care, what they need most is an acknowledgement of the error, an apology, and to know what happened and how it can be prevented from happening again (Lamb, 2004). Effective communication between practitioners and consumers and their families, and open disclosure about the causes and effects of the incident, is a vital part of the process of dealing with consumer safety incidents (National Patient Safety Agency, 2009; Health and Disability Commissioner, 2009b). Legally and ethically, it is the right thing to do (Lamb, 2004). Open disclosure is not a single conversation but rather a process of ongoing communication that continues until the consumer has all the information and support needed. The therapeutic relationship—characterised by trust, empathy, and honest and open discussion—is key to open disclosure.

CASE STUDY 26.3

Examples of things going wrong

The following examples are drawn from complaints letters to the Health and Disabilities Commissioner.

Complaint about surgical complications

A consumer who complained after surgical complications said: 'My surgeon made a fleeting visit after I was discharged from the intensive care unit and that was the last I saw of him ... What happened and who is responsible? I feel a mistake is being covered up.'

Silence after husband's death

'I still do not know what happened to my husband. The hospital is not giving me detailed facts ... nobody is letting me know what happened.'

Suicide following son's plea for care

The family of a man who unsuccessfully sought help from his doctor before taking his own life visited the doctor to discuss what had happened. They said: 'He was totally uncaring and arrogant, shrugged us off and showed us out of his rooms ... he didn't seem to care about us. He lacked empathy and was annoyed that we as a family expected him to discuss anything.'

Bismark and Paterson (2005)

Studies show that being open can decrease the trauma felt by consumers following an incident (Vincent, Pincus & Scurr, 1993), and that consumers are more likely to forgive medical errors when they are discussed in a timely and thoughtful manner (Vincent & Coulter, 2002).

Consumers often want to know what action has been taken as a result of the error or adverse event, as many want to ensure that the same thing does not happen to anyone else (Bismark et al., 2006). In numerous cases, adverse events are the result of one or more errors in the systems that underpin delivery of care in hospitals or medical practices. In these cases, frank discussion among practitioners fosters open and honest professional relationships, and enables systems to change to improve service quality and consumer safety (Health and Disability Commissioner, 2009b).

Openness also has benefits for practitioners, as it may help to reduce the burden of guilt or the fear of being found out, and also help them understand the incidents from the perspective of the consumer and their families. Further, it can help to prevent harmful events becoming formal complaints and the subject of litigation claims (Vincent & Coulter, 2002).

The principles of open disclosure are becoming valued and recognised worldwide, with organisational policies and standards being developed to promote them. In Aotearoa New Zealand, several pieces of legislation act together to promote a culture of openness in which practitioners feel safe to talk about things that have gone wrong.

First, accident compensation legislation (such as the Accident Compensation Act 2001) makes provision for consumers who experience treatment injury to be eligible for taxpayer-funded insurance cover for rehabilitation and care, with such compensation not dependent on the requirement to prove fault on the part of the person(s) who provided the treatment. Furthermore, the legislation bars injured consumers from bringing actions for negligence against a practitioner in a civil claim. Practitioners who make mistakes are free from the threat of legal action.

Second, the Health and Disability Commissioner Act 1994 enables a focus on learning from mistakes, along with changes in systems and policies as a means of improving the quality and safety of health care. Publication of the name of an individual practitioner who has failed to meet his or her responsibilities under the *Code of Health and Disability Services Consumers' Rights* is rare. In this environment, practitioners need not feel fearful of talking about errors or adverse events.

Third, provider organisations, such as residential care facilities and hospitals, have legal responsibilities to take steps to ensure that open disclosure is practised by staff and supported by management, both under the *Health and Disability Services Standards* (Ministry of Health, 2008) and the *Code of Health and Disability Services Consumers' Rights*, where several of the rights are relevant to open disclosure (Health and Disability Commissioner, 2009a).

{ SUMMARY }

Therapeutic engagement underpins all aspects of health care. It provides the context within which practitioners and consumers can relate openly and freely. Within it, rapport is developed, empathy is evident, information is shared and participants are equally and actively involved in a partnership through an effective communication process. It also provides space for solutions to problems to be discussed and a course of action to be agreed upon. Appreciating communication as an opportunity for therapeutic engagement promotes resolution for both consumers and practitioners, and opens the way for improvements in practices and systems to improve the safety and quality of health care.

REFLECTION POINTS

26.1 Intention (motivation, message, meaning, emotion)

The *Code of Health and Disability Services Consumers' Rights* sets out the right of health services consumers to effective communication (Right 5). What are the characteristics of effective communication?

26.2 Reception (received message, response, feedback)

This Code also states that communications need to occur in a 'form, language, and manner that enables the consumer to understand the information provided'. Thinking about communicating across the lifespan, what implications will this have for your practice?

26.3 Perception (style, manner, impression, analysis)

In addition, the Code states that 'an environment that enables both consumer and provider to communicate openly, honestly and effectively' is required. What implications does this have for your practice?

QUESTIONS FOR REVIEW

1 What are some barriers to effective communication?
2 For each of the barriers you listed, what are the ways in which these might be reduced?
3 In recognising that errors sometimes occur, what steps are recommended to redress harm to consumers that may have occurred?

REFERENCES

Bismark, M. M. & Paterson, R. L. (2005). 'Doing the right thing' after an adverse event. *New Zealand Medical Journal, 118*(1219), 55–60.

Bismark, M., Dauer, E., Paterson, R. & Studdert, D. (2006). Accountability sought by patients following adverse events from medical care: The New Zealand experience. *Canadian Medical Association Journal, 175*(8), 889–94.

Bolstad, R., Hamblett, M., Ohlson, T. & Hardie, J. (1992). *Communicating caring. A guide for health workers and caregivers*. Auckland, NZ: Longman Paul Ltd.

Canter, R. (2001). Patients and medical power. *British Medical Journal, 323*, 414.

Cartwright, S. (1988). *The report of the committee of inquiry into allegations concerning the treatment of cervical cancer at National Women's Hospital and into other related matters*. Auckland, NZ: Government Printing Office.

Davis, P., Lay-Yee, R., Briant, R., Schug, S. & Scott, A. (2001). *Adverse events in New Zealand public hospitals: Principal findings from a national survey*. Wellington, NZ: Ministry of Health.

Finn, E. A. (2003). Communicative effectiveness in pharmacy consultations: An investigation of advice-giving and recipiency in the New Zealand consumer-focused health environment. Unpublished PhD thesis. University of Otago, NZ.

Health and Disability Commissioner. (2008). *Decision 08HDC06165*. Retrieved from www.hdc.org.nz/decisions--case-notes/commissioner's-decisions/2008/08hdc06165.

Health and Disability Commissioner. (2009a). *Code of health and disability services consumer's rights*. Retrieved from www.hdc.org.nz/media/24833/leaflet%20code%20of%20rights.pdf.

Health and Disability Commissioner. (2009b). *Guidance on open disclosure policies*. Wellington, NZ: Author.

Heritage, J. (1997). Conversational analysis and institutional talk: Analysing data. In D. Silverman (ed.), *Qualitative research: Theory method and practice*. London, UK: Sage.

Kravitz, R. L. & Melnikow, J. (2001). Engaging patients in medical decision-making. *British Journal of Medicine, 323*, 584–5.

Laine, C. & Davidoff, F. (1996). Patient-centred medicine: A professional evolution. *Journal of the American Medical Association, 275*, 152–6.

Lamb, R. (2004). Open disclosure: The only approach to medical error. *Quality and Safety in Health Care, 13*, 3–5.

Landis, T. N. (1996). Lessons from medicine and nursing for pharmacist-patient communication. *American Journal of Health System Pharmacy*, *53*, 1306–14.

Ley, P. (1982). Satisfaction, compliance and communication. *British Journal of Clinical Psychology*, *21*, 241–54.

Maguire, T. (2001). More clarity, less dogma in our approach to pharmacy practice. *Pharmaceutical Journal*, *266*, 651–3.

McGregor, G. (1994). *Third person interpretation and the sociolinguists of verbal communication*. Unpublished PhD thesis. University of Newcastle, Newcastle upon Tyne, UK.

Ministry of Health. (2008). *Health and Disability Services Standards*, NZS 8134. Retrieved from www.moh.govt.nz/moh.nsf/pagesmh/8656/$File/81340-2008-nzs-readonly.pdf.

Morrow, D. (1997). Improving consultations between health care professionals and older clients: Implications for pharmacists. *International Journal of Ageing and Human Development, 44*(1), 47–72.

National Patient Safety Agency. (2009). *Being open policy*. National Reporting and Learning Service, UK: National Health Service.

Nettleton, S., Harding. G. & Taylor, K. (1994). The concept and context of social pharmacy. In G. Harding, S. Nettleton & K. Taylor (eds), *Social pharmacy: Innovation and development*. London, UK: The Pharmaceutical Press.

Parasuraman, A., Zeithaml, V. A. & Berry, L. L. (1988). SERVQUAL: A multiple-item scale for measuring consumer perceptions of service quality. *Journal of Retailing, 4*, 12–40.

Sclar, D. A., Robison, L. M. & Skaer, T. L. (1996). Pharmacy consultations and over-the-counter purchasing outcomes. *Journal of Clinical Pharmacy and Therapeutics*, *21*, 177–84.

Vincent, C. A. & Coulter, A. (2002). Patient safety: What about the patients? *Quality and Safety in Health Care, 11*, 76–80.

Vincent, C. A., Pincus, T. & Scurr, J. H. (1993). Patients' experience of surgical accidents. *Quality and Safety in Health Care, 2*, 77–82.

WEBSITES

Accident Compensation Corporation: www.acc.co.nz/about-acc/index.htm

Being Open: Communicating Patient Safety Incidents With Patients, their Families and Carers, National Patient Safety Agency: www.nrls.npsa.nhs.uk/resources/?entryid45=65077

Center for Healthcare Communication, USA: www.communicatingwithpatients.com

Open Disclosure, Health and Disability Commissioner: www.hdc.org.nz/decisions--case-notes/open-disclosure

{27}

Care at a Distance

Susan Shaw

CHAPTER OVERVIEW

This chapter covers the following topics:

+ Physical location
+ Technology
+ Making connections
+ Impact on practitioners
+ Communicating across time and space.

KEY TERMS

Expertise
Rural
Context
Access
Telemedicine
Interpreter
Cultural heritage
Locum

Changes in knowledge and technology have altered the way services are offered and this is particularly evident in terms of access to care and **expertise** for people who live or work at a considerable distance from those providing the care. At first glance, innovations in the provision of care may seem transformational, but there are several considerations that must be taken into account when services are provided in ways that are fundamentally different from face-to-face interactions between service provider and recipient. At the very core of these considerations is how the difference in time and space impacts on the communication that may, or should, take place between people.

Expertise Expert skills and knowledge.

Physical location

One of the most obvious challenges in terms of providing care across time and space is physical distance. Technological innovations have addressed many of the challenges associated with this, but there are distinct differences in terms of distance provision according to the needs of communities. In Australia, extensive distances have led to the development of a significant level of expertise in such provision. Remote or **rural** health-care provision has seen the development of 'flying doctor' services. This in turn has influenced the expertise of practitioners who need to respond to emergencies in ways that differ from colleagues who work in jurisdictions that do not routinely experience long delays in access to high-level care or expertise. The degree of remoteness influences service provision and outcomes, and may substantially contribute to negative health and outcomes (Phillips, 2009).

Rural Outside of urban centres.

Meeting the needs of people in remote areas is not simply about trying to speed up access to experts or tertiary health-care services. One of the fundamental challenges for practitioners in remote areas is to appreciate the cultural **context** of the community. The need to engage with people's history and experience in order to think and practice with a degree of creativity has been acknowledged in an Australian study (Wood, 2010). If practitioners are not accepted and trusted within the community, their level of skill or access to services will be largely irrelevant to health outcomes and the experiences of service users.

Context The range of elements that affect people and situations, including political, social and cultural issues.

Access is an important factor in health care and disability support services, and is about much more than distance (Sutherns & Bourgeault, 2008). True access is about choice, economics, information and experiences. This is only achieved when consumers rate the care they receive as effective and appropriate (including culturally suitable). Flexible and responsive delivery of mobile services contributes to accessibility in distant and remote areas. Large physical distances between practitioners and services mean that while care is available, individuals may not have as much choice as their counterparts in urban centres. This leads to a lack of consistent interaction with

Access The ability to seek and receive information and services without barriers.

health practitioners of their choice (Voyle & Simmons, 1999), suggesting that true access is compromised.

Technology

Technological developments in health care include new and improved medical and surgical procedures, tests, drugs, prosthetics and information technology (including record management) (National Center for Health Statistics, 2009). Technology provides obvious solutions to challenges of distance and scarcity of expertise. Quantitative analyses of costs have identified health information technology as contributing to efficiency (Chaudhry et al., 2006). However, assumptions that all practitioners and patients like, understand, trust or are comfortable with technology are problematic.

Telemedicine The use of technology to connect clinical staff with colleagues and patients at a distance.

The benefits of technology in terms of health care are obvious, but high-quality services are essential and this includes excellent clarity (bandwidth), rather than just basic connections. **Telemedicine** is not an easy technology (Whitehall et al., 1998) as the use of it requires practitioners to extend their skills and change their practice. People receiving services via technology also need to adapt. The primary communication route is removed from face-to-face communication, and for people in the generation that had to adjust to telephone technology, the emergence of video- and internet-based communication is a further challenge. People prefer face-to-face contact (Turnbull et al., 2010) and it is naive to assume that patients view telephone contact as a panacea for accessing services: 'Those already disadvantaged by geography or socioeconomic circumstances may continue to be at a disadvantage when services are provided by telephone' (Turnbull et al., 2010, p. 27.)

Technology is also a major cause of cost escalation in health care, including increased need for services as people live longer. Simplistic approaches to resource management and constraints may put services to rural and remote communities at risk.

CASE STUDY 27.1

IT in diabetes management

Providing support for people living with diabetes is a considerable cost to health-care services. A review of published information about type 2 diabetes and the use of telemedicine revealed that information technology can be used to provide support and information for patients and practitioners, and therefore to contribute to better quality care.

Adaji, Schattner and Jones (2008)

Making connections

Making connections is a huge part of human communication. In social settings, conversation often centres on individuals talking and questioning each other as they search for links such as shared images, experiences and understandings.

Communication between colleagues and service users occurs constantly and is also needed to make connections between various pieces of information. Good communication takes place when received messages are understood in the way that the sender intended them to be. The provision of health and disability services (including front-line and support services such as laboratories and imaging) is dependent on high-quality communication. In addition to being one of the foundations of good-quality care, good communication has a therapeutic benefit in and of itself. Poor communication can be linked to poor-quality care and outcomes (see, for example, Table 25.3 on serious and sentinel events).

People tend to communicate best with those from similar backgrounds, as they share language, experiences, codes and ways of making sense of information and situations. This is natural human behaviour, but it can be a challenge in terms of health and disability service provision. This is because practitioners are often more privileged, by way of their education and roles, than those receiving services from them. A number of professional groups in the health and disability support sector identify care as a key component of their identity, role and interaction with service users. Interacting with 'difficult' people requires that practitioners understand the challenges experienced by the people they interact with (Huynh, Alderson & Thompson, 2008).

There are several elements that may impact on experiences of communication, including language, cultural and comprehension barriers. Language is a particularly difficult barrier in terms of communicating about health and disability issues, as professionals often have specialised language (codes and jargon) that they use. When the service user does not understand the predominant language as well as the specialised language, they are at a significant disadvantage and this creates an environment for poor communication. People are entitled to understand information and decisions that relate to them; therefore, if they do not speak the predominant language (for example, English), they should be provided with an **interpreter** (Garrett, Dickson & Whelan, 2008).

Cultural heritage and experience has a profound impact on the way that people understand their health and well-being (Weerasinghe & Mitchell, 2007). Practitioners are responsible for ensuring that they carefully consider the cultural backgrounds of people. They also must appreciate that the culture of medical institutions and professions themselves are powerful and may confuse and offend service users.

Interpreter A skilled communicator who is able to translate information for two parties who do not share the same language.

Cultural heritage The history of cultural understanding that informs individuals' understanding and perspectives.

In any given situation, there are a number of perspectives that may be considered. In terms of communicating with patients and service users, the primary focus should be on understanding the situation and communication from their perspective. It is common for practitioners to have different understandings from service users. For example, incidents of aggression and violence may be considered by clients to be caused by environmental conditions and poor communication, while staff may consider the same incidents to be linked to the mental state of the service users (Duxbury & Whittington, 2005). Caldwell (2006) describes imitating body language to create a conversation based on gestures as a way of communicating. Interacting from a distance may reduce the immediate risks or concerns of aggression, but may also lessen the opportunities for subtle elements of human interaction (such as body language), which can assist in a positive way when people are in the same space.

CASE STUDY 27.2

Sense of place

Differences in status and outcomes between people living in rural and metropolitan areas are obvious inequities. Health promotion and prevention activities have been identified as of particular importance for Australians living in rural and remote areas.

Despite apparent health inequities, the sense of connection to place is of enormous importance to people and features strongly among reasons why people live and work in rural and remote areas.

The most advanced health promotion and prevention initiatives will fail if they are not accompanied by this appreciation of place, and the spiritual and cultural connections that are valued by Indigenous communities.

Wakerman (2008)

Impact on practitioners

Providing care at a distance requires a rethinking of professional boundaries, as spreading the load has been identified as one of the strategies in developing remote services (Kildea, Kruske & Bowell, 2006). Such approaches involve sharing expertise and blending roles to some degree. This requires an appreciation of the importance of interdisciplinary and interprofessional practice and communication (see Chapter 25) and challenges traditional boundaries and territories between groups of practitioners and defined scopes of practice. Engaging multidisciplinary therapy assistants (Lin et al., 2007) is an example of reconsidering scopes of practice and blending areas of expertise that have traditionally been clearly demarcated.

CASE STUDY 27.3

Big brother and practice

Technological innovations require a good deal of analysis in terms of how they reflect or impact on the practice of professionals. There are many examples in the world of health-care practice where the work of one group encroaches on that of another. A clear example of this is the introduction of automated dispensing technology.

Pharmacy and management perspective	*Clinical nursing perspective*
Drugs are safely and accurately dispensed	Lack of trust in terms of dispensing
Accountancy systems are automated	Unnecessarily time-consuming

The apparent lack of trust among professional groups, and the assertion that technology can somehow address these issues, has implications for providing services across distances. Opinions about how dispensing technology impacted on nursing practice have been published (see, for example, Shaw, 2002). Subsequent letters to the editor provided insights into how colleagues had interpreted the message and the issues, and particularly the different values placed on dispensing technology by nursing and pharmacy colleagues.

Within rural and remote environments there may be an apparent lack of evidence for practice, as knowledge from other settings is not necessarily transferrable (Parsons et al., 2003). This is problematic within the current health and disability service provision environment, as there is such a strong emphasis on evidence. Problems with evidence or resources are exacerbated in remote practice contexts because of lack of time, poor access to reliable technology and inconsistent (or **locum**) staffing. Practitioners need specific tools to assist them to cope with difficult situations (Blomberg & Sahlberg-Blom, 2007) when working at a distance. The way in which practitioners learn in rural and remote areas needs consideration, and this is a field in which simulation is used to develop skills, particularly in relation to emergency care (Walsh, 2010). The development of firm treatment protocols also limits variations in the provision of care, reducing differences in practice across distances (Allan, de Lacey & Payne, 2009).

Locum A casual employee providing a service that is unable to be met by regularly employed staff.

Despite the challenges, many practitioners choose to practice in remote areas. This type of work is often well paid but requires large adjustments for families

(Kruger & Tennant, 2005). The positive impact of adding rural experiences to the learning journey of professionals has been identified (Dowell, Crampton & Parkin, 2001) and some professions have offered benefits to individuals who choose to spend some of their time in rural communities.

Communicating across time and space

Interactions between practitioners and people using services should be mutually respectful and focused on a shared goal, such as identifying a problem or considering ways to address an issue. On one level, this could be considered a basic exchange of information between people. However, it is much more complex as it involves elements of stress and power dynamics. People who seek health care and disability support often have unanswered questions and are stressed or worried to some degree. The interactions they have with providers of services often take place in environments that are familiar to the professionals and less understood by the service user. Because communication is so fundamental to human interaction and occurring constantly, there are plenty of opportunities for mistaken interpretations, errors or confusion. It is important that individuals and organisations are able to accept that mistakes occur during communication and to have ways of identifying and addressing issues when they do occur.

TABLE 27.1 *Perspectives of practitioners and people seeking services in terms of communication*

Element	*Professional perspective*	*Client/patient perspective*
Physical environment	Familiar	Unfamiliar or intimidating
Specialised language	Familiar	Confusing, frightening or able to be misunderstood
Rules and culture of the encounter	Familiar	May not be understood
Emotional factors	Focus on role	Stressed or anxious

A number of elements have been identified as contributing to therapeutic relationships and communication. These include trust, respect, rapport, listening, honesty, sharing of information and confidentiality. However, patients have been found to place a greater emphasis on honesty and information sharing than practitioners do. One interpretation of this is that the intention behind the communication of nurses (for example) is to maintain control of the situation, therefore limiting opportunities for therapeutic communication (Tuckett, 2005).

CASE STUDY 27.4

Whitecoat hypertension

Whitecoat hypertension occurs when a patient who usually has 'normal' blood pressure experiences a significant increase in their blood pressure when they interact with health practitioners.

Many articles have been written about why this occurs and they are generally framed in terms of deficits that the patients have (for example, an anxiety disorder or poor ability to tolerate stress) and that it may be a pre-determinant of high blood pressure later in life. These analyses blame the patient for the elevated blood pressure.

The interesting thing about much of this literature is that it fails to address the fact that there are good reasons for people who may be otherwise well to experience stress when they interact with health practitioners. Some of these may be:

- past stressful experiences (for example, pain or discomfort)
- poor understanding of the situation or the information provided
- intimidating environments and people
- fear of bad news
- legitimate anxieties about health
- lack of familiarity with the processes
- the cost of the procedure or consultation.

A more respectful interpretation would be for health practitioners to acknowledge that their interactions with people are likely to cause stress. While white coats and stethoscopes are ubiquitous and relatively simple pieces of technology, the messages contained in the process of taking blood pressure are significant and can negatively impact on people.

The provision of care across distance can have the effect of creating a sense of space between practitioners and patients, affording more power to the patient within the encounter.

Good-quality communication can transcend the delivery and reception of messages, and make a positive contribution to the overall well-being of the service user. The social nature of human beings means that interaction with other people is considered important and, logically, positive interaction can have helpful effects. Only a small proportion of the message is conveyed between patients and practitioners in the spoken language that they use; the vast proportion of the message is embedded in expression, tone of voice and body language (Jones, 2009).

{ SUMMARY }

Developments in knowledge and technology have had an enormous impact on health care and disability support services. The understanding of, and responses to, challenges that people face are obviously impacted by knowledge, but access to that knowledge through technology has radically changed the role and power of those who consume these services.

While it may appear that technological advances are overwhelmingly positive, it must be remembered that they are costly and require specialised skill. When care or support is offered at a distance, the most fundamental aspects of communication and interaction between people are altered. This in itself can impact on the experience of those involved, and ultimately the outcome for the patient or service user.

REFLECTION POINTS

27.1 Intention (motivation, message, meaning, emotion)

Does the intent of a health-care service that is provided face-to-face alter when it is provided at a distance?

27.2 Reception (received message, response, feedback)

What limitations are there on an assessment of a client made either via teleconference or the internet? What steps might you take to ensure an assessment is accurate, given that there are fewer visual or (potentially) verbal cues?

27.3 Perception (style, manner, impression, analysis)

Providing care at a distance has benefit for the service provider as well as for a client. What might be these benefits? Do you think these benefits outweigh the costs?

QUESTIONS FOR REVIEW

1 What are the intended consequences of health-care services being provided at a distance? What might be unintended consequences?

2 How might you reduce the risks involved?

REFERENCES

Adaji, A., Schattner, P. & Jones, K. (2008). The use of information technology to enhance diabetes management in primary care: A literature review. *Informatics in Primary Care, 16*, 229–37.

Allan, H., de Lacey, S. & Payne, D. (2009). The shaping of organisational routines and the distal patient in assisted reproductive technologies. *Nursing Inquiry, 16*(3), 241–50.

Blomberg, K. & Sahlberg-Blom, E. (2007). Closeness and distance: A way of handling difficult situations in daily care. *Issues in Clinical Nursing, 16*, 244–54.

Caldwell, P. (2006). Speaking the other's language: Imitation as a gateway to relationship. *Infant and Child Development, 15*, 275–82.

Chaudhry, B., Wang, J., Wu, S., Maglione, M., Mojica, W., Roth, E., Morton, S. C. & Shekelle, P. G. (2006). Systematic review: Impact of health information technology on quality, efficiency, and costs of medical care. *Annals of Internal Medicine, 144*, 742–52.

Dowell, A., Crampton, P. & Parkin, C. (2001). The first sunrise: An experience of cultural immersion and community health needs assessment by undergraduate medical students in New Zealand. *Medical Education, 35*, 242–9.

Duxbury, J. & Whittington, R. (2005). Causes and management of patient aggression and violence: Staff and patient perspectives. *Journal of Advanced Nursing, 50*(5), 469–78.

Garrett, P. W., Dickson, H. G. & Whelan, A. K. (2008). Communication and healthcare complexity in people with little or no English: The communication complexity score. *Ethnicity and Health, 13*(3), 203–17.

Huynh, T., Alderson, M. & Thompson, M. (2008). Emotional labour underlying caring: An evolutionary concept analysis. *Journal of Advanced Nursing, 64*(2), 195–208.

Jones, L. (2009). The healing relationship. *Nursing Standard, 24*(3), 64.

Kildea, S., Kruske, S. & Bowell, L. (2006). Maternity emergency care: Short course in maternity emergencies for remote area health staff with no midwifery qualifications. *Australian Journal of Rural Health, 14*, 111–15.

Kruger, E. & Tennant, M. (2005). Oral health workforce in rural and remote Western Australia: Practice perceptions. *Australian Journal of Rural Health, 13*, 321–6.

Lin, I., Goodale, B., Villanueva, K. & Spitz, S. (2007). Supporting an emergency workforce: Characteristics of rural and remote therapy assistants in Western Australia. *Australian Journal of Rural Health, 15*, 334–9.

National Center for Health Statistics (2010). *Health, United States 2009: With special feature on medical technology*. Hyattsville, MD: Author.

Parsons, J. E., Merlin, T. L., Taylor, J. E., Wilkinson, D. & Hiller, J. E. (2003). Evidence-based practice in rural and remote clinical practice: Where is the evidence? *Australian Journal of Rural Health, 11*, 242–8.

Phillips, A. (2009). Health status differentials across rural and remote Australia. *Australian Journal of Rural Health, 17*, 2–9.

Shaw, S. M. (2002). Nursing and pharmacy—clash of professional values. *Nursing New Zealand, 8*(10), 16–19.

Sutherns, R. & Bourgeault, I. L. (2008). Accessing maternity care in rural Canada: There's more to the story than distance to a doctor. *Health Care for Women International, 29*, 863–83.

Tuckett, A. G. (2005). The care encounter: Pondering caring, honest communication and control. *International Journal of Nursing Practice, 11*, 77–84.

Turnbull, J., Pope, C., Martin, D. & Lattimer, V. (2010). Do telephones overcome geographical barriers to general practice out-of-hours services? Mixed-methods study of parents with young children. *Journal of Health Services Research and Policy, 15*(1), 21–7.

Voyle, J. A. & Simmons, D. (1999). Community development through partnership: Promoting health in an urban indigenous community in New Zealand. *Social Science and Medicine, 49*, 1035–50.

Wakerman, J. (2008). Rural and remote public health in Australia: Building on our strengths. *Australian Journal of Rural Health, 16*, 52–5.

Walsh, M. (2010). Using a simulated learning environment. *Emergency Nurse, 18*(2), 12–16.

Weerasinghe, S. & Mitchell, T. (2007). Connection between the meaning of health and interaction with health professionals: Caring for immigrant women. *Health Care for Women International, 28*, 309–28.

Whitehall, J., Blignault, I., French, C., Carson, V. & Patole, S. (1998). Telemedicine in neonatology: Lessons from North Queensland. *Australian Journal of Rural Health*, *6*, 140–3.

Wood, P. J. (2010). Historical imagination and issues in rural and remote area nursing. *Australian Journal of Advanced Nursing, 27*(4), 54–61.

WEBSITES

International Society for Telemedicine & eHealth: www.isft.net/cms/index.php?id=1

Royal Flying Doctor Service: www.flyingdoctor.org.au

Telehealth—Where are we Heading? Health Infomatics New Zealand: www.hinz.org.nz/page/seminars_telehealth/Telehealth-4-Dec-2009

Glossary

Abandonment theory
The perspective that ageing is linked to decreased social engagement and increased isolation.

Abbreviations
Brief or shortened form of words or phrases.

Aboriginal and Torres Strait Islanders
The indigenous people of what is now known as Australia.

Access
The ability to seek and receive information and services without barriers.

Active listening
The process of listening with the intention to understand and to treat the communication with respect.

Activity theory
A deterministic approach that sees the older person as responsible for making their own decisions and adjustments to their changing situation.

Adolescence
A developmental phase between childhood and maturity.

Ageism
Discrimination on the basis of age.

Agenda-setting
The process of managing information to achieve political impact.

Antenatal
The period of time before birth.

Aphasia
Reduced ability to comprehend language or articulate ideas.

Apraxia of speech
Physical difficulty in speaking.

Assimilation
The process of attempting to make all people similar in terms of their beliefs and practices.

Attachment
Emotional affection and social bonds between people.

Attuned
The state of being particularly aware of the needs of others.

Base reaction
The fundamental human drive to survive (survival instinct).

Behaviour
Observable activities, conduct and responses.

Behavioural empathy
Actions that demonstrate an understanding or genuine appreciation of the experience of others.

'Being with'
The process of supporting (being present with and for) people, which is not dependent on physical tasks or being busy.

Bereavement
The experience of losing a person who was emotionally close.

Birth
The process of a baby leaving the mother's body.

Body language
Communication conveyed through posture and other non-verbal expressions.

Boundary
The area between territories that marks the difference between them.

Broadcast
Transmission to the general population, as in television or radio.

Business model
The concepts that underpin the ideals to make money.

Candid
Honest and without affectation.

Cataract
Opaqueness of the eye causing impaired vision or blindness.

Censorship
Judgments about the suitability of, and access to, information and media content.

Childbearing
The process of pregnancy and birth.

Citizen journalism
The involvement of members of the public (rather than journalists) in the process of reporting and presenting information to others.

Cognitive
Relating to thought and thinking.

Cognitive communication disorders
Impaired ability to transform thoughts into meaningful language or gestures.

Colloquial
Relating to acceptable casual language that is used in everyday settings by particular groups of people (it is not as informal as slang).

Colonisation
The movement to a new place by a group of people who maintain strong ties with their place of origin in the process of establishing a settlement.

Conception
The point during the reproductive cycle at which an egg is fertilised.

Conductive hearing loss
Hearing loss resulting from inability to conduct sound.

Congruence
When all messages that are conveyed (verbal, physical and emotional) agree.

Consumerism
Viewing human interaction with an emphasis on access to goods and services.

Consumers
People who use goods and services.

Context
The range of elements that affect people and situations, including political, social and cultural issues.

Continuity theory
The view that ageing is a continuation of the earlier part of life, a component of the natural cycle of life.

Continuum of care
The provision of appropriate services over a period of time, which is relevant to the needs of individuals.

Convergence
The point at which ideas meet or come together.

Conversation
An informal exchange of ideas.

Crisis
A significant point of change with potential risks of loss or harm.

Critical listening
The process of listening with the intention to evaluate and form an opinion.

Critique
Critical comment, appraisal or evaluation.

Crowning
When the top of the baby's head becomes visible during birth.

Crystal intelligence
The ability to think and reason based on experience acquired during life.

Cultural awareness
A basic understanding that cultural difference exists and requires consideration and appropriate responses.

Cultural blindness
The apparent inability to see cultural differences.

Cultural competence
The concept that practitioners have the skills to interact in a culturally appropriate manner.

Cultural difference
The variations between groups that relate to their fundamental understandings about themselves, those around them and the communities of which they are a part.

Cultural domination
When one cultural group assumes superiority over others.

Cultural heritage
The history of cultural understanding that informs individuals' understanding and perspectives.

Cultural imposition
The deliberate establishment of one set of cultural beliefs over those from other groups.

Cultural safety
A concept, closely associated with health practitioners in Aotearoa New Zealand, relating to the expectation that people receiving services should experience security and respect in terms of their cultural identity.

Culture
Beliefs, traditions and rituals originating within the family and community into which a person is born and raised, and transmitted from one generation to the next through a common language.

Democracy
A system of government in which the majority of the people hold the power to decide.

Development
The process of progressive change and growth.

Digital divide
The gap between people with electronic (internet) access and those that do not have it.

Digital revolution
The radical change to digital technology enabling widespread access to information and technology.

Disengagement theory
A belief that ageing involves withdrawal and severing of ties between a person and others in society.

Documentation
Written information that often follows a prescribed format.

Dualistic thinking
A tendency to see things as binary opposites; for example, as black and white, good or bad, or right or wrong. In addition, such ways of seeing assume that these are permanent states and are independent of one's own thinking.

Dysarthria
Difficulty with articulation of speech.

Emotional intelligence
Insight into emotional needs and skills of self and others.

Empathy
The ability to appreciate the thoughts, feelings and perspectives of others.

Engagement
Being genuinely involved.

Epistemic thinking
Reflecting on how one arrives at facts, beliefs and ideas.

Ethics
A system of values or principles, which outlines conduct.

Ethnicity
A group of people united by cultural or national heritage but residing in a place different from their place of origin.

Expertise
Expert skills and knowledge.

Fact
Information that is based on apparent truth.

Family
A close social grouping of people who are related genetically, emotionally or culturally and who provide basic support for one another.

First stage of labour
The period of time from when contractions become established until the cervix is fully dilated.

Fluid intelligence
The in-born ability of an individual to think and reason quickly and responsively.

Foucauldian
In the spirit of French philosopher Michel Foucault and therefore with an interest in critique of institutions and power.

Freedom
Living with choice and without fear, coercion or restraint on beliefs or behaviour.

Geriatrics
The study of diseases of ageing.

Gerontology
The study of social, psychological and biological aspects of ageing.

Glaucoma
High pressure within the eye, which leads to damage and impaired vision.

Grief
The journey of coming to terms with loss.

Haptic
Relating to the sense of touch.

Holistic
An emphasis on the whole person, rather than separate parts.

Hospice
An approach to palliative and end-of-life care that emphasises holism and healing but does not focus on cure.

Identity
The sense of self and individual character that a person has in relation to others.

Impulsivity
The tendency to act without prior analysis.

In-depth
Detailed and thorough.

Inappropriate touch
Touch that is unwanted or of questionable intent.

Indigenous
The natural or native people of the land; the original inhabitants and carers of the place.

Information triage
The process of analysing and refining information that is received in order to discern what is of value.

Institutional racism
Racism that is accepted and allowed within an organisational or powerful framework.

Integumentary system
Skin and related structures.

Intention
A deliberate attempt to behave in a certain way.

Interaction
Mutual influence or reciprocal action between people.

Internet
The electronic means (and protocols) to connect computer users to information from a vast array of sources.

Interpersonal racism
When individuals treat others in a prejudiced manner based on judgments about their race.

Interpreter
A skilled communicator who is able to translate information for two parties who do not share the same language.

Interprofessional
Interaction between two or more professionals.

Language
Words and the way they are used by groups of people to communicate with each other.

Latent phase
The period of time prior to labour becoming established.

Lead Maternity Carer (LMC)
The qualified professional identified as providing primary care for a woman during pregnancy, labour and the post-partum period.

Learning
The process of acquiring skills and knowledge.

Life events
Situations or experiences that are significant for the change related to it.

Life roles
The set of rights, obligations and behaviours associated with various tasks and positions (for example, learner, parent and employee).

Light-hearted
Relaxed, happy and without fear.

Linguistics
The study of language.

Locum
A casual employee providing a service that is unable to be met by regularly employed staff.

Macular degeneration
Progressive deterioration of the central visual field.

Mainstream media
The prevailing information sources that are available to and are accessed by the public, including network television and large-circulation newspapers.

Māori
The indigenous people of Aotearoa New Zealand.

Maternity care
The care of the woman and her child through pregnancy and for a period beyond birth (postnatal).

Meaning
The significance of the message and its delivery and context.

Meaningful
A sense of significance, relevance, purpose or importance.

Message
The information contained within communication.

Multimedia
The combined use of various types of media (text, graphics and animation) in any given context or situation.

Music
The organised composition and presentation of sound.

Narrative
An account or story of an experience or journey.

Narrowcast
Transmission to an identified or limited group within the general public, as in digital platforms.

Nativist perspective
The view that children build on their innate understanding as they move through developmental processes.

Neonatal
Relating to the period of life from birth to 28 days.

Neuroplasticity
The ability of the nervous system to respond to insult or injury by building new pathways or connections (previously, it was believed that nerve tissue could not regenerate or modify its function).

Neurological
Involving the nervous system.

News values
The criteria used to identify the merit of a story (for example, proximity, novelty and negativity).

Norms
That which is considered average or usual for a group of similar people.

Ontology
Concerned with the nature of being or existence.

Opinion
A belief based on knowledge and considered information.

Oppression
The unfair or unjust exercising of power over others.

Pacific People
People indigenous to the islands of the Pacific region.

Palliative
Relating to the alleviation of symptoms rather than the cause of them.

Patient handover
The process of health practitioners giving information and giving or taking responsibility for the care of patients.

Person-centred
An emphasis within relationships that focuses on the person receiving or seeking support, rather than the people, systems or organisations providing it.

Play
Interaction and activity that is relaxed and entertaining.

Poetry
The construction of language in an artistic manner.

Post-formal thought
Cognitive processes that emphasise relativism and the non-absolute nature of information.

Post partum
The period following birth.

Power
The exercise of strength or control.

Pregnancy
Carrying a child from conception to birth.

Presence
The state of accompanying others in a meaningful way.

Professional accountability
The expectations that professionals should be able to defend or account for their actions.

Propaganda
Information designed to further a cause, while damaging another one.

Purposeful touch
Touch that has a meaningful and honourable intent.

Race
A group of people who share distinctive characteristics.

Racism
Treating people in a discriminatory manner based on their heritage or race.

Rapport
The basis for mutually respectful interactions between people.

Records
Documented information about what has occurred.

Relativistic thinking
Considering information according to its relationship with other known facts.

Reproductive technologies
The use of medical and surgical techniques to assist with fertility and conception.

Resilience
The ability to recover from stress or injury.

Risk
The possibility of injury, loss or death.

Risky behaviour
Actions that may lead to injury or death.

Role
A socially accepted way of behaving and carrying specific responsibilities.

Rural
Outside of urban centres.

Scientific communication
The formal conventions for conveying scientific information.

Second stage of labour
The part of labour between full dilation of the cervix and the birth of the baby.

Sensitive period
A developmental period where particular impressions are most likely to occur and therefore relevant behaviour learnt.

Sensorineural hearing loss
Hearing loss resulting from damage to the inner ear or acoustic nerve.

Serious and sentinel events
Incidents that lead to unexpected outcomes such as injury (serious) or death (sentinel).

Slang
Informal and popular use of language.

Social networking
The process of people interacting, often through the medium of technology.

Social networks
Relationships between people as they interact within groups or organisations, which include virtual locations.

Social rules
The accepted boundaries of behaviour within any particular group.

Socialisation
The process by which people learn to modify their behaviour to conform to the expectations of groups to which they belong.

Socio-environmental theory
An understanding of ageing based on the assumption that the environment of older adults is built on interrelationships between individual and social context.

Spiritual
Of belief and understanding beyond physical and cognitive experience.

Stereotypes
Beliefs held about a particular group that influence the way people respond to and treat people belonging to that group.

Story
The explained perspective of an individual.

Surveillance
The act of keeping watch over people and their actions.

Systematic
Following a planned and accepted pathway.

Talking past
The tendency for people to assume they agree with one another when their messages appear consistent but the intention or meaning differ.

Talking with
Genuinely engaging in conversation and interaction with another person (rather than talking to or at that person).

Technology
Tools that enable communication and access to information.

Telemedicine
The use of technology to connect clinical staff with colleagues and patients at a distance.

Therapeutic touch
Touch that is deliberate and intended to help and heal, and is understood accordingly.

'The state'
The politically organised leadership (or government) of groups of people or populations.

Transactional analysis
An approach to psychotherapy that emphasises interactions and relationships between people.

Transition
The part of labour between the first and second stages; also the journey from one place or position to another.

Trimester
A period of three months within a pregnancy of nine months.

Truth
Information that is considered honest and accurate.

Uncorrected refractive error
When the lens of the eye loses the ability to change shape in order to focus light directly onto the retina, which results in reduced accuracy of vision.

Vibe
An informal description for the sense of meaning conveyed between people when they communicate.

Vocabulary
The collection of words and symbols that people use to communicate.

Whānau
Either family and extended family and significant others, or to be born or give birth.

Index

abandonment theory 91
abbreviations, interpretations of 301
Aboriginal and Torres Strait Islander people 159–61, 168
Aboriginal Health Workers 168–9
access 124–39
  care challenges 323
  digital divide 208–9
accident compensation legislation 318–19
active listening 248
activity theory 89
adolescents *see* teenagers
adrenalines 19
adults *see* early adulthood; middle years; senior years
adverse events 302–4
  therapeutic engagement and 317–19
advice giving 252–3
age groups
  adults *see* adults; early adulthood; middle years; senior years
  babies *see* babies; neonates
  children *see* children; teenagers
ageing 89–91, 93–5 *see also* senior years
  communication and 96–8
ageism 96
agenda-setting 208
alcohol use 62
amyotrophic lateral sclerosis 134–5
analytical responses to messages 252
antenatal care 9–13
anxiety 180–1
aphasia 125–6
appropriate boundaries *see* boundaries
apraxia of speech 125–6
artwork 291–2
assessment
  applying SBAR 183
  of young children 42–3
assimilation 158
asthma 55–6
attachment 34
attuned relationships 26
auditory process hearing loss 132
Australasian colloquialisms *see* slang
autism and immunisation case study 225
awareness *see* cultural awareness

babies *see also* neonates
  age of communication 36
  assumptions about 32
  communication and 23–6, 29–46, 53–7
  crying 35–6
  sign language and 38–9
bad news 178–9, 218
  communicating to children 54
barriers to effective communication *see* communication failures
base reactions 114
behaviour, emotional 53
behavioural empathy 22
'behaviourist' perspective to learning language 52
'being with' someone 181
bereavement 102–10
birth 19–22 *see also* pregnancy
  consumer case study 148–52
  continuous support for mothers during 21–2
  first communication with baby following 23
blindness 128–30
blogs 277–9
body language 116, 312, 325
boundaries
  appropriateness of 174–7
  communicating with peers 182
Bowlby, John 34
brain development
  adolescent 61–2
  early adulthood 73
breastfeeding 27
brevity *see* abbreviations
broadcasting 202
Bruner's theory 51
business models for mass media 203–6

candid conversations 213–14
care *see also* maternity care
care at a distance 322–32
casual communication
 slang 68, 228–30, 301–2
 'small talk' 240–1
cataracts 129–30
catecholamines 19
censorship 206–7 *see also* freedom of the press
cervical cancer treatment case study 225
chat 214
'chemical restraint' case study 232
childbearing: defined 11
childbirth *see* birth
childhood: social and cultural contexts 31–2
children 31–2 *see also* babies
 communication and 53–7
 disciplining 33–4
 language and vocabulary 41–2
 parents of 34–5, 42–3
 physical development 48–9
 pre-school children 29–46
 psychosocial development 49
 school-age children 47–59
 terminally ill children 54
 touch and 190
children's rights 32–3, 56–7
choice in childbirth case study 150–2
Chomsky, Noam 52
citizen journalism 208–9
clients *see* patients
cochlear implants 134
Cochrane Reviews 21–2
Code of Health and Disability Services Consumers' Rights 259, 262, 312, 316, 319
codes for communication 300–1
codes of ethics 119
cognitive communication disorders 126
cognitive development 74–5
cognitive theories 48
colloquial communication (slang) 68, 228–30, 301–2
colonisation 27, 158, 170
Colquhoun, Glenn 284–7
communication 3–8, 328–9 *see also* casual communication; conversation; professional communication
 with babies and children 23–7, 29–46, 53–7
 delivering information 216–18
 effective 313–15
 flexible styles of 238–9
 in health-care settings 55–7, 312–13
 impairments and 126–8, 130–1, 133–4
 interprofessional 306
 with older people 95–8
 with peers 182–3
 with practitioners 26–7, 53–5, 314–15, 328–9
 in social settings 325–6
 supportive 22–3, 182
 survival and 113–23
 with teenagers 67–9
 written 223–4, 258–68
communication codes 300–1
communication devices case study 135
communication failures 231–3, 302–4
 barriers to effective communication 120–1, 315–17
 dysfunctional styles 242–5
'communicative intent' *see* intention
competence *see* cultural competence
complaints 178, 254–6
comprehension of technical language 136
conception 11
conductive hearing loss 132
congruence 118
connections in social settings 325–6
consent forms 262–3
consumerism 147
consumers 310
 adverse events and 318
 case studies about 148–52, 314–15
 communication and satisfaction of 314
 involvement in health care 148, 152–3, 310–11
context: defined 323
continuity theory 91–2
continuum of care 216

Convention on the Rights of the Child 32–3, 56
convergence of media platforms 201
conversation 213–15, 226–7, 273
 children 41–2
 health-care settings 312
 texting 273
 as two-way process 311–12
coping strategies 180
cortisol 23
counselling using text messaging 66, 274
creative messages 283–96
crisis situations 85, 116–18
critical listening 249
critical social theory 143
critiques of power 142
cross-cultural communication skills 169
crossing boundaries 176–7
crowning 21
crying by babies 35–6
crystal intelligence 75, 98
cultural difference 158–62
 cultural competence 164–5
 cultural context of childhood 31–2, 36–7
 cultural domination 158–9
 cultural heritage 325
 cultural safety 166, 168–70
 culturally appropriate support 162–4
 dying, grief and bereavement 104
 stereotyping 160–1
culture 157–72

Deaf Community 133
'death with dignity' 103
decolonisation 170
delivering information 215–19
democracy: defined 198
development 3–8, 48
developmental delay 135–6
developmental theories 31–2, 48–50
devices to enhance hearing 134
diabetes management case study 324
dialogue *see* conversation; feedback
difficult messages 178–9, 218
digital divide 208–9
digital revolution 203
disability 125 *see also* neurological impairments; visual impairments
disability support sector 136
disciplining of children 33–4
discourses of empowerment 147–8, 152–3
discussion boards 277
disengagement theory 90
distance *see* care at a distance; physical location
documentation 223–4, 260
 elements of consent forms 262–3
domination *see* cultural domination
drug use 62
dual relationships 177
dualistic thinking 74
dying, grief and bereavement 102–9
dysarthria 126
dysfunctional communication styles 242–5

early adulthood 72–9 *see also* teenagers
 cognitive development 74
 emotional adjustment 77–8
 physical development 73
 social development 75–6
economic models *see* business models for mass media
effective communication 313–17
electronic messages 269–82
electronic support for visual challenges 131
elements of communication 5–6, 14
elimination communication 36–7
emergency situations 116–18
emotional behaviour 53
emotional intelligence 77–8
empathy 22, 248, 313 *see also* behavioural empathy
empowerment 145–7
 models and discourses of 147–8, 152–3
end-of-life situations *see* dying, grief and bereavement
endorphins 19
engagement 4 *see also* therapeutic engagement
epistemic thinking 74

Erikson's theory 49, 63
  adulthood 75–7, 81
  as a continuity theory 91–2
error reporting case study 259
ethics 119
ethnicity 158
evaluating the message 249–50
events *see* serious and sentinel events
evidence-based medicine 327
expertise: defined 323
eye contact 25

facts: defined 225
families 29, 31
  disciplining of children in 33–4
family planning clinic case study 69–70
feedback 253–4
fertility 77
first stage of labour 20
fluid intelligence 97
formal communication *see* professional communication
formal language 230–1
formal submissions 264–5
Foucauldian critiques 142, 144
fracture treatment case study 228
Frame, Janet 288–9
freedom: defined 198
freedom of the press 200
  censorship 206–7
Freud, Sigmund 49

'generativity' 81
genuineness 68
geriatrics 89
gerontology 89
glaucoma 129–30
glossary 333–40
'good death' 103
gossip 214–15
Grace, Patricia 288–9
grief 102–10

handover *see* patient handover
haptic communication 188
health information on the internet 276
Health Information Privacy Code case study 263
health practitioners *see* practitioners
Health Practitioners Competence Assurance Act 255, 260
health promotion case study 69–70
health-care settings 75
  communication in 55–7, 312–13
  consumer involvement in 148, 152–3, 310–11
  engagement when things go wrong 317–19
  institutional racism in 162
  virtual reality and 279–80
hearing, newborn 25
hearing aids 134
hearing impairments 131–4
'helping skills' 6
holistic views 48, 52, 160
honesty *see* truth telling
hormones 19
hospices 103
hospital experience survey 56–7
human development *see* development
human rights 32–3

identity 61, 63, 65, 68
images 291
immunisation and autism case study 225
impairment *see also* neurological impairments; visual impairments
  communication and 126–8, 130–1, 133–4
  vs disability 125
impulsivity 62
inadequate communication 302–3
inappropriate touch 193
in-depth conversations 213
Indigenous people 160 *see also* Aboriginal and Torres Strait Islander people; Māori; Pacific People
infants *see* babies
informal communication *see* casual communication; slang
information giving 215–18
information processing 51
information technology *see* technology
information triage 249
informed consent 150–2, 262–3
injuries in early adulthood 73

institutional racism 161
integrity 242 *see also* genuineness; truth telling
integumentary system 190
intellectual disabilities 135–6
intention 4, 223, 305
interaction 26–7, 242
internet 204, 276–8 *see also* social networking
interpersonal dynamics 173–86 *see also* engagement
interpersonal racism 159
interpretation 226–7, 248–9, 293–4
interpreters 325
interprofessional communication 306
intimacy 65, 241–2
IT *see* technology

journalism *see* citizen journalism; media; news

karakia 51
Kaupapa Māori (health-care providers) 104, 168
knowledge and power 300
Kübler-Ross, Elisabeth 103–4

labour *see* birth
language 222–36 *see also* sign language; slang; vocabulary
  babies 35–40
  children 41–2
  formal language 230–1
  interpreters 325
  technical or specialised language 136
  text messaging 66, 274
  theories of development of 52–3
latent phase 20
Lead Maternity Carers 20, 149
learning
  about people and communication 4–5, 243–4
  learning disabilities 135–6
  learning theories 49–51
  social context and 33
legal issues in written communication 259–60
liberational framework 143
life events 85
life roles 81
lifestyle changes 311
light-hearted conversations 213
limits *see* boundaries
linguists 160
listening 13–14
location *see* care at a distance; physical location
locums 327
lying *see* truth telling

macular degeneration 129–30
mainstream media 198
management theories 143–4
manner and style 237–46
Māori 159
  cultural differences 104, 160, 166
  health-care providers 104, 168
  perspectives on birth 27–8
  perspectives on development 51–2
mass media: business model for 203–6
maternal phases 11
maternity care 10 *see also* Lead Maternity Carers
meaning 5, 224–6
meaningful interactions 4
media 197–211
  business models for 203–6
  principles of openness 198–201
medical slang 229–30
mental illness case study 145–7
message boards *see* discussion boards
messages 223
  creative 283–96
  difficult 178–9, 218
  electronic 269–82
  evaluating 249–50
  interpreting 120–1
  receiving 247–57
  responding to 250–3
  slang 302
  types of 212–21
messaging *see* text messaging
microblogging 278–9
middle years 80–7
  roles in 83–4
mid-life transitions/crises 82, 85

midwifery case study 148–52
mindfulness 14
misrepresentation, professional 223–4, 305
mobile phones 271–5
models of communication 5–6
models of empowerment 147–8, 152–3
modified phones 134
motherhood 11–12, 34–5
motor neurone disease case study 134–5
Moules, N 288
multimedia 202
music 292–3

narratives of pregnancy 12–15
narrowcast publishing 203
nativist perspective 52–3
natural childbirth 152
neonates (newborns) 18–29 *see also* babies
    communication with 24–7
    touch and 190
Neufeld, Michael 293
neurological changes in adolescence 62
neurological impairments 125–6, 128
    communication and 126–8
New Zealand Relay service 134
New Zealand Sign Language 133
newborns *see* neonates
news *see* media
news, bad *see* bad news
news values: defined 207
non-verbal communication 24–6 *see also* body language; sign language
norms 114

Official Information Act 199
older people *see* senior years
ontology 293–4
openness
    media openness 198–201
    therapeutic engagement 317–19
operating theatres case study 233
opinion 225
oppression 141–2
oral history 118
organisational communication 306–7
organisational theories 143–4
over-involvement zone 175–6
oxytocin 19, 23

Pacific People 76, 159–60, 162–4
paediatric care *see* children
pain: communication regarding 55
palliative care 103
parallel messages 306
Parten's theory 43–4
partial blindness 125
patient empowerment 145–8, 152–3
patient handover 216
patient-centred medicine 311
patients 328–9 *see also* consumers; therapeutic engagement
    poems about 284–7
patterns of engagement 159
peer affiliation 63–4, 74–5
peers: communication with 182–3
person-centred communication 301
pharmacy dispensing case study 327
phones 134, 271–5
physical development
    children 48–9
    early adulthood 73
    teenagers 65–6
physical location 323–4, 326
Piaget's theory 39, 43, 49–50, 61, 74
pictures 291–2
play 43–4
poetry 284–8
political process 264–5
poor communication *see* communication failures
post partum: defined 27
post-formal thought 74
post-structuralist theories 144
power 141–3, 300
power relations 140–56
practitioners *see also* professional communication; therapeutic engagement
    care at a distance and 326–8
    communication by 26–7, 53–5, 314–15, 328–9
    responses to death 104–5
    touch and 193–4
pragmatism 74
pregnancy 10–13 *see also* birth
presence/present 238
press freedoms *see* freedom of the press

private speech 50
professional accountability 307
professional communication 239–40, 297–308 *see also* care at a distance; practitioners; therapeutic engagement
  academic writing 265–6
  misrepresentation 223–4, 305
professional responsibilities 305–6
prolactin 19
propaganda: defined 207
psychosocial development *see also* social development; social psychological theories
  adolescence 62–4
  ageing 89–90
  children 49
  early adulthood 75, 77
puberty 65
purposeful touch 192

race 158
racism 159, 161
rapport 68, 313
reassurance 180–2
receiving messages 247–57
record keeping 260–2
records: defined 260
recovery model 145–7
relativistic thinking 74–5
remote health-care provision 323–4, 327–8
report-writing 265–6
reproductive technologies 77
resilience 68
responding to complaints 256
responding to messages 250–3
responsibilities 233, 305–6
  truth and 118–20
responsible communication 253
rewards 62
risks: defined 63
risky behaviour 62–3, 73
roles 61, 83–4
rules *see* norms; social rules
rural health-care provision 323–4, 327–8

safety *see* cultural safety
satisfaction: communication and 314
Saunders, Cicely 103
SBAR (Situation, Background, Assessment and Recommendation) 183–4
scaffolding 50
school-age children 47–59
scientific communication 224–5
second stage of labour 21
senior years 88–94
  communication in 95–8
sensitive period 23
sensorineural hearing loss 132–3
serious and sentinel events 302–4
sexual maturation 65
short message service (SMS) 272–5
sign language 133
  baby sign language 38–9
simulations: virtual reality and health care 279–80
Situation, Background, Assessment and Recommendation (SBAR) 183–4
Skinner, BE 52
skin-to-skin contact (SSC) 23–4
slang 68, 228–30, 301–2
'small talk' 240–1
social and interpersonal dynamics 173–86
social contexts of childhood
  ageing 92, 95
  childhood 31–3
social development 75–6 *see also* psychosocial development
social networking 276–8
social networks: defined 115
social psychological theories 144
social rules 114
social settings 325–6
social theory, critical 143
socialisation 114
sociocultural theory of development 50
socio-environmental theory 94–5
sound 292–3
specialised language 136
speech impairment 127–8
speech synthesisers 135
spiritual harm 105
stages of life *see* age groups
'state, The': defined 141
stereotypes 160–1

story 288–90
strengths-based approaches 68–70
stress 329
  neonates 23
style and manner 237–46
submissions 264–5
support for people with impairments 127–8, 131, 133–4
support workers 136
supportive communication
  communicating with peers 182
  during labour 22–3
surveillance 141
survival: communication and 113–23
systematic approach to communication 216

tactile communication 188 *see also* touch
talking past or with another person 227–8, 306
taonga 52
technical language 136
technology 270–2 *see also* reproductive technologies
  case studies 324, 327
  remote health provision 324–5
  vision support 131
teenagers 60–6 *see also* early adulthood
  communication with 67–9
telemedicine 324
telephones 134, 271–5
terminally ill people 226
  children 54
terminology 228–30
text messaging 272–5
theories of language development 52–3
therapeutic engagement 309–21 *see also* patients; practitioners
  message interpretation in 120–1
  when things go wrong 317–19
therapeutic touch 191
tools for communication *see* technology
Torres Strait Islanders *see* Aboriginal and Torres Strait Islanders
touch 187–96
  communication and 191–3
  professional practice and 193–5
transactional analysis 241
transition (in childbirth) 20–1
transition (mid-life crisis) 82
transition to motherhood 11–12
Treaty of Waitangi 168
trimesters of pregnancy 12
truth telling 179–80 *see also* genuineness; integrity
  professional misrepresentation 223–4, 305
  responsibility and 118–20
  in scientific communication 225
Twitter 278–9
types of messages 212–21

uncorrected refractive error 129–30
under-involvement zone 175
understanding 64–5
  language and 35–40
  newborns 25
  as ontology 293–4
United Nations Convention on the Rights of the Child 32–3, 56–7

vibe: defined 227
virtual reality and health care 279–80
visual impairments 128–31
  impact on communication 130
vocabulary 222–36 *see also* slang
  babies and children 39–42
  talking with and past each other 227–8, 306
  understanding terminology 228–30
Vygotsky's theory 43

whānau (family) 19, 160
whenua (placenta and land) 27–8
women's narratives *see* narratives of pregnancy
words *see* language; vocabulary
written communication 258–68
  case studies 223–4, 259

young adults *see* early adulthood
young children 29–46
  assessing 42–3
Youthline 66, 274

zone of helpfulness 175–6
zone of proximal development 50